Drugs Affecting Leukotrienes And Other Eicosanoid Pathways

NATO ASI Series

Advanced Science Institutes Series

A series presenting the results of activities sponsored by the NATO Science Committee, which aims at the dissemination of advanced scientific and technological knowledge, with a view to strengthening links between scientific communities.

The series is published by an international board of publishers in conjunction with the NATO Scientific Affairs Division

A	**Life Sciences**	Plenum Publishing Corporation
B	**Physics**	New York and London
C	**Mathematical and Physical Sciences**	D. Reidel Publishing Company Dordrecht, Boston, and Lancaster
D	**Behavioral and Social Sciences**	Martinus Nijhoff Publishers
E	**Engineering and Materials Sciences**	The Hague, Boston, and Lancaster
F	**Computer and Systems Sciences**	Springer-Verlag
G	**Ecological Sciences**	Berlin, Heidelberg, New York, and Tokyo

Recent Volumes in this Series

Series A: Life Sciences

Drugs Affecting Leukotrienes and Other Eicosanoid Pathways

Edited by

B. Samuelsson

Karolinska Institute
Stockholm, Sweden

F. Berti

G. C. Folco

University of Milan
Milan, Italy

and

G. P. Velo

University of Verona
Verona, Italy

Plenum Press
New York and London
Published in cooperation with NATO Scientific Affairs Division

Proceedings of a NATO Advanced Study Institute entitled
Drugs Affecting Leukotrienes and Other Eicosanoid Pathways,
held September 9–20, 1984,
at the Ettore Majorana Center, Erice, Sicily, Italy

Library of Congress Cataloging in Publication Data

Main entry under title:

Drugs affecting leukotrienes and other eicosanoid pathways.

   (NATO ASI series. Series A, Life sciences; v. 95)
   Based on presentations at the International School of Pharmacology on
"Drugs Affecting Leukotrienes and Other Eicosanoid Pathways," held in Erice,
Sicily, at the Ettore Majorana Center, Sept. 9–20, 1984.
   "Published in cooperation with NATO Scientific Affairs Division."
   Includes bibliographies and index.
   1. Arachidonic acid—Metabolism—Congresses. 2. Leukotrienes—Metab-
olism—Congresses. 3. Arachidic acid—Metabolism—Congresses. I.
Samuelsson, Bengt. II. North Atlantic Treaty Organization. Scientific Affairs
Division. III. International School of Pharmacology on "Drugs Affecting
Leukotrienes and Other Eicosanoid Pathways" (1984: Ettore Majorana Center)
IV. Title: Eicosanoid pathways. V. Series. [DNLM: 1. Arachidonic Acid—
metabolism—congresses. 2. Drug Therapy—congresses. 3. Eicosanoid Acids
—metabolism—congresses. 4. Leukotrienes B—metabolism—congresses. 5.
SRSA—metabolism—congresses. QU 90 D794 1984]
QP752.A7D78   1985   615.7   85-19217
ISBN 0-306-42090-2

©1985 Plenum Press, New York
A Division of Plenum Publishing Corporation
233 Spring Street, New York, N.Y. 10013

Printed in the United States of America

PREFACE

This volume, the fourth in the series "The Prostaglandin System", contains most of the presentations at the International School of Pharmacology on "Drugs Effecting Leukotrienes and other Eicosanoid pathways" held in Erice, Sicily, at the "Ettore Majorana Center" on 9-20 September 1984.

The discovery of a new class of biologically active compounds is always exciting even if at the present time knowledge is advancing very rapidly; this is particularly true for the eicosanoids. Evidence for a pivotal role of arachidonic acid as a precursor of mediators and modulators of various cell functions is now well established. This broad knowledge has stimulated the search for drugs capable of interfering with the eicosanoid system and since the discovery of the mechanism of action of Aspirin, new drugs have become available in order to act more specifically not only at the level of different enzymes involved in arachidonic acid conversion but also more selectively at the receptor sites where the active metabolites are effective. In addition to this, several stable synthetic derivatives of endogenous unstable prostanoids mimicking their functions in a variety of physiopathological processes are also of potential therapeutic interest.

This volume will certainly help scientists and students with different interests related to those diseases that stem from arachidonic acid metabolites interactions in hypersensitivity phenomena and in host defence mechanisms.

We like to take this opportunity to expresse our gratitude to all the speakers for their important contributions and to NATO ADVANCED STUDY INSTITUTE for making this Course possible.

B. Samuelsson
F. Berti
G.C. Folco
G.P. Velo

CONTENTS

INTRODUCTION

Bengt Samuelsson

Dept. of Physiological Chemistry
Karolinska Institutet
S-104 01 Stockholm, Sweden

Prostaglandin research has developed rapidly especially during the past two decades. The elucidation of the chemistry, biosynthesis and metabolism of the prostaglandin system as well as advances concerning the biological effects and physiological roles of prostaglandins and related compounds are important areas in this development (1). The new knowledge has formed the basis for understanding the role of prostaglandins in many pathophysiological processes and for the therapeutic use of prostaglandins in various diseases.

After the elucidation of the chemistry of the prostaglandins and their biosynthesis from polyunsaturated fatty acids, studies on the mechanism of prostaglandin biosynthesis demonstrated the existence of unstable endoperoxide intermediates as PGG_2 and PGH_2. The finding that the endoperoxides had unique biological effects indicated that additional biologically active derivatives were formed from the endoperoxides (2). These considerations formed the basis for the discovery of thromboxane A_2 and subsequently also prostacyclin (3,4).

The leukotrienes constitute another group of biologically active derivatives formed from polyunsaturated fatty acids. They were originally discovered in leukocytes (LTB_4), however, studies on their mechanism of biosynthesis resulted in the recognition of an unstable intermediate (LTA_4). This finding formed the basis for the elucidation of the chemistry of slow reacting substance of anaphylaxis (LTC_4, LTD_4, LTE_4) (5). The leukotrienes have potent biological effects related to inflammation and allergy.

More recently, the importance of other lipoxygenase catalyzed reactions has been recognized. Thus, the dihydroxy acids 14,15-DHETE and 5S,12S-DHETE can modulate various neutrophil functions of importance in inflammation. Furthermore, a new group of arachidonic acid derived products, the lipoxins, has been discovered (6). These compounds, formed by multiple interactions of lipoxygenases, have biological effects related to the immune system and inflammation.

The discovery of the inhibition of prostaglandin biosynthesis by non-steroidal anti-inflammatory drugs has been important not only in the development of new therapeutic agents but also in the understanding of the biological roles of the prostaglandins (7). Our knowledge of the mechanism of action of corticosteroids is also developing rapidly (8,9).

Arachidonic acid plays a unique role as a precursor molecule which is transformed into a large number of mediators with far-

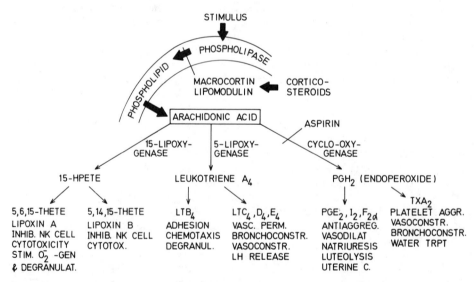

Fig. 1. Formation and biological effects of derivatives of arachidonic acid

ranging effects. The recognition of the importance of arachidonic acid in the regulation of various cell functions under physiological and pathological conditions has stimulated the interest in finding new specific inhibitors with novel mode of actions. Thus extensive work is in progress to develop thromboxane synthetase inhibitors, 5-lipoxygenase inhibitors and inhibitors of more distal transformations of arachidonic acid. With the advancing knowledge about the transformation of arachidonic acid into biologically active compounds it should also be of interest to reinvestigate the mode of action of existing drugs.

References

1. Bergström, S. and Samuelsson, B. (1965) Ann. Rev. Biochem. 34, 101-108.
2. Samuelsson, B., Goldyne, M., Granström, E., Hamberg, M., Hammarström, S. and Malmsten, C. (1978) Ann. Rev. Biochem. 47, 997-1029.
3. Hamberg, M., Svensson, J. and Samuelsson, B. (1975) Proc. Natl. Acad. Sci. USA, 72, 2994-2998.
4. Moncada, S., Gryglewski, R.J., Bunting, S. and Vane, J.R. (1976) Nature, 263, 663-665.
5. Samuelsson, B. (1983) Science, 220, 568-575.
6. Serhan, C., Hamberg, M. and Samuelsson, B. (1984) Proc. Natl. Acad. Sci. USA, 81, 5335-5339.
7. Vane, J.R. (1978) In: Advances in Prostaglandin and Thromboxane Research (Eds. F. Coceani and P.M. Olley), Raven Press, New York, vol. 4, pp. 27-44.
8. Blackwell, G.J., Carnuccio, R., DiRosa, M., Flower, R.J., Ivanyi, J., Langham, C.S.J., Parente, L., Persico, P. and Wood, J. (1983) In: Advances in Prostaglandin, Thromboxane and Leukotriene Research (Eds. B. Samuelsson, R. Paoletti and P. Ramwell), Raven Press, New York, vol. 11, pp. 65-71.
9. Hirata, F. (1983) In: Advances in Prostaglandin, Thromboxane and Leukotriene Research (Eds. B. Samuelsson, R. Paoletti and P. Ramwell), Raven Press, New York, vol. 11, pp. 73-78.

MEASUREMENT OF THROMBOXANE PRODUCTION IN VIVO:

METABOLIC AND ANALYTICAL ASPECTS

E. Granström, P. Westlund, M. Kumlin and
A. Nordenström

Department of Physiological Chemistry
Karolinska Institutet
Stockholm, Sweden

INTRODUCTION

In studies aiming at establishing a role for thromboxanes in various physiological or pathological conditions, it is often desirable to measure the endogenous thromboxane production. Since TXA_2 is difficult to measure as such, a common approach in such studies is to monitor its stable hydrolysis product, TXB_2, instead, and to compare obtained TXB_2 levels in, for example, plasma samples in patient and control groups. Numerous such studies have been published to date; however, even the so called "basal" TXB_2 levels reported therein vary widely. Not infrequently, "basal" TXB_2 levels were found to be around 100-200 pg/ml plasma or even higher, however, others claim to find values below 15, 10 or even 2 pg/ml (e.g., refs. 1-6). It is difficult to explain such differences between studies where identical assay methods have been used (for example a commercially available TXB_2 radioimmunoassay); that is, if the obtained data really reflect the endogenous situation.

One explanation for these discrepancies is that thromboxane was actually formed during the sampling procedure, for example due to the inevitable mechanical damage done to the blood cells. Such artifactual formation of arachidonate metabolites is well known in the prostaglandin field, where it was realized already in the early 1970's, that measured peripheral plasma levels of primary prostaglandins were far too high to be the true ones[7]. Since the thromboxanes are by far the dominating cyclooxygenase products in platelets, it may be safely assumed that at least similar quantities of thromboxane may be formed and released as artifacts, in parallel with the prostaglandins, when the samples are collected and/or processed.

5

THROMBOXANE FORMATION DURING BLOOD SAMPLING

So far, very few attempts have been made to estimate the extent of artifactual thromboxane production during sampling. The few studies addressing this aspect have generally reported figures which show differences in blood collected into tubes with or without a cyclooxygenase inhibitor (e.g., Refs 5,8,9). Such differences indicate that some further biosynthesis may indeed occur in the test tube. However, most inhibitors, especially aspirin, require several minutes for complete effect[10], and thromboxane biosynthesis is a very rapid process[11]. Thus, it would be of considerable interest to estimate also the artifactual biosynthesis <u>during</u> collection of the blood sample. The importance of this is further borne out by the fact that the platelets have a very high capacity for TX biosynthesis, and even an activation of <0.1% of this capacity would lead to biosynthesis of several 100 pg of thromboxane[12].

To examine how much the stimulation caused by the sampling procedure contributes to the later measured level of TXB_2, blood was collected into Vacutainer tubes containing either heparin or citrate, and then centrifuged to obtain platelet rich plasma (PRP). The PRP was then repeatedly drawn through a syringe into new Vacutainer tubes, without anticoagulant, at 30 min intervals. After each passage, an aliquot of the sample as well as of a control (part of the PRP left standing on the lab bench) were subjected to addition of indomethacin and later assayed for TXB_2 by radioimmunoassay.

As expected, the TXB_2 level increased with each passage of the PRP through the syringe. In the corresponding control, the amounts of TXB_2 rose only slightly with time. However, sometimes a large increase in TXB_2 was seen also in the controls after 2-3 hrs. This phenomenon may not be of any great importance but emphasizes the necessity for rigourously standardized procedures for handling of blood samples.

The amount of TXB_2 produced by the mechanical stimulation caused by the sampling process varied between individuals and also from time to time in PRP from the same individual. Thus, calculation of this artifactual contribution in a "normal" sample seems impossible.

During the sample collection, the blood cells are exposed to two types of mechanical trauma: the shearing when passing through the syringe and the impact when hitting the bottom of the Vacutainer tube. Thus, a milder method which could be expected to give less activation is the free flow sampling technique, especially when a wide syringe is used. On the other hand, collection of the blood sample with this technique takes longer time, and particularly when large samples are taken the possible contribution by the beginning coagulation may seriously disturb the results. Blood coagulation is known to lead to the production of large amounts of TXB_2: usually serum TXB_2 levels are about three orders of magnitude higher than plasma levels,[5,8,13,14] and thus, even a minor clot formation in a sample may completely overshadow the "true" amounts of TXB_2.

To examine the importance of the time factor during sampling using the free flow technique, blood was taken from the marginal ear vein from a rabbit, and was collected in 1 ml portions until the flow stopped because of the coagulation process. This usually happened after 5-6 min, and the last few samples were then clearly viscous. Time was noted for each sample: during the first few minutes the blood flow was roughly constant and the collection of each sample took about 10-15 sec. The last sample usually took about 1 min or more to get, and a small clot was seen. Each sampling tube contained indomethacin to prevent further TXB_2 formation.

Typical results are shown in Fig. 1. As expected, there was a dramatic rise in TXB_2 levels in the last few samples, when coagulation had started. More interesting, however, was the finding that the TXB_2 level actually rose already from the start, during the time when the blood flow was rapid and constant.

That the measured thromboxane was formed locally was seen by the fact that blood obtained from the opposite ear immediately after the blood flow had stopped had as low concentration of TXB_2 as the initial aliquot from the first ear.

The origin of the measured TXB_2 in the early phase of the experiment is likely to be the growing platelet plug at the puncture site (cf. Ref. 15). Judging from Fig. 1, it is obvious that with this comparatively slow sampling technique the finally measured TXB_2 levels to a great extent depend on the sample volume, smaller samples, thus giving lower values. Again, it can thus be emphasized that measured TXB_2 levels do not necessarily reflect the endogenous situation.

Apparently, there is no satisfying way to avoid the formation of thromboxane during blood collection, nor can the sampling procedure be standardized to the extent that one can predict the amount of thromboxane artifactually produced at each occasion.

It could be expected that such problems will be solved if a metabolite of thromboxane can be identified, which represents a major and constant fraction of thromboxane formed in vivo and which is not formed as an artifact during sample collection. In the prostaglandin area, these conditions were met by the 15-keto-13-14-dihydro metabolites and their β-oxidized tetranor dioic acid

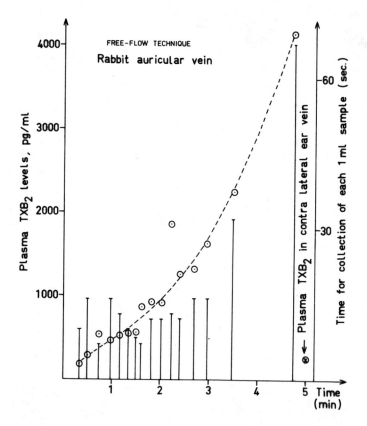

Fig. 1 TXB$_2$ amounts measured in a series of blood samples collected by free flow from a rabbit ear (o-----o). Bars denote time necessary for collection of each sample (1 ml).

counterparts,[7] all of which occur in blood in comparatively high concentrations and with longer half-lives than the parent compounds (Refs. 7,16,17). The latter compounds are also the dominating prostaglandin metabolites in urine.[7]

In the thromboxane field, however, matters are more complex. First, metabolic studies with the most relevant compound, TXA_2, cannot be conducted, due to lack of purification methods for the substance, its extremely short half-life and its biological potency. Most metabolic studies have instead been done with its stable hydrolysis product, TXB_2. There are however other possible metabolic fates known for TXA_2, such as covalent binding to albumin and conversion into the corresponding 15-keto-13,14-dihydro product (for review, see Ref. 18). The relative importance of these pathways in comparison with hydrolysis to TXB_2 is not known at present, and thus, in our attempts to identify a reliable thromboxane parameter in vivo, we have employed TXB_2 as the starting material; always keeping in mind, however, that this may represent only a small fraction of the TXA_2 actually released.

METABOLISM OF THROMBOXANE B_2 IN VIVO

The metabolic pathways for TXB_2 in man have been extensively elucidated by Roberts et al.[19,20] They identified twenty metabolites in human urine. The major urinary metabolites have also been identified in a few other species.[18] The predominant steps involved in TXB_2 degradation are β- and ω-oxidation as well as dehydrogenation at C-11 and C-15. A minor pathway leading to acyclic compounds with alcohol groups at the C-11 and C-12 positions is also known (Fig. 2). The metabolites identified so far are formed in various in vitro systems or excreted into urine. Nothing has so far been known about circulating metabolites of TXB_2, and the following study was thus undertaken to identify dominating TXB_2 metabolites in blood in two different species, viz. man and rabbit; the latter species a commonly used model for thrombosis studies.

$[^3H_8]$-TXB_2 or unlabeled TXB_2 were administered i.v. to New Zealand white rabbits and to a human volunteer.[21,22] Blood samples were taken at different times for 90 min, and urine was collected for 48 hrs after the administration. For the purification and identification of metabolites several techniques were used, i.v. XAD-2, Sep-Pak, Polygosil C_{18} open column chromatography, straight and reversed phase HPLC, 2D TLC with autoradiography, radio-GLC and GC/MS of several derivatives.

In the rabbit the injected TXB_2 was rapidly removed from the circulation and converted to several metabolites.[21] Already after about 2 min, only 10-20% of the radioactivity was left in blood; this figure continued to decrease to about 2% about 1 hr after the injection. Thirty to 40 min after the injection the total lipophilic

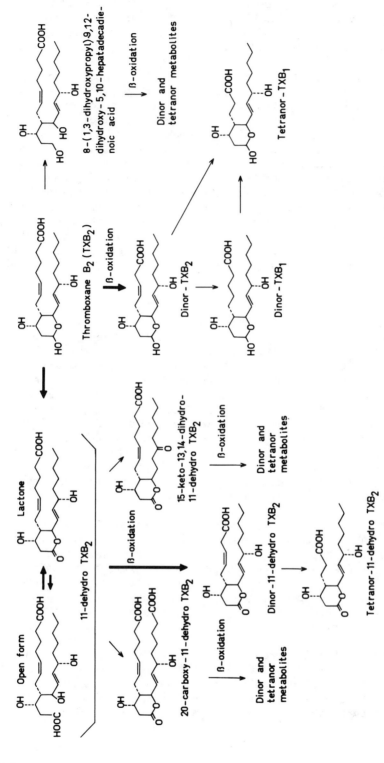

Fig. 2 Metabolic pathways for degradation of TXB$_2$ in vivo.

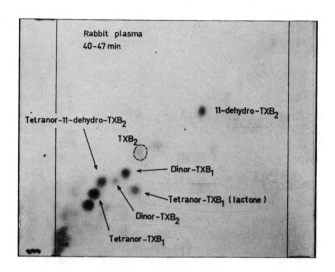

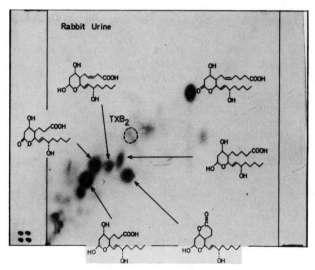

Fig. 3 Metabolic profile of [^{3}H$_8$]-TXB$_2$ in the rabbit as analyzed
by two-dimensional thin layer chromatography. Upper panel:
Blood sample taken 40-47 min after i.v. injection of the
compound. Lower panel: Urine collected until 48 hrs after
the injection (From Ref. 21).

radioactivity in blood consisted of metabolites: no unconverted TXB_2 could be detected at all. In all the blood samples (2-90 min), a prominent metabolite was identified as 11-dehydro-TXB_2.[21] Several other products appeared with time (Fig. 3). Most of these had undergone β-oxidation. In the later blood samples the metabolic profile was dominated by 11-dehydro-TXB_2, tetranor-TXB_1 and tetranor-11-dehydro-TXB_1, and the picture at this stage was almost identical to the urinary profile (Fig. 3). Smaller amounts of dinor metabolites (dinor-TXB_2 as well as dinor-TXB_1) were also identified.

In the human the metabolic profile was quite different.[22] As reported by Roberts et al.,[19,20] the major metabolite in the urine was found to be dinor-TXB_2, which in abundance was followed by 11-dehydro-TXB_2 (Fig. 4). The radioactivity was removed from the human circulation as fast as in the rabbit, but only a minor part of the products formed were polar metabolites (Fig. 4). The final metabolic profile in blood thus did not resemble the urinary profile, as is generally the case with prostaglandins.[16,17] Unconverted TXB_2 dominated the blood profile for about 30 min, and the three major metabolites were all less polar (Fig. 4). Two of these were identified as 11-dehydro-TXB_2 and 11,15-diketo-13,14-dihydro-TXB_2.[22] The third one was tentatively identified as 15-keto-13,14-dihydro-TXB_2, judged from chromatographic data.

The metabolism of TXB_2 in the rabbit and the human thus differs considerably both in the blood and urinary metabolic profile. However, 11-dehydro-TXB_2 seems to be a major metabolite in both species in urine as well as in the circulation, and may therefore serve as a better target for measurement of thromboxane production in vivo than the parent compound. A radioimmunoassay for 11-dehydro-TXB_2 was therefore developed.

DEVELOPMENT OF A RADIOIMMUNOASSAY FOR 11-DEHYDRO-TXB_2

Both synthetically produced (a generous gift of F.A. Fitzpatrick, The Upjohn Comp.) and biosynthetically prepared 11-dehydro-TXB_2 was used. The latter was obtained from guinea pig liver cytosol incubated with TXB_2 and 5 mM NAD. The compound was purified on SP-HPLC and the conversion into 11-dehydro-TXB_2 was approximately 50% under these conditions.

Antibodies were then raised in rabbits against two conjugates with BSA, obtained using two different coupling methods: one with N,N-carbonyldiimidazole[23] (antibody I) and the other with carbodiimide[24] as the coupling reagent (antibody II). Each conjugate was injected subcutaneously into rabbits and the blood was collected into heparinized Vacutainer tubes 10 days after the final injection.

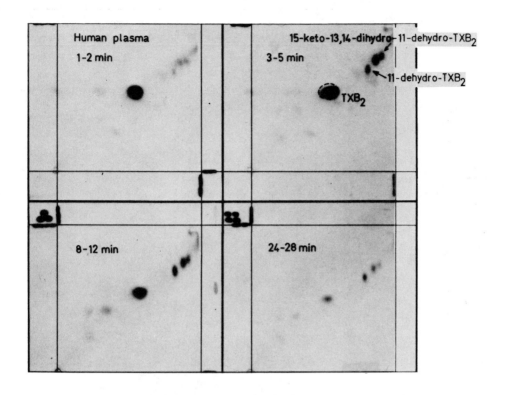

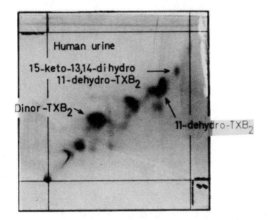

Fig. 4   Metabolic profile of [³H₈]-TXB₂ in the human as analyzed
by two-dimensional thin layer chromatography (HPTLC).
Upper panel: Blood samples collected 2-28 min after i.v.
injection of the compound. Lower panel: Urine collected
until 5 hrs after the injection (From Ref. 22).

Preparation of $[^3H_7]$-11-dehydro-TXB$_2$ of high specific activity for use as tracer in the assay was done with the incubation procedure described above, employing $[^3H_8]$-TXB$_2$ (spec. act., 140 Ci/mmol, NEN) as substrate.

The titer of the two antibody preparations was tested. Both antiplasmas bound tritium labeled 11-dehydro-TXB$_2$ to give a B_0 of 0.5 at a dilution of about 1:1000.

The chemical stability of the molecule was tested at various pH, ion strength and temperature. 11-Dehydro-TXB$_2$ was shown to occur in two forms (Fig. 5). One is the δ-lactone form with an intact thromboxane ring. The other has an open ring structure, with a second carboxyl group at C-11 in the molecule.

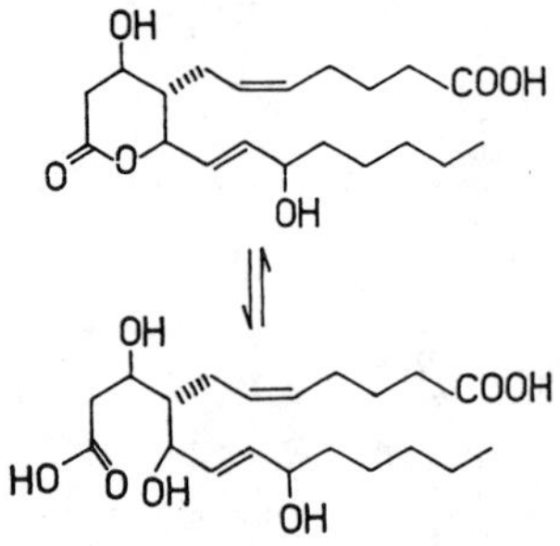

Fig. 5 Structures of the two forms of 11-dehydro-TXB$_2$.

The two antibody preparations showed different behavior in the assay, with regard to binding of these two forms, viz. one antibody (II) bound either form with equal avidity (raised against CDI coupled conjugate), whereas the other (antibody I, raised against the carbonyldiimidazole coupled conjugate) preferred the lactone form.

A further difference between the two antibody preparations was seen when standard curves were analyzed. The methyl ester of the compound was used as the unlabeled ligand: normally, prosta-

noid antibodies do not discriminate between free and esterified
C-1 carboxyls, since coupling to the carrier protein is done at
this position. However, antibody II did not show a 100% displace-
ment of tritium even with high concentration of unlabeled ligand.
This indicated that the antibody was capable of discriminating between the free and esterified C-1 carboxyl, in contrast to antibody
I. Taken together, these data suggested that the CDI coupling might
to some extent have taken place at the ring (C-11) carboxyl, whereas
the coupling with carbonyldiimidazole seemed to have occurred exclusively at C-1.

An experiment was performed where unlabeled TXB_2 (500 µg) was
injected intravenously to a rabbit and blood samples were collected
from the contralateral ear vein at different times. TXB_2 and the
metabolite 11-dehydro-TXB_2 were measured in the plasma before and
after the injection. Measured TXB_2 peaked immediately (1 min after
the injection) and then the level rapidly decreased to the "basal"
concentration. The levels of 11-dehydro-TXB_2 showed a different
pattern. The peak appeared later (after 5-10 min) and the level remained considerably elevated even after 5 hrs.

This study thus indicated that 11-dehydro-TXB_2, a major, stable,
long-lived metabolite, may be more suitable than TXB_2 for measuring
release of thromboxane into the circulation. The excretion of 11-
dehydro-TXB_2 in urine during this experiment was also measured.
Also in this fluid 11-dehydro-TXB_2 was found to be a better parameter than urinary TXB_2, the origin of which is somewhat uncertain.[25,26]

Acknowledgements

This study was supported by grants from the Swedish Medical
Research Council (projs. no. 03P-5804 and 03X-05915), and
Petrus and Augusta Hedlund´s Foundation.

References

1. R. Lorenz, U. Spengler, S. Fischer, J. Duhm and P.C. Weber,
    Platelet function, thromboxane formation and blood
    pressure. Control during supplementation of the western
    diet with cod liver oil, Circulation, 67:504 (1983).
2. R.J.T. Ouwendijk, F.J. Zijlstra, J.H.P. Wilson, I.L. Bonta and
    J.E. Vincent, Raised plasma thromboxane B_2 levels in
    alcoholic liver disease, Prostaglandins Leukotrienes Med.
    10:115 (1983).
3. R.M. Graham, M.B.W. Campbell and E.K. Jackson, Effects of short-
    term betablockade on blood pressure plasma thromboxane B_2
    and plasma and urinary prostaglandins E_2 and $F_{2\alpha}$ in nor-
    mal subjects, Clin. Pharmacol. Ther. 31:324 (1982).

4. G.A. FitzGerald, A.K. Pedersen and C. Patrono, Analysis of prostacyclin and thromboxane biosynthesis in cardiovascular disease, Circulation, 67:1174 (1983).

5. H.G. Morris, N.A. Sherman and F.T. Shepperdson, Variables associated with radioimmunoassay of prostaglandins in plasma, Prostaglandins, 21:771 (1981).

6. K. Andrassy, J. Koderisch, B. Kern and E. Ritz, Does arachidonic acid interfere with measurements of thromboxane B_2? Thromb. Haemost., 47:185 (1982).

7. B. Samuelsson, E. Granström, K. Gréen, M. Hamberg and S. Hammarström, Prostaglandins, Annu. Rev. Biochem., 44:669 (1975).

8. L. Viinikka and O. Ylikorkala, Measurement of thromboxane B_2 in human plasma or serum by radioimmunoassay, Prostaglandins, 20:759 (1980).

9. Y. Hayashi, N. Ueda, K. Yokota, et al., Enzyme immunoassay of thromboxane B_2, Biochim. Biophys. Acta, 750:322 (1983).

10. G.J. Roth, N. Stanford and P. Majerus, Acetylation of prostaglandin synthetase by aspirin, Proc. Natl. Acad. Sci. USA, 72:3073 (1975).

11. J. Svensson, M. Hamberg and B. Samuelsson, On the formation and effects of thromboxane A_2 in human platelets, Acta Physiol. Scand., 98:285 (1976).

12. C. Patrono, This symposium.

13. D.S. McCann, J. Tokarsky and R.P. Sorkin, Radioimmunoassay for plasma thromboxane B_2, Clin. Chem., 27:1417 (1981).

14. C. Patrono, G. Ciabattoni, E. Pinca, F. Pugliese, G. Castrucci, A. DeSalvo, M.A. Satta and B.A. Peskar, Low dose aspirin and inhibition of thromboxane B_2 production in healthy subjects, Thromb. Res., 17:317 (1980).

15. M. Thorngren, S. Shafi and G.V.R. Born, Thromboxane A_2 in skin bleeding-time blood and in clotted venous blood before and after administraiton of acetylsalicylic acid, Lancet, i:1075 (1983).

16. E. Granström, H. Kindahl and M.-L. Swahn, Profiles of prostaglandin metabolites in the human circulation: Identification of late-appearing long lived products, Biochim. Biophys. Acta, 713:46 (1982).

17. E. Granström and H. Kindahl, Species differences in circulating prostaglandin metabolites: Relevance for the assay of prostaglandin release, Biochim. Biophys. Acta, 713: 555 (1982).

18. E. Granström, U. Diczfalusy and M. Hamberg, The thromboxanes, in: "Prostaglandins and Related Substances", C.R. Pace-Asciak and E. Granström, eds., New Comprehensive Biochemistry, vol. 5, Elsevier, Amsterdam (1983), pp. 45-94.

19. L.J. Roberts, II, B.J. Sweetman, N.A. Payne, and J.A. Oates, Metabolism of thromboxane B_2 in man: identification of the major urinary metabolite, J. Biol. Chem., 252:7415 (1977).

16

20. L.J. Roberts, II, B.J. Sweetman, and J.A. Oates, Metabolism of thromboxnae B_2 in man: Identification of twenty urinary metabolites, J. Biol. Chem., 256:8384 (1981).
21. P. Westlund, M. Kumlin and E. Granström, Metabolism of thromboxane B_2 in the rabbit: Urinary and blood metabolic profile, to be published.
22. P. Westlund, A. Nordenström, M. Kumlin and E. Granström, Circulating metabolites of thromboxane B_2 in the human, to be published.
23. U. Axen, N,N´-carbonyldiimidazole as coupling agent for the preparation of bovine serum albumine, Prostaglandins, 5:45 (1974).
24. B. Caldwell, S. Burstein, W. Brock and L. Speroff, Radioimmunoassay of the F prostaglandins, J. Clin. Endocrinol. Metab. 33:171 (1971).
25. C. Patrono, G. Ciabattoni, P. Patrignani, P. Filabozzi, E. Pinca, M.A. Satta, D. Van Dorne, G.A. Cinotti, F. Pugliese, A. Perucci, and B.M. Simonetti, Evidence for a renal origin of urinary thromboxane B_2 in health and disease, Adv. Prostaglandin Thromboxane Res., 11:493 (1983).
26. R.D. Zipser, G.H. Radvan, I.J. Kronborg, R. Duke and T.E. Little, Urinary thromboxane B_2 and prostaglandin E_2 in the hepatorenal syndrome: Evidence for increased vasoconstrictor and decreased vasodilator factors, Gastroenterology, 84:697 (1983).

HIGH PRESSURE LIQUID CHROMATOGRAPHY-[125]J-RIA, A SENSITIVE AND SPECIFIC PROSTAGLANDIN ASSAY

T. Mourits-Andersen, R. Jensen and
J. Dyerberg

Department of Clinical Chemistry, Aalborg
Hospital, Section North, 9100 Aalborg, Denmark

INTRODUCTION

The interest in the biological influence of prostaglandins on different physiological and pathophysiological conditions in man has led to the development of several methods for measuring prostaglandins in biological materials.

The methods most frequently applied include bioassay, gas chromatography/mass-spectrometry (GS/MS) and radioimmunoassay (RIA).

The reported levels of prostaglandins (PGs) and their metabolites (PGMs) in human plasma have been markedly different, obviously due to the methodological problems (2,6,9,12,19,20).

When RIA is used, the primary extraction and separation of PGs and their metabolites from other plasma constituents and the isolation of the assay component are crucial steps as even a small cross reactivity with substances present in vaste excess may result in falsely elevated results (7). The lack of this precaution seems to be the major reason for variations invalidating the comparison between studies and making the physiological interpretations difficult.

In order to circumvent these problems we have used a SEP-PAK$_{C18}$^{R} extraction and a reverse-phase high pressure liquid chromatography system (rp-HPLC) to isolate some of the most important prostaglandins and metabolites in plasma: 6-keto-PGF$_{1\alpha}$ (the stable metabolite of prostacyclin), TXB$_2$ (the stable metabolite of thromboxan A$_2$) and prostaglandin E$_2$ prior to a RIA-determination of these components. In this way the major cause of analytical errors by RIA has been avoided.

APPARATUS

Extraction of PGs and PGMs from plasma was performed on a SEP-PAK$_{C18}$^{R} cartridge from Waters Associates, Milford, Massachusetts, U.S.A.

Isolation of the components was carried out by use of HPLC delivery system, model 6000A^R, with a universal injector model U-6K^R. The chromatography column was radial compression reverse-phase$_{C18}$ (Radial Pack^R, 10 μm, 8 x 100 mm) fixed with precolumn Guard-PAK$_{C18}$^{R}. All from Waters Associates, Milford, Massachusetts, U.S.A.

The HPLC fractions were collected on a LKB-2211 super Rack^R, Bromma, Sweden. Flow pressure was continously recorded on a pen-recorder.

^{125}J-tracers used in the RIA-assays were counted on a Gambyt CS$_{10}$^{R}, Wilj International, Ashford, Kent, UK. ^{3}H-tracers were measured on a Packard Tri-carb Liquid Scintillator spectrometer model 3375^R, with Insta-GEL^R as scintillator liquid, both from Packard Instrument Company, Downers Grove, Illinois, U.S.A.

REAGENTS

^{3}H-labelled prostaglandins: ^{3}H-6-keto-PGF$_{1\alpha}$ (120 Ci/mmol), ^{3}H-TXB$_2$ (163 Ci/mmol) and ^{3}H-PGF$_{2\alpha}$ (150 Ci/mmol) were purchased from New England Nuclear (NEN), Boston, U.S.A. ^{3}H-labelled prostaglandins: ^{3}H-PGE$_2$ (160 Ci/mmol), ^{3}H-PGD$_2$ (130 Ci/mmol) were purchased from Amersham International, Amersham, Great Britain. The ^{3}H-labelled standards were all purified by HPLC before use. Radioimmunological measurements of 6-keto-PGF$_{1\alpha}$, TXB$_2$ and PGE$_2$ were performed with commercial ^{125}J-kits from New England Nuclear International, Boston, U.S.A. The sensitivity of the RIA-kits, defined as twice the standard deviation at zero binding was 0.5, 2.0 and 0.1 pmol/l for 6-keto-PGF$_{1\alpha}$, TXB$_2$ and PGE$_2$ respectively.

Water was glass distilled, acetonitril and methanol
were of HPLC grade (Rathburn Chemicals Walkerburn,
Peebleshire, Scotland) and acetic acid was of analytical
grade (Merck. Damstadt, West Germany). These solvents
were filtered through a 0.5 µmillipore filter (Water
Associates, Milford, Massachusetts, U.S.A.). The other
reagents were: Methylformat (97% v/v), Janssen Chemica
Beerse, Belgium. Hexan (laboratory Chemical) May and
Baker, Dagenham, England. Ethanol (99.3% v/v). The
danish Distillery, Aalborg, Denmark.

ASSAY CONDITIONS

After discarding the first 2 ml blood, venous blood
was drawn from a cubital vein with 50 mmHg of stasis
into a precooled 12 ml polyprophylen tube containing
200 µl of a mixture of K_2EDTA 95 mg/ml and indomethacin
1.8 µg/ml.

The blood was kept on ice until centrifugation for
10 minutes at 2000 g at 4°C to obtain platelet free
plasma (6-8 ml) which was enriched with 1-2 pg/ml of a
mixture of ^{3}H-labelled 6-keto-PGF$_{1\alpha}$, TXB$_2$ and
PGE$_2$ as internal standards.

Immediately after this the samples were adjusted to
pH 3.5 with 1 mol/1 HCl to get the prostaglandins in a
non-ionic state. After preparation of SEP-PAK$_{C18}$^{R}
cartridge with ethanol and water the sample was slowly
passed through the cartridge which was then eluted with
20 ml water, 20 ml ethanol: water (15:85 v/v), 20 ml hexan and 10 ml methylformat as described by Powell (11).
The methylformat fraction was evaporated at 0°C under
nitrogen and stored at -21° until further processing.
Before the high pressure liquid chromatography the
sample was redisolved in 150 µl solvent of which 140 µl
was injected on HPLC-column. The solvent was water,
acetonitril, acetic acid (71.5; 28.5; 0.5 v:v) degassed
with two volumes helium (16).

The eluation was isocratic, flow rate: 2 ml/min.,
solvent flow pressure: 35 kg/cm^2 and radial column
pressure: 200 kg/cm^2 at ambient temperature.

The different prostaglandins were individually
sampled after programming of the fraction collector with
data from the retention volumes of the ^{3}H-labelled
prostaglandins. All fractions were lyophilized and
re-dissolved in 500 µl RIA phosphate buffer of which 2 x
100 µl were assayed with the relevant ^{125}J-RIA-kit.

2 x 50 μl were counted by liquid scintillation for recovery determination. After each chromatography the column was washed with 200 μl acetonitril and 200 μl methanol: H_2O (1:1 v/v) followed by 100 ml solvent.

A blank plasma sample (charcoal treated) was rutinely chromatographied in series with the biological samples.

Subjects

13 volunteers, mainly technicial staff members participated in the study. Venipuncture was performed in the morning in a fasting state and again 1 1/2 hours after breakfast (postprandial).

RESULTS

As the prostaglandins in biological quantities can not be detected by conventional methods for HPLC (UV-detection or electro-chemical detection) the collection of the fractions containing the individual prostaglandins was based on a determination of the retention volume of the relevant ^{3}H-labelled prostaglandins. Fig. 1 shows a typical control chromatogram of a mixture of ^{3}H-labelled 6-keto-PGF$_{1\alpha}$, TXB$_2$ and the prostaglandins of the 2-serie: PGF$_{2\alpha}$, PGE$_2$ and PGD$_2$. Obviously 6-keto-PGF$_{1\alpha}$, TXB$_2$ and PGE$_2$ are well separated by a single chromatography run without interference from the interjacent prostaglandins, PGF$_{2\alpha}$ and PGD$_2$. The chromatography is completed within 30 minutes.

The capacity(K), selectivity (S) and resolution (R) factors for 6-keto-PGF$_{1\alpha}$, TXB$_2$, PGF$_{2\alpha}$ PGE$_2$ and PGD$_2$ by the present method are given in Table I.

To check the stability of the column the variation of the peak retention volume of 15 control runs was recorded during one month in which 70 sample runs were carried out. The results are given in Table II.

The recovery of the prostaglandins in the assay system was found by the determination of the ^{3}H-activity from the internal standards in the HPLC eluate, corrected for quenching and purity.

The total recovery and variation after SEP-PAK extraction, HPLC and lyophilisation determined in the

Table I. Capacity (K), Selectivity (S) and Resolution
(R) Factors for 6-Keto-PGF$_{1\alpha}$, TXB$_2$, PGF$_{2\alpha}$
PGE$_2$ and PGD$_2$.

Prostaglandin	Capacity factor	Selectivity factor	Resolution factor
6-keto-PGF$_{1\alpha}$	4,7		
TXB$_2$	10,1	2,2	2,9
PGF$_{2\alpha}$	12,7	1,3	1,3
PGE$_2$	15,1	1,2	1,5
PGD$_2$	17,5	1,2	1,5

$$K = \frac{V_S - V_O}{V_O}$$

V_S = Peak retention volume of solute

V_O = The void volume of the column

$$S = \frac{K^N}{K^{N-1}}$$

K = Capasity factors of the solute (N = 2-5)

$$R = \frac{V_{S_N} - V_{S_{N-1}}}{1/2 \ (W_N + W_{N-1})}$$

W_2 = Basic width volume of solute (N = 2-5)

RIA-buffer at 3 different biological realistic concentrations are given in Table III. (The marked variation
at the highest TXB$_2$ level is due to one abnormly low

Table II. The mean, SD and coefficient of variation for peak retention volumen (in ml) of 15 control runs during 1 month comprising 70 runs with 344 ml plasma.

	6-keto-PGF$_{1\alpha}$	TXB$_2$	PGF$_{2\alpha}$	PGE$_2$	PGD$_2$
Mean ml	16,1	31,6	39,1	44,9	51,9
SD ml	0,35	0,63	0,96	1,33	1,66
CV%	2,1	2,0	2,5	3,0	3,2

Table III Total recovery of ^{3}H-labelled 6-keto-PGF$_{1\alpha}$, TXB$_2$ and PGE$_2$ after SEP-PAK extraction, HPLC and lyophilisation.

Prostaglandins	Added to 8 ml plasma PG		Recovery PG $\pm$ 1 SD	Recovery % mean	
^{3}H-keto-PGF$_{1\alpha}$	10,8	N=5	8,4 $\mp$ 0,7	78	
	43,8	N=5	33,3 $\mp$ 2,8	76	75
	87,5	N=5	62,6 $\mp$ 9,5	72	
TXB$_2$	7,9	N=5	6,9 $\mp$ 0,4	87	
	31,6	N=5	25,7 $\mp$ 1,5	81	80
	96,9	N=4	69,5 $\mp$17,1	72	
PGE$_2$	11,5	N=5	8,9 $\mp$ 0,3	77	
	66,0	N=5	47,4 $\mp$ 2,6	72	75
	125,3	N=5	94,1 $\mp$ 4,4	75	

value. Without this value the mean recovery was 78.0 pg $\pm$ 3.3 at this level.

The fasting and postprandial plasma levels of 6-keto-PGF$_{1\alpha}$, TXB$_2$ and PGE$_2$ in 13 healthy non-smoking laboratory technicians, mean age: 33 years (range 22-48 years) are given in Table IV.

The intra series precision (CV%) of the assay procedure (including the variation of the extraction, HPLC-procedure and RIA) was 6-8%, determined as the sum of the variation in recoveries of the internal standards

Table IV. Fasting and postprandial plasma levels (pmol/l) of 6-keto-PGF$_{1\alpha}$, TXB$_2$ and PGE$_2$ in 13 healthy non-smoking laboratory technicians, age 21-48 years.

pmol/l	Fasting	Postprandial	
	Median range	Median range	
6-keto-PGF$_{1\alpha}$	3,7 (0,8-12,9)	3,6 (0,7-7,0)	NS P > 0,05
TXB$_2$	47,7 (14,1-185,3)	30,5 (< 2,0-82,5)	NS P > 0,05
PGE$_2$	0,4 (< 0,1-3,1)	0,5 (< 0,1-2,4)	NS P > 0,05

in 13 samples and the variation of the RIA per se.

The coefficients of correlation between fasting plasma levels of 6-keto-PGF$_{1\alpha}$, TXB$_2$ and PGE$_2$ are given in Table V.

To check the importance of the HPLC-procedure to remove substances interacting with the radioimmunoassay the prostaglandin level in a plasma pool after SEP-PAK extraction and after supplementary HPLC-isolation were determined. The results are given in Table VI.

DISCUSSION

High pressure liquid chromatography (HPLC) for isolation of prostaglandins in plasma was first described by Carr and Frölich in 1976 (4).

Since then this method has been used by several authors to separate prostaglandins in different biological materials (1,5,8,10,13,15,17).

Reverse-phase HPLC preceeded by SEP-PAK$_{C18}$ column extraction has been reported for experimental separation of the metabolites of prostacyclin in plasma (14).

Table V.   Correlation coefficiens between fasting plasma
            levels of 6-keto-PGF$_{1\alpha}$, TXB$_2$ and PGE$_2$ in
            13 healthy non-smoking laboratory technicians.

	PGE$_2$	TXB$_2$
Keto-PGF$_{1\alpha}$	- 0,06 NS	0,16 NS
TXB$_2$	0,72 P < 0,01	

Table VI.   Median and range levels (pmol/l) in pooled
             plasma of 6-keto-PGF$_{1\alpha}$, TXB$_2$ and PGE$_2$
             estimated by RIA after SEP-PAK extraction
             and after supplementary HPLC separation.

	6-keto-PGF$_{1\alpha}$	TXB$_2$	PGE$_2$
SEP-PAK	148,7	140,1	9,7
N=6	134,4 - 162,1	129,9 - 174,0	8,5 - 10,8
SEP-PAK+HPLC	< 0,5	72,0	1,4
N=5		63,8 - 73,5	0,8 - 1,5

    In our study we used a reverse-phase$_{C18}$ column for
the HPLC separation of 6-keto-PGF$_{1\alpha}$, TXB$_2$, PGF$_2$,
PGE$_2$ and PGD$_2$ at non-ionic form preceeded by a
SEP-PAK$_{C18}$ cartridge extraction.

    By this method we obtained satisfactory separation
of plasma prostaglandins and metabolites with resolution
factors ranging from 1.3 - 2.7. The chromatography was
performed in a single isocratic eluation completed
within 30 minutes with a solvent consumption of less
than 60 ml. This in contrast to the method reported by
Worton (18), who used a -Bonde Pak fatty acid column,
preceeded by a silica acid column chromatography, and
had longer retention times and insufficient separation
of PGE$_2$ and PGD$_2$.

The variation in the capacity factors during 1 month was less than 3.4%. The high recovery of the present method means that we can use plasma samples of 6-8 ml in contrast to the method reported by Siess (14), where a plasma sample of 50 ml was needed.

The low basal and postprandial levels (pg/ml) of 6-keto-PGF$_{1\alpha}$, TXB$_2$ and PGE$_2$ in plasma as determined with the present method are in accordance with the values obtained by gas chromatography/mass-spectrometry (2,12). This means that the SEP-PAK extraction in combination with the HPLC procedure has minimized the amount of cross reacting substances present in plasma which gives rise to the falsely high and variating plasma levels so often reported in radioimmunoassay studies. In one recent RIA study(6) where a non commercially available antibody was used, very low levels of 6-keto-PGF$_{1\alpha}$ comparable with results of GC/MS was reported.

The sampling technique is another important factor which may give rise to variation in plasma levels of prostaglandins in man (3). In order to standardize the sampling procedure we used venous stasis standardized at 50 mmHg for a few seconds, discarded the first 2 ml blood in which the platelets often are activated and stopped the synthesis of PG immediatly with EDTA/-indometacin and cooling. Polyprophylen tubes were used to minimize the bindings of PG to the tubes. However it can not be excluded that the stasis has stimulated the prostaglandin production so that the reported levels are not true basal levels.

The use of high pressure liquid chromatography for purification and isolation of prostaglandins before radioimmunoassay makes it possible to determine the circulating levels of different prostaglandins in plasma. This is a necessity for the investigation of interrelations between different prostaglandins in physiological and pathophysiological conditions. The correlation between plasma thromboxan and PGE$_2$ as found in this study obviously reflect production in the platelets.

The very low levels of 6-keto-PGF$_{1\alpha}$ and PGE$_2$ found by this method makes any generation of hypothesis including reduced basal levels of the plasma 6-keto-PGF$_{1\alpha}$ and PGE$_2$ in relation to pathophysiological conditions unrealistic.

ACKNOWLEDGEMENTS

The technical assistance of Ulla Jakobsen and Edith Christiansen is highly appreciated.

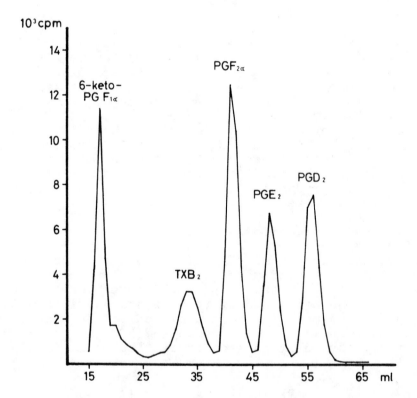

Fig. 1. A typical reverse-phase HPL-chromatogram of a mixture of ^{3}H-labelled-6-keto-PGF$_{1a}$, TXB$_2$, PGF$_{2a}$, PGE$_2$ and PGD$_2$. Flow rate 2 ml/min, solvent composition: Acetonitril, H$_2$O, acetic acid (28.5; 71.5; 0.15) isocratic elution.

Suzanne Ekelund, Terkel Arnfred and Niels Hjørne are acknowledged for fruitful discussions.

The secretarial assistance of Susanne Randrup and Helle Krigslund are greatfully acknowledged.

This study was supported by a grant from the fund of the county of North Jutland for Medical Research.

REFERENCES

1   Benzoni, D., 1982, A new technique for the measurement of urinary 6-keto-prostaglandin $F_{1\alpha}$: normal values in adults, Clin Chem Acta, 126:283.
2   Blair, I. A., 1982, Prostacyclin is not a circulating hormone in man, Prostaglandins, 23:579.
3   Butt, R. W., 1983, Basal 6-keto-$PGF_{1\alpha}$ levels: Influence of sampling techniques, Thromb Res, 29:469.
4   Carr, K.,1976, High performance liquid chromatography of prostaglandins: Biological applications, Prostaglandins, 11:3.
5   Fischer, S., 1982, Prostacyclin metabolites, in urine of adults and neonates, studied by gas chromatography-mass-spectrometry and radioimmuno-assay, Biochi et Biophys Acta, 710:493.
6   Forder, R. A., 1983, Measurement of human venous plasma prostacyclin and metabolites by radioimmunoassay, Prostaglandins Leukotrienes and Medicine, 12:323.
7   Greaves, M., 1982, Plasma 6-keto-prostaglandin $F_{1\alpha}$: Fact or fiction, Thromb Res, 26:145.
8   Hubbard, W. C., 1976, Determination of 15-keto-13, 14-dihydro-metabolites of PGE_2 and PGE_2 in plasma using high performance liquid chromatography and gas chromatography-mass spectrometry, Prostaglandins, 12:21.
9   Myatt, L., 1981, Metabolism of prostacyclin and 6-Oxo-$PGF_{1\alpha}$ in man, Clin Pharm of Prostacyclin, Raven Press.
10 Ody, C., 1982, 6-ketoprostaglandin $F_{1\alpha}$, prosta-glandins E_2, $F_{2\alpha}$ and thromboxane B_2 production by endothelial cells, smooth muscle cells and fibro-blasts cultured from piglet aorta, Biochem et Bio-phys Acta, 712:103.
11 Powell, W. S., 1980, Rapid extraction of oxygenated metabolites of arachidonic acid from biological samples using octadecylsilyl silica, Prostaglandins, 20:947.

12 Ritter, J. M., 1983, Release of prostacyclin in vivo and its role in man, The Lancet, February, 317.

13 Rollins, M. V., 1983, High-pressure liquid chromatography of underivatized fatty acids, hydroxy acids, and prostanoids having different chain lengths and double-bond positions, Methods in enzymology, 86: 518.

14 Siess, W., 1982, Very low levels of 6-keto-prostaglandin $F_{1\alpha}$ in human plasma, J Lab Clin Med, 99: 388.

15 Skrinska, V., 1983, High-performance liquid chromatography of prostacyclin, J of Chromatography, 277: 287.

16 Snyder, L. R., 1983, Solvent degassing for HPLC, J of Chromatographic Sience, 21:65.

17 Sraer, J., 1982, In vitro prostaglandin synthesis by human glomeruli and papillae, Prostaglandins, 23: 855.

18 Whorton, A. R., 1979, Reverse-phase high-performance liquid chromatography of prostaglandins - biological applications, J of Chromatography, 163:64.

19 Ylikorkala, O., 1982, The effect of age on circulating 6-keto-prostaglandin $F_{1\alpha}$ in humans, Prostaglandins Leukotrienes and Medicine, 9:569.

20 Yoshio, U., 1983, Plasma levels of 6-keto-prostaglandin $F_{1\alpha}$ in normotensive subjects and patients with essential hypertension, Prostaglandins Leukotrienes and Medicine, 10:455.

ENZYME IMMUNOASSAYS OF ICOSANOIDS USING ACETYLCHOLINESTERASE

P. Pradelles[1], J. Maclouf[2] and J. Grassi[1]

[1]Section de Pharmacologie et Immunologie
Commissariat à l'Energie Atomique C.E.N. Saclay
91191 Gif/Yvette Cèdex, France
[2] U 150 INSERM, LA 334CNRS Hospital Lariboisiere
75474 Paris Cèdex 10, France

In the early seventies, the need for the development of
sensitive and quantitative assay methods for the analysis of the
prostanoids became obvious. Two major complementary methods were
selected by the scientists : gas-chromatography combined with mass
spectrometry and radioimmunoassay (RIA) techniques. Both methods
were improved throughout the years in regard of their specificity
and sensitivity. The introduction of deuterated carriers for the
first one and the use of low-bleeding fused glass capillary column
with high efficiency allowed the detection of a few picograms. The
RIA techniques improved their specificity after gradually avoiding
the classical pitfalls that result from a mishandling of the
assay. The gain in sensitivity was related to the increase of
specific radioactivity of the tracers. From the early days of (^{3}H)
prostaglandins (PG) with 5-10 Ci/mmole (1) these tracers presently
range from 50-200 Ci/mmole. In 1975, we introduced the ^{125}I
labeling of these substances after coupling of their carboxyle to
the amino group of a potential iodine receptor (e.g. histamine,
tyramine or tyrosylmethyl ester) (2). Such an approach allowed us
to reach for these tracers the theoretical specific radioactivity
of the iodine, i.e. 2,000 Ci/mmole. The gain in sensitivity was
x5-10 as compared with the corresponding tritiated systems ;
further these tracers provided the advantages intrinsic to the
iodinated labels (absence of quenching, low cost, rapidity of
counting...). More recently, non isotopic immunoassay methods for
PG have emerged : they involve enzyme immunoassay (EIA) or
chemiluminescence immunoassays. These methods should gain a
widespread use due to the reinforcement of the regulation on the

use of radioactive substances and because of environmental and
pollution requirements. However, until now, these methods are
rather disappointing because their sensitivity is still poor (3,
4) especially as compared to iodinated tracers.
We have developped an EIA for various icosanoids (PG,
thromboxane-TX-, and leukotriene C_4-LTC_4-) coupled to an enzyme.
This technique is based on the use of acetylcholinesterase (AChE)
(EC-3-1-1-7) extracted from the electric organs of an electric eel
("Electrophorus Electricus"). The assay is performed using 96
wells microtiter plates coated with second antibodies. The use of
this solid phase allows a semi-automatization of the procedure.
The sensitivity was equal or superior to that obtained with
corresponding iodinated tracers.

MATERIALS AND METHODS

AChE - X (AChE-icosanoid conjugate)
AbX (specific antiserum)   50 ul each
Standard, or unknown or buffer

96 well microtiter plate coated
with piganti-rabbit immunoglobulins

|

overnight incubation (4°C)

|

washing of the plate (<u>automatic</u>) 60 sec

|

removal of unbound fraction

addition of Ellman's reagent (enzyme substrate) (<u>automatic</u>) 15 sec

|

enzymatic reaction (30-45 min)

|

measurement of absorbance (414 nm) (<u>automatic</u>) 90 sec

|

CALCULATIONS

Figure 1 : Scheme of the different steps for the enzyme
immunoassay of the various icosanoids. (X = icosanoid)

The preparation of all antisera was done in the laboratory,
unless otherwise stated, according to previously described
procedures (5). All standards were kind gifts of Dr. J.E. Pike
(The Upjohn Company, USA) or Dr. J. Rokach (Merck-Frosst
Laboratories Canada). Our purification of AChE from "Electrophorus
Electricus" electric organs was done in a one step affinity
chromatography as previously described (6). The preparation
contains essentially the heaviest molecular forms of the enzyme
(A8 and A12) for a review, see ref. 7. The enzyme activity was
measured by the method of Ellman et al (8). The preparation of the
PG-, TX- or LTC_4-AChE conjugates will be described elsewhere (9).
After coupling of the ligands to the enzyme, a gel filtration

chromatography was used to separate the conjugates from the unreacted molecules of hapten. The enzyme did not suffer any noticeable loss of activity. For some studies, iodinated TX has been used ; its preparation has been described elsewhere (2). The assay procedure is described in figure 1. It involves the use of 96-well microtiter plates coated with pig anti-rabbit IgG purified by affinity chromatography. The reaction is performed in a total of 150 ul. After overnight incubation at 4°C, solid phase is intensively washed using a Titertek Multiwash apparatus. The Ellman's reagent is automatically dispensed in each well using a Titertek Autodrop equipment. After 30-45 min., the absorbance at 414 nm of each well is measured using a Titertek Multiskan spectrophotometer. Calculations performed on the bound fraction are done following classical procedures using a linear log transformation and a microcomputer.

RESULTS AND DISCUSSION

Since RIA cannot be performed in 96 wells-microtiter plates we first made a comparison between the performances obtained with either the radioactive or the enzymatic tracer. This experiment was performed in test tubes using second antibody immunoprecipitation as described previously (10).

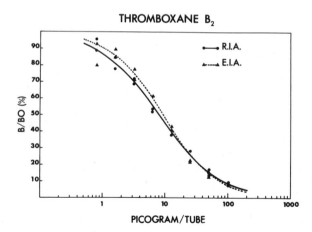

Figure 2. Comparison of dose response curves for TXB_2 using ^{125}I -Histamine or AChE as labels.

Results are presented in figure 2 : similar sensitivities were obtained with both systems (IC 50 $\simeq$ 9 pg/tube ; practical detection limit 2 pg). The sensitivity of EIA could be significantly improved by the use of 96 wells microtiter plates coated with the second antibody. In this system the IC 50 and

33

practical detection limit are 2 pg and 0.3 pg, respectively
(figure not shown). This improvement in sensitivity was
essentially due to a lowering of the non specific binding (<0.1 %)

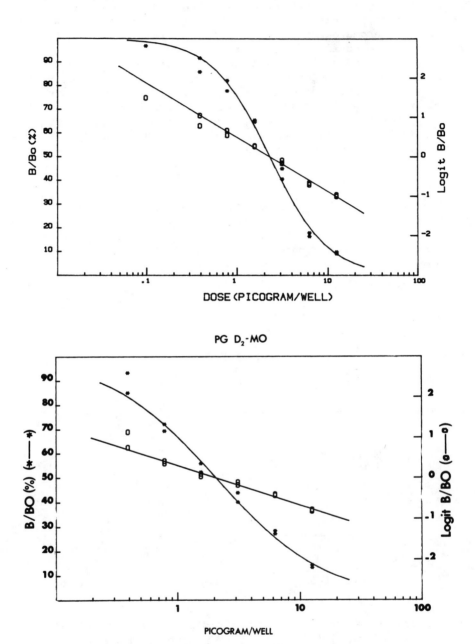

Figure 3. Dose response curves for 6-Keto PG $F_{1}\alpha$ PG
D_2-methoxamine, using AchE label.

and an increased precision. Further details will be given in réf.9.

Similar standard curves have also been obtained with other icosanoids such as 6-keto $PGF_{1\alpha}$, or PGD_2-methoxamine, (figure 3). For most of the compounds, the sensitivity was in the same range as what was already observed with the TX-AChE tracer. We could also extend the use of AChE as a label for LTC_4. Figure 4 shows the performance of such tracer as compared with ^3H LTC_4 using a specific antiserum (kind gift of Drs. Rokach and Young, Merck-Frosst Laboratory). The enzyme tracer provided a dramatic gain in sensitivity as compared to ^3H .

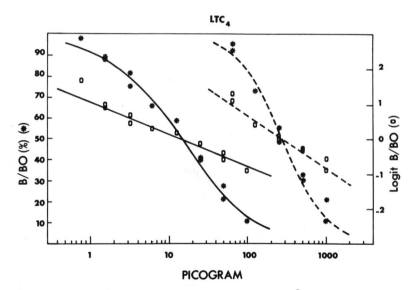

Figure 4. Dose response curves for LTC_4 using ^3H (--) or AChE (—⚫) as labels.

To demonstrate the practical applicability of AChE-PG -TX or LTC_4 as a tracer we have correlated the results obtained with 2 techniques. Figure 5a shows the correlation of EIA with RIA for

the determination of the TXB_2 content of 17 supernatants from
stimulated human platelets suspended either in plasma or in

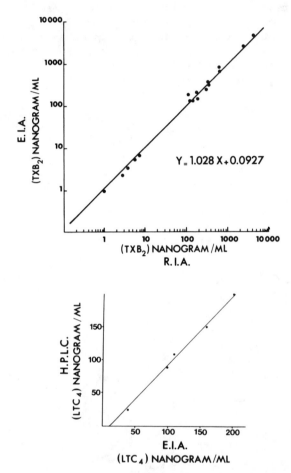

Figure 5. Determination of TXB_2 and LTC_4 concentrations in
different biological fluids : correlation with other analytical
methods. a) Correlation of TXB_2 values in unextracted supernatants
of stimulated human platelets in plasma or in buffer determined by
RIA or by EIA. (upper curve) b) Correlation of LTC_4 values in
unextracted supernatants of stimulated human neutrophils
determined by HPLC or by EIA. (lower curve)

buffer. Figure 5b shows the correlation of EIA with quantitative HPLC for the determination of the LTC_4 content of 5 supernatants from stimulated human neutrophils. As can be seen in those 2 examples, a linear regression analysis gives a good correlation between the different methods, thus demonstrating the possibility of performing the EIA analysis on unextracted samples from cell supernatants either in the presence or in the absence of proteins.

CONCLUDING REMARKS

The intensive use of assay methods to investigate the occurence of icosanoids in biological fluids from various pathological diseases or under pharmacological manipulations may help to clarify their exact role as autacoids. Radioimmunoassays represent the most favoured analytical methods in the icosanoid research because of their capacity to treat a large number of samples ; the impossibility of GC-MS to monitor the peptido-leukotrienes has reinforced their use. However, due to the extreme potency of action of these substances, the minute amounts that are found in biological fluids have to be monitored by highly sensitive technique because in such studies the amount of biological sample to monitor is limited. These requirements are a prerequisite for clinical investigations by which the improvement of our knowledge on the role of these substances should come.

The criteria of sensitivity can be circumvented by an increase of the specific activity of the tracer. Although the iodinated tracers were a first step in this direction, the intensive use of radioactivity raises a serious cost and environment problem ; further their relative short half-life requires the preparation of a new batch of tracer every 2 months. Therefore the use of non radioactive and long-life time tracers such as AChE-PG, -TX, -LT possessing specific activities that can match or even surpass that of the iodine is a major improvement. In addition the possible use of semi-automatized device combined with 96-well microtiter plates allows the treatment of a large number of samples in the minimum amount of time. In both these respects our technique has reached its goal. In spite of these improvements we should not forget the drastic rules that have to be followed in regard of specificity. Such rules which have been listed in the excellent review of Granström and Kindahl (10) should include a validation that has to be performed on the specific problem that has to be solved i.e. depending on the biological fluid, of the antiserum specificity as well as of the chemical stability of the compound(s) to be analyzed.

REFERENCES

1. Caldwell B.V., Burstein S., Brock W.A. and Speroff L., 1971, Radioimmuno-assay of the F prostaglandins, J. Clin. Endocr., 33:171.

2. Maclouf J., Pradel M., Pradelles P. and Dray F., 1976, ^{125}I derivatives of prostaglandins. A novel approach in prostaglandin analysis by radioimmuno-assay, Biochim. Biophys. Acta, 431:139.

3. Hayashi Y., Ueda N., Yokota K., Kawamura S., Ogushi F., Yamamoto Y., Yamamoto S., Nakamura K., Yamashita K., Miyazaki H., Kato K. and Terao S., 1983, Enzyme immuno-assay of thromboxane B_2, Biochim. Biophys. Acta., 750:322.

4. Weerasekera D.A., Koullapis E.N., Kim J.B., Barnard G.J., Collins W.P., Kohen F. and Lindner H.R., 1983, Chemiluminescence immuno-assay of thromboxane B_2, in Advances in Prostaglandin, Thromboxane and Leukotriene Research, Vol 11, B. Samuelsson, R. Paoletti and P. Ramwell, Raven Press, New York pp 185.

5. Dray F., B. Charbonnel and J. Maclouf., 1975, Radioimmuno-assay of prostaglandins F_α, E_1 and E_2 in human plasma, Eur. J. Biochem., 5:311.

6. Massoulié J. and Bon S., 1976, Affinity chromatography of acetylcholinesterase. The importance of hydrophobic interactions, Eur. J. Biochem., 68:531.

7. Massoulié J. and Bon S., 1982, The molecular forms of cholinesterase and acetylcholinesterase in vertebrates, Ann. Rev. Neurosci., 5:57.

8. Ellman G.L., Courtney K.D., Andres V. and Featherstone R.M., 1961, A new and rapid colorimetric determination of acetycholinesterase activity, Biochem. Pharmacol., 7:88.

9. Pradelles P., Grassi J. and Maclouf J., 1984, (submitted).

10. Marsh D., Grassi J., Vigny M. and Massoulié J., 1984, An immunological study of rat acetylcholinesterase : comparison with acetylcholinesterases from other vertebrates, J. Neurochem., 43:204.

11. Granström E. and Kindahl H., 1978, Radioimmuno-assay of Prostaglandins and Thromboxane. Adv. Prostaglandin Thromboxane Res., 5:119.

SYNTHESES AND BIOLOGICAL EFFECTS OF LEUKOTRIENES AND ANALOGS

Bernd Spur,* Attilio Crea,** and Wilfried Peters**

*Department of Chemistry, Harvard University, 12 Oxford
Street, Cambridge MA 02138
Department of Rheumatology and Immunology, Brigham and
Women's Hospital, Harvard Medical School, Boston, MA
02115

**Institut für Medizinische Mikrobiologie und Institut
für Anorganische Chemie I der Universität Düsseldorf
D-4000 Düsseldorf 1, F.R.G.

Polyunsaturated fatty acids such as arachidonic acid are transformed

via the cyclooxygenase pathway into three groups of biological active

compounds, the prostaglandins, the thromboxanes and the prostacyclins.

In the last years another family the leukotrienes was discovered.

These compounds are formed via the 5-lipoxygenase pathway and play

a major role as biological mediators in immediate hypersensitivity

reactions and inflammation [1-4].

The discovery of the leukotrienes as well as other hydroxy-eicosa-

tetraenoic acids synonym with the names B. Samuelsson and E.J. Corey

was a collaboration between medicals and organic chemists.

The metabolism of arachidonic acid in polymorphonuclear leukocytes from the peritoneal cavity of rabbits leads to the 5(S)-hydroxy-6,8,11,14-eicosatetraenoic acid (5-HETE) as the major metabolite. Minor products were later identified as the 5(S),12(R)-dihydroxy-6,8,10,14-eicosatetraenoic acid (leukotriene B_4, LTB_4) as well as two other 5(S),12-dihydroxy-6,8,10;14-eicosatetraenoic acids epimers in the position 12. Also the two isomers of 5,6-dihydroxy-7,9,11,14-eicosatetraenoic acid could be detected [5,6].

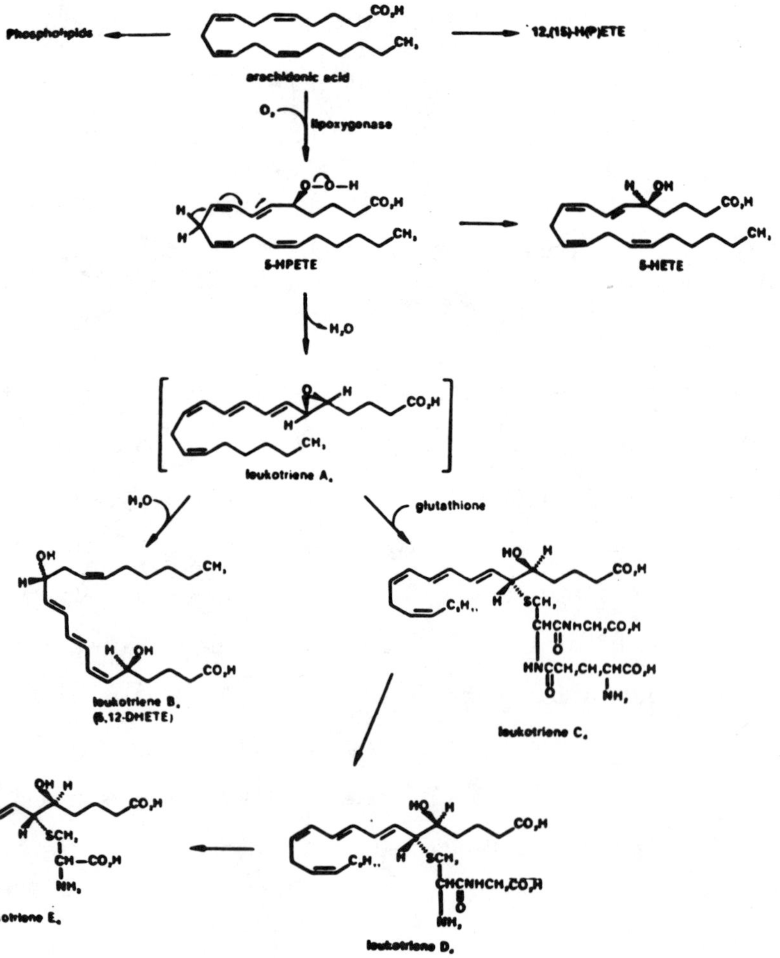

Figure 1.

The starting metabolite 5-HETE as well as other HETEs can be obtained
by singulett oxygenation or copper catalysed oxygenation of arachidonic
acid followed by reduction [7]. The first synthesis of 5-HETE in racemic
and later on in optical active form was achieved by iodo-lactonisation
of arachidonic acid followed by dehydroiodination and opening of
the δ-lactone with methanol / triethylamine in the presence of a
trace of water, otherwise the δ-lactone remains intact [8,9].
The racemic mixture of the 5-HETE methyl ester could be separated
into 5(S)-HETE (natural occuring form) and the 5(R)-HETE by chromatography of the diastereomeric urethanes followed by deprotection [10].
Another general approch to the racemic HETEs was described by Rokach [11]
et al. using the Rhodium catalysed addition of diazoketones to furan
yielding the trans,cis unsaturated ketone which upon reduction and
chain extension via Wittig reactions leads to the HETEs. It seems
to be possible to obtain the optical active forms directly without
a resolution step using the recently described optical active boranes
developed by H.C. Brown.
Another general approach to all optically active HETEs has been
developed from inexpensive d- or l-arabinose [12].
The scheme outlined in the following picture illustrate the flexibility
of these starting materials which are readily available in multigram
quantities. The two different leaving groups liberate an aldehyde
which can be transformed to the HETEs by standard Wittig reactions.
The same strategy was recently used for the syntheses of all possible
8,15-diHETEs and will be mentioned later [13].
The conversion of 5-HETE to 5-HPETE using lipoxygenase enzyme from
potato tubers as well as the conversion of 5-HPETE to LTA$_4$ has been
succeded chemically. The chemical conversion of 5(S)-HETE to 5-HPETE

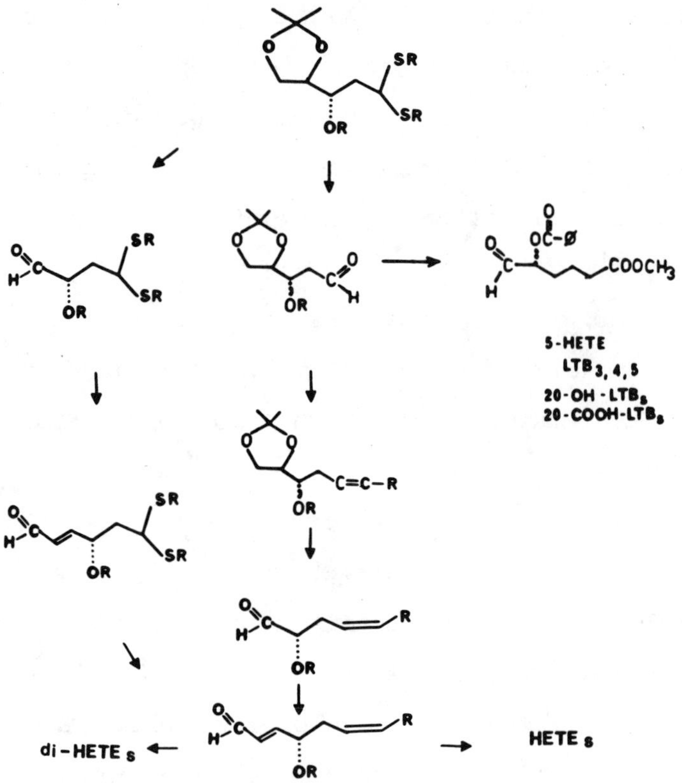

Figure 2.

via oxidation of the mesylate occurs via an S_N-1 type reaction
leading always to the racemic form of 5-HPETE[14].
The synthesis of the 15(S)-HETE or HPETE can be easily achieved
using the enzymatic oxidation of arachidonic acid in basic solution
with soybean lipoxygenase type I[15].

The connection between 5-HETE, 5-HPETE, LTA$_4$ and the "slow reacting
substance of anaphylaxis" (SRS-A) later named leukotriene C$_4$, D$_4$,
E$_4$, F$_4$ was suggested by the evidence that both species are metabolites
of arachidonic acid and can not be inhibited by aspirin or indomethacin
and both formation is stimulated by the calcium ionophore A23187.
The UV spectra as well as chemical degradation including the mobility
of these products by R.P. h.p.l.c. and by comparison with synthetic

materials led to the structure determination of the leukotrienes.
These products were shown to be identical with the "slow reacting
substances of anaphylaxis" first described by Feldberg and Kellaway
in 1938 obtained during perfusion of guinea pig lungs with cobra
venom. The same authors described the release of these compound
during the anaphylactic shock [16-17].

The biological data have been shown that these substances are potent
bronchoconstrictors in several species including humans with specific
efects on the periphal airways. Furthere more these products are
potent vasoconstrictors and show negative inotropic efects on the
cardiac contractions. The permeability of the postcapillary venules
are increased. Another leukotriene 5(S),12(R)-diHETE (leukotriene B_4)
is a potent chemotactic agent for eosinophils and neutrophils. The
leukotrienes are 1000 - 10000 times more potent than histamine on
the molar base. During the availability of synthetic leukotrienes
a large number of biological efects could be found with increasing
importance for deseases such as asthma, allergic disorders and
inflamation.

The first synthesis of the natural occuring leukotrienes LTA_4, LTC_4
was described by Corey starting from D-ribose. The absolute configuration and the stereochemistry was established for the first
time by chemical synthesis and by comparison with the natural derived
products by UV, h.p.l.c., reaction with soybean lipoxygenase and
bioassay and found identical in all aspects [18].

At the same time different syntheses have been developed for the
racemic and optically active LTs. The use of araboascorbic acid or
2-deoxy-ribose as a source for the required chirality has been
described [19].

The Methyl 5(S),6(R)-epoxy-6-formylhexanoate became the main target
molecule for a large number of research groups in the world. This
compound can easily be converted by two Wittig reactions into LTA_4.
In the meantime alternative and shorter routes to the optical active

key intermediates have been developed mainly based on the asymmetric epoxidation procedure of Sharpless starting from inexpensive achiral olefinic alcohols which differ only in the carboxyl equivalents [20-22]. The simple methyl 7-hydroxyhept-5-enoate proved to be difficult to convert directly to the chiral epoxide with respect to reaction and work up conditions. In the meantime a few other routes to LTA_4 have been described in the literature, for example via Emmons-Horner reaction of the epoxy aldehyde or the addition of an vinyl-lithium reagent to the aldehyde followed by mesylation and elimination with DBU [23,24].

The syntheses of LTC_4, LTD_4, LTE_4 from LTA_4 using protected thio-peptides under S_N-2 conditions (methanol/triethylamine) with subsequent cleavage of the protecting groups lead to the free SRS substances, Later on it was found that the free peptides can be used for the syntheses of the monomethyl esters which are hydrolysed more easily under mild conditions. In this case no isomerisation of the labile 11-cis double bond was observed [25].

Leukotriene B_4 5(S),12(R)-diHETE is formed enzymatically from LTA_4. The exact geometry of the double bonds of the conjugated triene system was established by total syntheses of all possible isomers and comparison by h.p.l.c. and bioassay. The first synthesis of Corey used 2-deoxy-ribose for the 5(S)-segment and d-mannose for the 12(R)-segment [26]. Later on Corey developed the most efficient stereoselective synthesis of LTB_4. The key step is a novel internally promoted elimination reaction of the epoxy ester using potassium isopropylate in isopropanol followed by hydrolysis with water and extraction of LTB_4 with ether at pH 6.0 [27]. The 5(S)-segment can be prepared from commercial available tri-)-acetyl-glucal [28]. Other syntheses of LTB_4 were developed using 2-deoxy-ribose as a source of chirality of both hydroxy-groups [19].

Following Corey's first synthesis the Sharpless epoxidation was succesfully used to construct the optical active phosphonium salt [19].

44

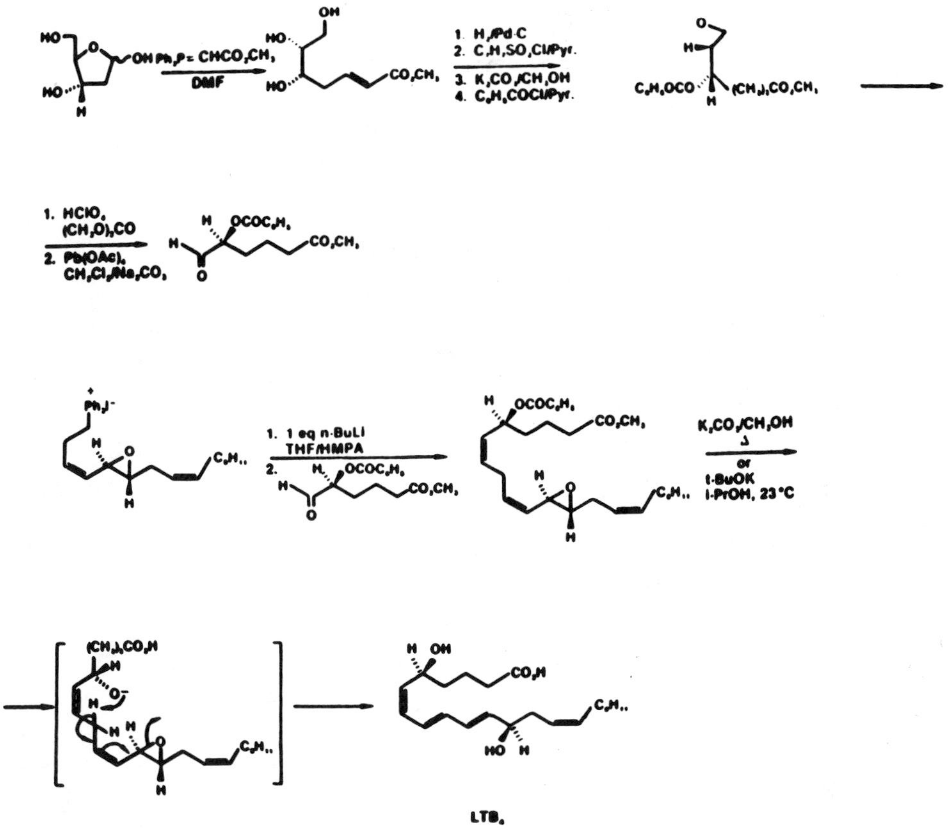

Figure 3. Synthesis of LTB$_4$ (Corey)

This route gives always a mixture of 6-cis and 6-trans isomers
which can be seperated by RP-h.p.l.c. .

Last not least d-arabinose and l-arabinose were used in the synthesis[29]
of leukotriene B$_3$ and its 6-trans isomer. It should also be possible
to establish the stereochemistry and the absolute configuration
of the new discovered lipoxines using derivates derived from
arabinose. The lipoxines are 5,6,15-trihydroxy-tetraenoic acids
of arachidonic acid and 5,14,15-trihydroxy-eicosatetraenoic acid
with uncertain assignment of the 6-hydroxygroup which can be in the
R or S configuration whereas the stereochemistry of rationally
reason of the four double bonds should be the same as described
in the publication of Serhan and Samuelsson [30].

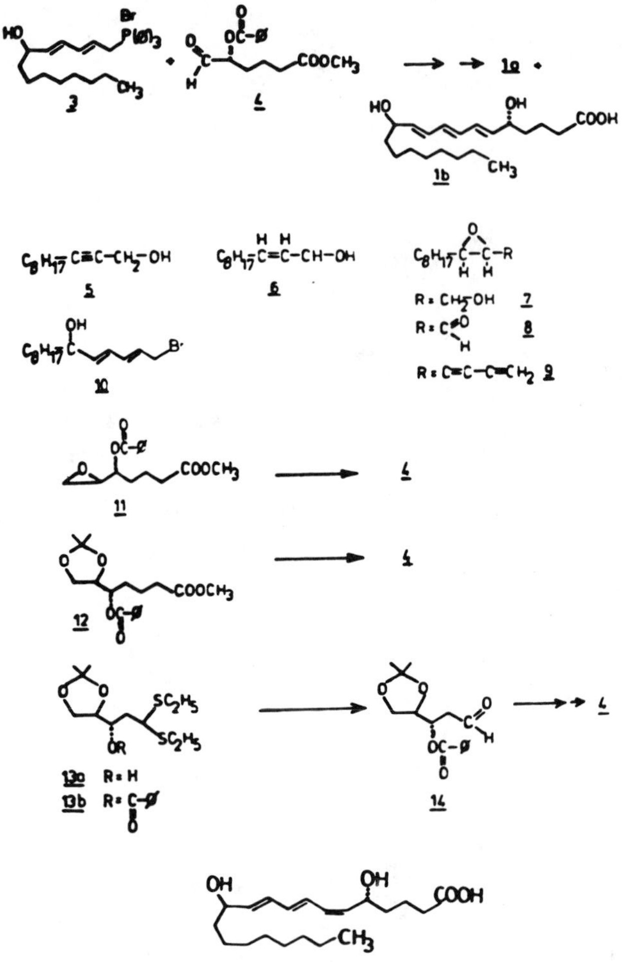

Figure 4. Synthesis of LTB$_3$

A large number of leukotriene analogs has been described in the literature in order to find the biological active sites and the antagonists. These analogs were synthesized using the general strategy of Corey's first syntheses. Among the large number of analogs only a few are briefly described. Thus the leukotrienes derived from eicosapentaenoic acid LTA$_5$, LTC$_5$, LTD$_5$, LTE$_5$ were synthesized stereospecifically and have biological activities [31] comparable with the natural leukotrienes whereas LTB$_5$ is only 1/10 as active as LTB$_4$ [28]. Another interesting finding is the nearly total loss of activity if the 7-trans double bond is changed to cis [32].

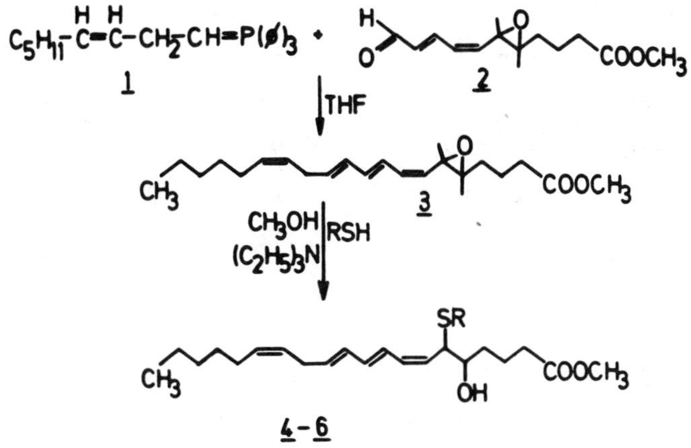

Figure 5. Synthesis of leukotriene analogs

If the total number of carbon atoms is over 20 or less than 20 a considerable activity remains. Larger differences resulted in the unnatural forms, but final remarks can only made when all investigations are completed [33-36].

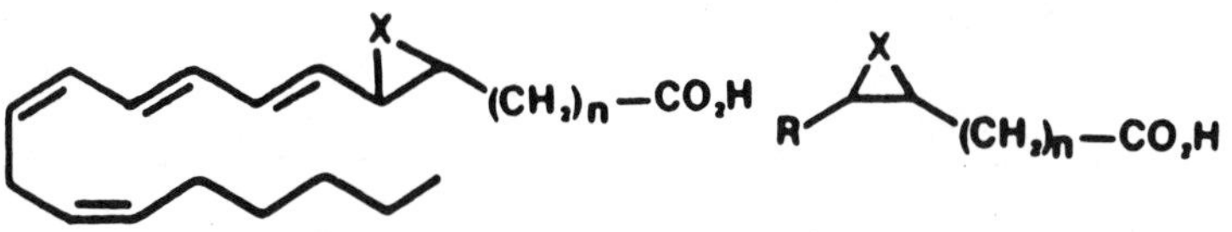

Methano LTA₄ X = CH₂, n = 1-4

Methano LTA$_4$ $X = CH_2$, n = 1-4
Thio LTA$_4$ $X = S$, n = 3
Aza LTA$_4$ $X = NH$, n = 3

$X = CH_2$, O
n = 1,3,4
$R = C_{14}$ alkyl: saturated
unsaturated
partially unsaturated
various geometrical isomers

Figure 6.

Another reason for the syntheses of analogs of LTA is the hope to block the conversion of LTA to the SRS compounds or to inhibit the 5-lipoxygenase enzyme. The first inhibitors such as thia-, aza-, and methano-leukotrienes were not very potent [37-41].
The substituted hydroxamic acids of arachidonic acid are very powerfull inhibitors of the 5-LO enzyme [42].

Up to this date a large number of unsolved problems remain; we have only little knowledge about the human enzymes, especially the 5-lipoxygenase which resists isolation and purification to homogenity, but hopefully new techniques can be used to achieve these goals. Our knowledge about the different receptors is increasing.

ACKNOWLEDGEMENTS

We wish to thank the Deutsch Forschungsgemeinschaft DFG and Dr. W.D. Busse, Bayer-Pharma AG Wuppertal for the financial support of this research.

REFERENCES

1. Samuelsson, B. (1982) The leukotrienes, highly biologically active substances involved in allergy and inflammation. Angew. Chem. Int. Ed., 21: 902-910.

2. Borgeat, P. and Sirois, P. (1981) Leukotrienes: A major step in the understanding of immediate hypersensitivity reactions. J. Med. Chem. 24: 121-126.

3. Samuelsson, B., Paoletti, R. and Ramwell, P. (1983) Advances in prostaglandin, thromboxane and leukotriene research. 11: Raven Press, New York.

4. Lewis, R.A., and Austen, K.F. (1984) Molecular determinants for functional responses to the sulfidopeptide leukotrienes.
    J. Allergy Clin. Immunol. 74: 369-372.

5. Corey, E.J. (1982) Chemical studies on the slow reacting substances leukotrienes.
    Experientia, 38: 1259-1281.

6. Radmark, O., Malmsten, C., Samuelsson, B., Goto, G., Marfat, A., and Corey, E.J. (1980) Leukotriene A: Isolation from human poly-morphonuclear leukocytes.
    J. Biol. Chem., 255: 11828-11831.

7. Boeynaems, J.M., Brash, A.R., Oates, J.A., and Hubbard, W.C.(1980) Preparation and assay of monohydroxy-eicosatetraenoic acids.
    Anal. Biochem., 104: 259-267.

8. Corey, E.J., Albright, J.O., Barton, A.E., and Hashimoto, S. (1980) Chemical and enzymic synthesis of 5-HPETE, a key biological pre-cursor of slow-reacting substance of anaphylaxis (SRS) and 5-HETE.
    J. Am. Chem. Soc., 102: 1435-1436.

9. Spur, B., Crea, A., Peters, W., and König, W. (1983) Formation and structure determination of 5,6-epoxy-8,11,14-Z-eicosatrienoic acid and 5-oxo-8,11,14-Z-eicosatrienoic acid.
    Tetrahedron. Lett. 24: 1755-1758.

10. Corey, E.J., and Hashimoto, S. (1981) A practical process for large scale synthesis of (S)-5-hydroxy-6-trans-8,11,14-cis-eicosatetraenoic acid (5-HETE).
    Tetrahedron Lett. 22: 299-302.

11. Rokach, J., Adams, J. and Perry, R. (1983) A new general method for the synthesis of lipoxygenase products: Preparation of 5-HETE
    Tetrahedron Lett. 24: 5185-5188.

12. Spur, B., Crea, A., and Peters, W. unpublished results

13. Fitzsimmons, B.J. and Rokach, J. (1984) The total syntheses of several 8,15-dihydroxy arachidonic acid derivatives (8,15, LTB's). Tetrahedron Lett. 25: 3043-3046.

14. Zamboni, R. and Rokach, J. (1983) Stereospecific synthesis of 5S-HETE, 5R-HETE and their transformation to 5(+)HPETE. Tetrahedron Lett. 24: 999-1002.

15. Baldwin, J.E., Davies, D.I., Hughes, L. and Gutteridge, N.J.A. (1979) Synthesis from arachidonic acid of potential prostaglandin precursors.
    J. Chem. Soc. Perkin I: 115-121.

16. Feldberg, W. and Kellaway, J.C.H. (1938) Liberation of histamine and formation of lysocithin-like substance by cobra venom.
    J. Physiol. (London), 94: 187-226.

17. Kellaway, C.H. and Trethewie, Q.J. (1940) The liberation of a slow reacting smooth muscle stimulating substance of anaphylaxis.
    Quart., J. Exp. Physiol., 30: 121-145.

18. Corey, E.J., Clark, D.A., Goto, G., Marfat, A., Mioskowski, C., Samuelsson, B. and Hammarström, S. (1980) Stereospecific total synthesis of a "slow reacting substance of anaphylaxis", leukotriene C-1 . J. Am. Chem. Soc., 102: 1436-1438,3663.

19. Green, R.H. and Lambeth, P.F. (1983) Leukotrienes. Tetrahedron, 39: 1687-1721.

20. Corey, E.J., Hashimoto, S. and Barton, A.E. (1981) Chirally directed synthesis of (-)-methyl-5(S),6(S)-oxido-7-hydroxyheptanoa key intermediate for the total synthesis of leukotriene C,D,E.
    J. Am. Chem. Soc., 103: 721-722.

21. Rossiter, B.E., Katsuki, T. and Sharpless, K.B. (1981) Asymmetric
    epoxidation provides shortest routes to four chiral epoxy alcohols
    which are key intermediates in the syntheses of methymycin, erythro-
    mycin, leukotriene C-1 and disparlure. J. Am. Chem. Soc. 103: 464.

22. Pridgen, N.L., Shilcrat, S.C. and Lantos, I (1984) Asymetric
    epoxidation of allylic alcohols employing 4,5-diphenyloxazole as
    masked ester functionality. Tetrahedron Lett. 25: 2835-2838.

23. Buck, J.C., Ellis, F. and North, P.C. (1982) A novel stereospecific
    synthesis of (+)-leukotriene A_4 (LTA_4), methyl ester.
    Tetrahedron Lett., 23: 4161-4162.

24. Corey, E.J., Mehrota, M.M. and Cashman, J.R. (1983) New synthetic
    routes to leukotrienes and other arachidonate derived epoxy eicosa-
    tetraenoic acids (EPETEs). Exclusion of the hydroxy epoxide pathway
    from leukotriene biosynthesis. Tetrahedron Lett. 24: 4917-4920.

25. Cohen, N. et al (1983) Syntheses of leukotrienes C_4, D_4 and E_4.
    J. Am. Chem. Soc., 105: 3661-3672.

26. Corey, E.J., Marfat, A., Goto, G. and Brion, F. (1980) Leukotriene
    B_4. Total synthesis and assignment of stereochemistry.
    J. Am. Chem. Soc., 102: 7984-7985.

27. Corey, E.J., Marfat, A., Munroe, J., Kim, K.S., Hopkins, P.B.
    and Brion, F. (1981) A stereocontrolled and effective synthesis
    of leukotriene B. Tetrahedron Lett., 22: 1077-1080.

28. Corey, E.J., Pyne, S.G.,and Su, W. (1983) Total synthesis of
    leukotriene B_5. Tetrahedron Lett., 24: 4883-4886.

29. Spur, B., Crea, A., Peters, W. and König, W. (1984) Synthesis of leukotriene B_3. Arch. Pharm.(Weinheim), 317: in press.

30. Serhan, C.N., Hamberg, M. and Samuelsson, B. (1984) Trihydroxy-tetraenes: A novel series of compounds formed from arachidonic acid in human leukocytes. B.B.R.C., 118: 943-949.

31. Spur, B., Crea, A., Peters, W. and König, W. (1984) Synthesis of Leukotriene C_5, D_5, and E_5. Arch. Pharm. (Weinheim) 317: 280-1.

32. Spur, B., Jendralla, H., Crea, A., Peters, W. and König, W.(1984) Syntheses of 7Z,9E,11E,14Z-leukotriene C_4, D_4, E_4. Arch. Pharm. (Weinheim), 317: 651-652.

33. Spur, B., Crea, A., Peters, W. and König, W. (1984) Synthese of leukotriene analogs. Arch. Pharm. (Weinheim) 317: 647-648.

34. Spur, B., Crea, A., Peters, W. and König, W. (1983) Synthesis of 11,12,14,15-Tetrahydro-leukotriene C, D, E, via A. Tetrahedron Lett., 24: 2135-2136.

35. Spur, B., Crea, A., Peters, W and König, W. (1983) Synthese und biologische Eigenschaften der 14,15-Didehydro-leukotriene und ihrer Methylester. Arch. Pharm. (Weinheim) 316: 968-970.

36. Spur, B., Crea, A., Peters, W. and König, W. (1983) Synthesis of 9,10,11,12,14,15-hexahydro-leukotriene E. Arch. Pharm. (Weinheim), 316: 572-574.

37. Corey, E.J., Park, H., Barton, A. and Nii, Y. (1980) Synthesis of three potential inhibitors of the biosynthesis of leukotriene A-E. Tetrahedron Lett., 21: 4243-4246.

38. Spur, B., Crea, A., Peters, W. and König, W. (1984) Synthesis of 5,6-thialeukotrienes, inhibitors of the leukotriene biosynthesis. Arch. Pharm. (Weinheim), 317: 84-85.

39. Zamboni, R. and Rokach, J. (1983) Synthesis of the aza analog of LTA_4. Tetrahedron Lett., 24: 331-334.

40. Nicolaou, K.C., Petasis, N.A. and Seitz, S.P. (1981) 5,6-Methano-leukotriene A_4. A stable and biologically active analog of leukotriene A_4. J. Chem. Soc. Chem. Commun., 1195-1196.

41. Spur, B., Crea, A. and Peters, W. (1984) Novel synthesis of Methyl-6-formyl-trans-5,6-methanohexanoate. Z. Naturforsch. (B) 125-125.

42. Corey, E.J., Cashman, J.R., Kantner, S.S. and S.W. Wright (1984) Rationally designed, potent competitive inhibitors of leukotriene biosynthesis. J. Am. Chem. Soc. 106: 1503-1504.

PHARMACOLOGIC MODULATION OF LEUKOTRIENE BIOSYNTHESIS BY

INCORPORATION OF ALTERNATIVE UNSATURATED FATTY ACIDS (20:5 and 22:6)

Robert A. Lewis,* Tak H. Lee,** and K. Frank Austen

Department of Medicine, Harvard Medical School
Department of Rheumatology and Immunology, Brigham and
Women's Hospital, Boston, MA 02115

INTRODUCTION

The 5-lipoxygenase pathway for oxidative metabolism of
unsaturated fatty acids was first recognized less than 10 years
ago with the definition of 5S-hydroxy-eicosatetraenoic acid (5-
HETE) as a product,[1] and its potential biological relevance to
inflammation was defined solely by the modest chemotactic activity
of 5-HETE.[2] However, major interest in this pathway did not occur
until 5 years ago when leukotriene B_4 (LTB$_4$), 5S,12R-dihydroxy-
6,14-cis-8,10-trans-eicosatetraenoic acid was first described[3] and
the elusive "slow reacting substance of anaphylaxis (SRS-A)," was
chemically defined as three additional leukotriene products of
this pathway: LTC$_4$, 5S-hydroxy-6R-S-glutathionyl-7,9-trans-11,14-
cis-eicosatetraenoic acid[4]; LTD$_4$, 5S-hydroxy-6R-S-cysteinylglycyl-
7,9-trans-11,14-cis-eicosatetraenoic acid[5-7]; and LTE$_4$, 5S-hydroxy-
6R-S-cysteinyl-7,9-trans-11,14-cis-eicosatetraenoic acid.[8] That
efforts to decrease the generation of the leukotriene compounds
could have a significant effect in down-regulating a variety of
inflammatory events has been strongly suggested by several types of
data developed over the past 5 years, with regard to the breadth of
proinflammatory effects manifested by these compounds, indications
that a variety are mediated via specific receptors that do not

*Recipient of Allergic Diseases Academic Award AI-00399 from the
National Institutes of Health
**Recipient of a Saltwell Fellowship, Royal College of Physicians,
London, U.K.
This work was supported in part by grants AI-07722, AI-20081,
HL-17382, and RR-05669 from the National Institutes of Health

recognize other naturally-occurring compounds, an expanding knowledge of the inflammatory cell types which serve as sources for the leukotrienes, and the demonstration that leukotrienes are recoverable from complex biological fluids in both in vivo models of inflammation and human disease. Although there is potential for antagonizing the biological effects of each leukotriene at the end-organ receptor level, the present discussion will focus mainly on regulation of leukotriene biosynthesis as an anti-inflammatory therapeutic approach. Furthermore, the potential of dietary alteration as an adjunct to developing pharmacotherapeutic inhibitors of the 5-lipoxygenase pathway will be specifically considered.

BIOLOGICAL EFFECTS OF THE LEUKOTRIENES

The primary indications that these naturally-occurring compounds might be major mediators of inflammatory events have been provided from assessments of their biological effects and potencies. The non-vascular smooth muscle spasm that occurs in asthmatic airways was thought to be effected by a major contribution of LTC_4, LTD_4, and LTE_4 even before they were chemically defined as components of SRS-A. This effect was first shown on human bronchi[9] and later on both tracheal and pulmonary parenchymal strips from the guinea pig, in vitro.[10] Once LTC_4, LTD_4, and LTE_4 were available as purified compounds, these in vitro observations were confirmed.[8,11] In vivo administration of the authentic compounds intravenously to guinea pigs[11,12] as well as by aerosol to guinea pigs[13] and lower primates[14] demonstrated the same predominant effects on peripheral versus central airways that had been previously shown with partially purified SRS-A.[15] That the absolute and relative in vitro potencies of LTC_4, LTD_4, and LTE_4 on airway tissue vary with the level of the airway from which the tissue derives was shown by comparision of the dose-dependent effects of each on guinea pig trachea, for which the 50% effective concentrations (EC_{50} values) are approximately 1×10^{-7} M, 1×10^{-7} M, and 1×10^{-8} M, respectively, and on guinea pig pulmonary parenchymal strips, for which EC_{50} values are 1×10^{-8} M, 6×10^{-10} M and 4×10^{-9} M, respectively.[16] Inhalation of aerosolized LTC_4 and LTD_4 by normal human subjects also effects bronchospasm, mainly of the peripheral airways, such that the relative bronchospastic potencies of each, as compared to histamine, is approximately 4000-fold on a molar basis.[17-19]

Since compromised airflow through asthmatic airways is presumed to reflect increased bronchial mucus secretion and bronchial mucosal edema, as well as muscular bronchospasm, enhancement of mucus secretion and vasopermeability was also sought and demonstrated. Bronchial mucosal explants responded in tissue culture by enhanced mucus secretion in the presence of as little as 10^{-9} M LTC_4 or LTD_4.[20,21] The augmented post-capillary venular permeability was first shown for dermal vascular beds of the guinea pig responding to locally injected LTC_4, LTD_4, and LTE_4 in concentrations as low as 10^{-7} M[8,11] and was later confirmed by the leakage of intravascular fluorescent dye into the tissue of the hamster cheek pouch after topical application of each leukotriene.[22] Further, the intradermal administration of LTC_4, LTD_4, and LTE_4 to normal human subjects produced a local wheal and flare response, in which the wheal, representing enhanced venopermeability, was sustained for 2-4 hr.[23] It is evident that the vascular permeability effects mediated by leukotrienes would logically extend to other organ systems beyond the pumonary compartment.

One additional vascular effect of LTC_4 and, to a lesser extent, LTD_4, is that of an arteriolar spasmogen. Vascular smooth muscle spasmogenicity was initially demonstrated in guinea pig skin at the site of intradermal administration of the leukotriene, requiring less than 10^{-7} M concentration of either compound[8,11], and was confirmed by the response to topical administration of the hamster cheek pouch[22] and by blanching at the injection site in normal human skin.[23] Coronary vasoconstriction in response to these molecules has been shown after direct infusion into a major coronary vessel of the sheep in vivo[24] and after infusion into the systemic venous circulation of the anesthetized rat.[25] In each case, myocardial contractility was compromised on a dose-dependent basis. The interpretation of which mechanisms underly the myocardial failure induced by LTC_4 or LTD_4 is somewhat controversial; however, a major effect is clearly indirect, whereby myocardial oxygen extraction becomes limited by diminished perfusion.[26] The in vivo administration of LTC_4 by intravenous infusion to the anesthetized rat also evoked renal vasoconstriction, which limited renal blood flow and secondarily decreases the glomerular filtration rate.[27] In this model, LTC_4 also increased systemic vasopermeability, which further compromised renal perfusion and augmented the direct effect on the renal artery. A contribution to decreased glomerular filtration via a direct effect of the leukotriene on the glomerular capillary bed was also suggested.[27]

LTB_4, like LTC_4, LTD_4, and LTE_4 is also spasmogenic for airway smooth muscle. However, unlike the SRS-A components, which directly effect bronchospasm, LTB_4 evokes the response indirectly, only via stimulated biosynthesis of constrictor cyclooxygenase products.[28] The more noteworthy effects of LTB_4 relate to the direct attraction (chemotaxis) of granulocytes into an area of inflammation. LTB_4 was first shown to be chemotactic for neutrophilic polymorphonuclear leukocytes (PMN) at concentrations as low as 10^{-9} M, using Boyden chambers in vitro,[29] and this was confirmed in vivo after intracutaneous injection into the skin of monkeys[30] and human subjects.[23] In the humans, 1.6 nanomoles of LTB_4 elicited infiltration of large numbers of PMN by 4-6 hr, as demonstrated histologically from biopsies.[23] The mechanism of evoked PMN infiltration of tissue in response to LTB_4 involves not only the response of the leukocyte, but also an increased capacity of the vascular endothelial cells to bind PMN in the marginated pool.[31] LTB$_4$ is also immunoregulatory, inducing increased numbers of suppressor T lymphocytes from precursors which largely possess the cell surface marker of helper cells[32] and thus inhibiting mitogen-induced T cell proliferation[33,34] as well as immunoglobulin synthesis.[32]

RECEPTOR-DEPENDENT MEDIATION OF LEUKOTRIENE EFFECTS

That spasmogenic effects of LTC$_4$, LTD$_4$, and LTE$_4$ are evoked via specific receptors was indicated both from physiologic studies and from the relative responsiveness of non-vascular smooth muscle to artificial chemical analogs of the natural leukotrienes. The demonstration that LTC$_4$ effected a monophasic increase in the contraction of a guinea pig pulmonary parenchymal strip that was not reproducibly altered by FPL55712, whereas LTD$_4$ evoked a biphasic response, of which the low-dose phase was selectively antagonized by this compound, indicated that the latter effect was separately mediated from the former and that at least two unique sulfidopeptide leukotriene receptors exist on this tissue.[11] Additionally, the preferential responsiveness of guinea pig tracheal spirals to LTE$_4$ versus LTD$_4$ and LTC$_4$ indicates that this recognition unit is different from that initiating the response on pulmonary parenchymal strips, where LTE$_4$ is a relatively weak agonist, as compared to LTD$_4$. Chemical analogs of the sulfidopeptide leukotrienes, synthesized for the purpose of varying the stereochemistry at optically active centers, demonstrated distinct stereospecificity for evoking responses of both guinea pig ileum and guinea pig lung parenchymal strips, with a marked recognition of the asymmetric centers at the fifth and sixth carbons of the eicosanoid backbone, to which are attached hydroxyl and sulfidopeptide domains, respectively.[35] The direct demonstration of a receptor for LTC$_4$ was provided by analysis of radioligand binding, including saturation and competition studies with unlabeled homoligand and heteroligands, on a smooth muscle cell line and on normal guinea pig ileum smooth muscle.[36,37] In each case, the LTC$_4$ receptor demonstrated a dissociation constant (K$_d$) for its homoligand of $5-8 \times 10^{-9}$ M. Comparable K$_d$ values for LTC$_4$ on a specific receptor have also been shown on sedimented materials obtained from disrupted lung tissue of guinea pig and rat.[38-40] That the receptor was specific for LTC$_4$ was indicated for each cell or disrupted tissue preparation by the relative ineffectiveness of LTD$_4$ and LTE$_4$ in competing with LTC$_4$ radioligand for binding; for each heteroligand, 50% inhibition of LTC$_4$ radioligand binding required a molar excess of 2 to 4 orders of magnitude.[36-40]

LTD$_4$ has also been shown to interact with a unique and specific receptor on disrupted guinea pig lung tissue, with a K$_d$ of 5×10^{-11} M.[41] Preliminary studies on guinea pig ileum have also suggested the presence of a specific LTD$_4$ receptor on that tissue.[42] Based upon the cited physiological observations, it is likely that radioligand binding will also demonstrate a tracheal LTE$_4$ receptor.

The demonstrations of receptors for specific sulfidopeptide leukotrienes support the judgment that the airway spasmogenicity mediated by each compound is dependent upon its unique chemical structure. That this also pertains to at least some vascular responses is indicated by the demonstration of an LTC$_4$ receptor on the rat glomerulus.[43] However, it is premature to conclude that all effects of the sulfidopeptide leukotrienes reflect such a degree of molecular specificity. The mucus secretion response is exemplary in that it has few apparent requirements for the molecular domains of lipid agonists.[21]

Specific receptors for LTB$_4$ on PMN were first suggested by studies in which natural and artificial 5,12-diHETE isomers were compared with LTB$_4$ for PMN chemotaxis and the response was shown to be highly stereospecific[44-46], as was the PMN aggregating response to the same series of agonists.[46] Direct radioligand binding studies with ^{3}H-labeled LTB$_4$ have demonstrated the presence of a specific receptor, with a K$_d$ of 11-14 x 10^{-9} M, the occupation of which correlates on a dose-dependent basis with chemotaxis[47]; a second receptor of 3 orders of magnitude lower affinity has been suggested to mediate other PMN responses to LTB$_4$, including the lysosomal secretion which occurs in the presence of cytochalasin B.[48]

GENERATION OF LEUKOTRIENES FROM HUMAN CELLS

The human cells that are capable of biosynthesizing large quantities of leukotrienes are each derived from known or presumed bone marrow precursors. They include the PMN, which, on a per 10^6 cell basis, generates an average of 50 ng LTB$_4$ but only 4-6 ng LTC$_4$ in response to the calcium ionophore A23187;[49,50] the normal eosinophil, which generates an average of 38 ng LTC$_4$ and only 6 ng LTB$_4$, in response to A23187;[49] and the pulmonary alveolar macrophage, which can synthesize 100-400 ng LTB$_4$ and 5-20 ng LTC$_4$ in response to A23187 as well as relatively large quantities of LTB$_4$ (50 ng, 80 ng) in response to zymosan and opsonized zymosan, respectively.[53] The human peripheral blood monocyte also generates both LTB$_4$ and LTC$_4$ (70 ng and 30 ng/10^6 cells, respectively) in response to the calcium ionophore and synthesizes each compound (10 ng LTB$_4$, 2 ng LTC$_4$) after activation by zymosan, but not after incubation with opsonized zymosan.[54] Human pulmonary mast cells, isolated after enzymatic tissue dispersion and purified by counter-current elutriation, generate about 25 ng LTC$_4$/10^6 cells, on average, after activation by an IgE-dependent stimulus; little or no authentic LTB$_4$ is generated under these circumstances.[55] The capacity of a cell type to generate these products is highly variable among donors, as

particularly noted in comparing ionophore-stimulated LTC$_4$ generation from eosinophils of various hypereosinophilic subjects, where
the range for LTC$_4$ generation/10^6 cells was 6 ng to 155 ng among
5 donors.[49] Likewise, for IgE-mediated mast cell generation of
LTC$_4$, the range has been over two orders of magnitude.[55,56]

Leukotriene biosynthesis proceeds from 5-lipoxygenation of
arachidonic acid to generate 5S-hydroperoxy-6-trans-8,11,14-cis-
eicosatetraenoic acid (5-HPETE) and then, perhaps, via a second
catalytic activity of the same 5-lipoxygenase enzyme, as shown for
the potato 5-lipoxygenase[57], to 5,6-oxido-7,9-trans-11,14-cis-
eicosatetraenoic acid, leukotriene A$_4$ (LTA$_4$).[58] The latter product
serves as a substrate for both the epoxide hydrolase(s) which produces LTB$_4$[59] and for the glutathione-S-transferase which generates
LTC$_4$.[60] The conversion of LTC$_4$ to LTD$_4$ and LTE$_4$ is effected by
§-glutamyl transpeptidase and by a variety of dipeptidases, respectively (reviewed in 61).

INTRODUCTION OF DIETARY ALTERNATIVE FATTY ACIDS

On the basis of the accumulated understanding of the biological
functions of each leukotriene, at least some of which are mediated
by specific receptors, and of the stepwise biosynthesis of each product by recognized enzymes in mammalian cells, it would be rational
to attempt in vivo regulation of leukotriene proinflammatory effects
by altering either biosynthesis or response. Approaches to the
regulation of biosynthesis have included the use of compounds with
a variety of chemical structures, of which 5,6-dehydro-arachidonic
acid[62,63] and U-60,257, a prostacyclin analog[64] are two examples.
Attempts to alter response at the receptor level have been generally
less successful although, in addition to FPL55712, a 2-nor-LTD$_4$
analog has provided a promising lead.[65] The possibility of de-
creasing leukotriene-mediated inflammation at both levels, by
introducing marine-derived dietary fatty acids, is considered not
as an alternative, but as an adjunct, to other pharmacotherapies.
The first consideration of this approach was carried out by feeding
mice, which bore mastocytoma cells as an ascites tumor, on a fish
oil-enriched diet for 6 weeks before and 2 weeks after the introduction of the tumor cells, and then removing the mastocytoma cells
and activating them ex vivo with the calcium ionophore A23187.[66]
These mastocytoma cells, as compared to cells carried in peritoneal
cavities of mice on control diets, could generate only 5-10% of the
sulfidopeptide leukotrienes and dihydroxy-leukotrienes.[66] The 5-
lipoxygenase products generated under the alternative dietary conditions included not only those derived from arachidonic acid, but
also those synthesized from eicosapentaenoic acid (EPA) (20:5, N-3),
a major constituent of the triglycerides in the fish oil supplement.
The metabolism of EPA in this cascade, by analogy with that of
arachidonic acid (Fig. 1), proceeds via action of the 5-lipoxygenase

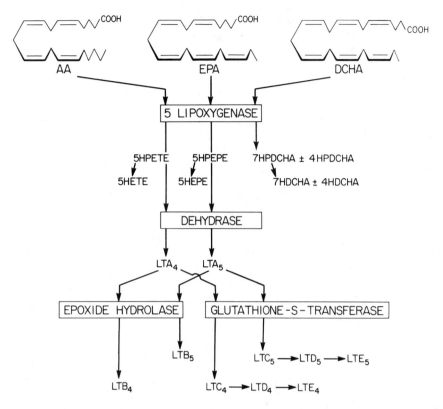

Fig. 1. Metabolism of arachidonic acid (AA), eicosapentaenoic acid (EPA), and docosahexaenoic acid (DCHA) via the 5-lipoxygenase pathway to specific enzymatic products.

enzyme to generate the 5-hydroperoxy-derivative, 5-hydroperoxy-eicosapentaenoic acid (5-HPEPE), of which some is directly reduced to its alcohol (5-HEPE) and the rest of which is converted to the pentaene epoxide, LTA$_5$. Again, consistent with the metabolism of arachidonic acid-derived LTA$_4$, LTA$_5$ is converted via epoxide hydrolase(s) to LTB$_5$ and via a glutathione-S-transferase to LTC$_5$; LTD$_5$ and LTE$_5$ are presumably derived from $\overline{\text{LTC}}_5$ in the same manner as are the SRS-A peptide cleavage products from LTC$_4$. In the cited study of mouse mastocytoma cells which were activated ex vivo by A23187, the cells from animals with fish oil dietary supplements generated LTB$_5$:LTB$_4$ in a ratio approximating the relative tissue concentrations of EPA and arachidonic acid; the relative generation of sulfidopeptide leukotrienes from LTA$_4$ exceed that from LTA$_5$ by a ratio of 10:1, despite the tissue concentration ratio of precursor fatty acids.[66]

That the relevance of these observations to in vivo inflammatory models should be pursued was indicated from studies on a murine
model for systemic lupus erythematosus (NZB-NZW/F$_1$ hybrids) and a
rat model for rheumatoid arthritis (Type II collagen arthritis), in
which fish oil enriched diets inhibited and enhanced inflammation,
respectively.[67,68] Although the limitation of cyclooxygenase product generation by fish oil fatty acids, including docosahexaenoic
acid (DCHA) (22:6, N-3) as well as EPA,[69] was likely, the presumed
alteration in vasopermeability to immune complexes in each case
suggested possible regulation of factor(s) which would not derived
from prostaglandin endoperoxides, but rather from epoxide leukotrienes. Since the historical standard model for immunologically
generating the vasopermeability effector SRS-A components was IgG/
antigen immune complex-dependent inflammation in the rat peritoneal
cavity,[70] this model was initially explored.

After feeding weanling rats for 8-10 weeks on standard lab
chow supplemented with menhaden fish oil (containing 13.8% EPA and
5.7% DCHA, as a percentage of total fatty acid content), or, as a
control, beef tallow (mainly saturated fatty acids and virtually
lacking EPA or DCHA), the animals were passively sensitized with rat
anti-ovalbumin antiserum and then challenged intraperitoneally with
antigen. Harvested, extracted and chromatographically resolved (on
reverse phase-high performance liquid chromatography) leukotrienes
from peritoneal exudate fluids were not decreased overall by the
fish oil supplement, but the preponderant dihydroxy-fatty acid
leukotriene was LTB$_5$, rather than LTB$_4$, in ratios varying from
2-7:1, and in keeping with the incorporated tissue ratios of EPA
to arachidonic acid (2.5:1) in lungs and spleens of these animals.
A smaller quantity of LTC$_5$ and its peptide cleavage products were
generated at the expense of arachidonic acid-derived sulfidopeptide
leukotrienes, but the ratio of pentaene to tetraene sulfidopeptide
leukotrienes was 1:1.[71] That the altered 5-lipoxygenase product
profile could affect the level of inflammation in this model would
therefore have to depend upon an altered pro-inflammatory potential
for the EPA products relative to those derived from arachidonic acid.
Indeed, the capacity of LTB$_5$ to effect either PMN chemotaxis or
aggregation was reduced by at least an order of magnitude relative
to that of LTB$_4$ and for each function, the EPA product was additionally only a partial agonist.[71,72] At least with respect to their
potential for smooth muscle spasmogenicity on guinea pig pulmonary
parenchymal strips in vitro, LTC$_5$ and LTC$_4$ were comparable[71,73,74],
but the relative vasoactivities of sulfidopeptide leukotrienes in
each series are not known. Further, the interaction of any of the
EPA-derived leukotrienes with cell or tissue receptors, as compared
to the ineractions of the analogous products derived from arachidonic acid has not been evaluated.

A comparable study of marine fatty acid dietary supplements for their effects on antigen-induced systemic anaphylaxis in guinea pigs has also demonstrated modulation of the inflammatory response. Like the rats in the previous study, weanling guinea pigs were fed for 9-10 weeks in two groups, on diets supplemented with menhaden oil or beef tallow. The guinea pigs were then passively sensitized with a long-acting antibody to ovalbumin and challenged approximately 4 days later by intravenous injection of the antigen. Monitoring the dynamic lung compliance and specific airways conductance in each animal before and for 10 min after antigen challenge demonstrated that when the major histamine effect was removed with an H-1 antagonist, the animals on a fish oil dietary supplement had significantly greater worsening of each airway functional parameter following anaphylactic challenge, as compared to the animals on the beef tallow-supplemented diet.[75] These differences correlated with minute-by-minute measurements of LTB_4 and LTB_5 (where generated) in the arterial plasma, wherein the synthesized quantities of dihydroxy-leukotrienes were relatively increased 2-fold for the animals on a fish oil-enriched diet and the predominant product in that group was LTB_4.[75] Pretreatment of the animals with indomethacin (in addition to the H-1 blocker) caused worsening of pulmonary dysfunction and increased LTB_4 generation in anaphylaxing animals on the beef tallow-enriched diet, relative to animals in the same group that were not treated with the cyclooxygenase inhibitor; however, indomethacin affected neither pulmonary functions nor LTB_4/LTB_5 generation in anaphylaxing fish oil-fed guinea pigs.[75] It was therefore suggested that the menhaden diet worsened the anaphylactic response to intravenous antigen challenge by more than one mechanism, possibly including inhibition of biosynthesis for bronchodilator prostaglandins and the removal of the capacity to generate prostaglandin inhibitors of leukotriene biosynthesis.[76] The presumption also exists that the measured plasma levels of LTB_4/LTB_5 could also reflect relative generation of sulfidopeptide leukotrienes, direct measurements of which in plasma are still confounded by interfering background "noise" in the only assay of adequate sensitivity, the radioimmunoassay.[77,78]

As a substrate for the 5-lipoxygenase enzyme, EPA is comparable to arachidonic acid, whereas DCHA is poorly metabolized; the ratios for product generation at equimolar substrate concentrations are 125:100:1, respectively, using cell-free 5-lipoxygenase preparations from guinea pig PMN or human PMN.[79,80] Further, whereas EPA and arachidonic acid are converted via 5-HPEPE and 5-HPETE to their respective leukotriene epoxides (LTA_5 and LTA_4), DCHA is metabolized only as far as its monohydroperoxide products, 7-hydroperoxy-DCHA and 4-hydroperoxy-DCHA, in a ratio of 10:1 in RBL-1 or human PMN; these compounds are then reduced to their respective alcohols.[81,82]

More detailed _in vitro_ studies, assessing the activation of human PMN by A23187 in the presence of varying concentrations of each fatty acid have identified additional effects of EPA on the 5-lipoxygenase pathway. In this model, lower concentrations of EPA (5-10 μg/ml) enhance the 5-lipoxygenase enzyme activity, higher concentrations (20-40 μg/ml) inhibit it, and all concentrations tested (5-40 μg/ml) inhibit the epoxide hydrolase.[82] Slightly preferred metabolism of endogenous EPA versus arachidonic acid by extracted human PMN 5-lipoxygenase reflects a favorable V_{max} for the former, since K_m for arachidonic acid is lower than for EPA.[80] Inhibition of the LTA_4 epoxide hydrolase in the presence of EPA probably represents competitive interaction of LTA_5 with the enzyme. The presumed lesser efficiency of LTA_5 as a substrate for this enzyme must be overridden by mass action in the _in vivo_ demonstrations of LTB_5:LTB_4 ratios >1.

There is considerable evidence that fish oil enriched diets can substantially modulate the generation and biological activities of arachidonic acid-derived mediators _in vivo_. In addition to the evidence in experimental models, it is known that Eskimo populations, who have a high ratio of EPA and DCHA to arachidonic acid in their platelets and plasma lipids, also have a low incidence of both myocardial infarction and bronchial asthma.[83,84] The former statistics have been attributed to the inhibitory effect of N-3 fatty acids on the cyclooxygenase and, to a lesser extent, on the generation of a thromboxane compound (thromboxane A_3) with attenuated activity, such that platelet aggregation, vasospasm, and the incidence of coronary occlusive disease are reduced.[69,85-87] However, the proinflammatory effects of the menhaden oil-enriched diet on certain mammalian models, e.g., type II collagen arthritis of the rat and guinea pig anaphylaxis, suggest that interactions occurring among metabolites of the cyclooxygenase and 5-lipoxygenase pathways may not always be favorable to the organism. It is therefore appropriate that alternative fatty acid supplementation be evaluated cautiously and critically in each inflammatory disease and that concurrent basic science evaluations consider not only the product ratios and biologic effects of EPA versus arachidonic acid metabolites, but also the conditioning by alternative fatty acids of the cell membranes and potential effects on membrane receptors of target cells and tissues.

REFERENCES

1. P. Borgeat, M. Hamberg, and B. Samuelsson, Transformation of arachidonic acid and homo-gamma-linolenic acid by rabbit polymorphonuclear leukocytes. Monohydroxy acids from novel lipoxygenases, _J. Biol. Chem._ 251:7816 (1976), and correction: 252:8772 (1977).

2. E.J. Goetzl, A role for endogenous mono-hydroxy-eicosatetra-
    enoic acids (HETEs) in the regulation of human neutrophil
    migration, Immunology. 40:709 (1980).
3. P. Borgeat and B. Samuelsson, Arachidonic acid metabolism in
    polymorphonuclear leukocytes: effects of ionophore A23187,
    Proc. Natl. Acad. Sci. USA. 76:2148 (1979).
4. R.C. Murphy, S. Hammarström, and B. Samuelsson, Leukotriene C:
    a slow reacting substance from murine mastocytoma cells,
    Proc. Natl. Acad. Sci. USA. 76:4275 (1979).
5. R.A. Lewis, K.F. Austen, J.M. Drazen, D.A. Clark, A. Marfat,
    and E.J. Corey, Slow reacting substances of anaphylaxis:
    identification of leukotriene C-1 and D from human and rat
    sources, Proc. Natl. Acad. Sci. USA. 77:3710 (1980).
6. L. Örning, S. Hammarström, and B. Samuelsson, Leukotriene D:
    a slow reacting substance from rat basophilic leukemia
    cells, Proc. Natl. Acad. Sci. USA. 77:2014 (1980).
7. H.R. Morris, G.W. Taylor, P.J. Piper, and J.R. Tippins,
    Structure of slow reacting substance of anaphylaxis from
    guinea pig lung, Nature. 285:104 (1980).
8. R.A. Lewis, J.M. Drazen, K.F. Austen, D.A. Clark, and E.J.
    Corey, Identification of the C(6)-S-conjugate of leukotri-
    ene A with cysteine as a naturally occurring slow reacting
    substance of anaphylaxis (SRS-A). Importance of the 11-cis
    geometry for biological activity, Biochem. Biophys. Res.
    Commun. 96:271 (1980).
9. W.E. Brocklehurst, The release of histamine and formation of
    a slow reacting substance of anaphylaxis (SRS-A) during
    anaphylactic shock, J. Physiol. 151:416 (1960).
10. J.M. Drazen, R.A. Lewis, S.I. Wasserman, R.P. Orange, and
    K.F. Austen, Differential effects of a partially purified
    preparation of slow reacting substance of anaphylaxis on
    guinea pig tracheal spirals and parenchymal strips, J.
    Clin. Invest. 63:1 (1979).
11. J.M. Drazen, K.F. Austen, R.A. Lewis, D.A. Clark, G. Goto, A.
    Marfat, and E.J. Corey, Comparative airway and vascular
    activities of leukotrienes C-1 and D in vivo and in vitro,
    Proc. Natl. Acad. Sci. USA. 77:4354 (1980).
12. J.M. Drazen C.S. Venugopalan, K.F. Austen, F. Brion, and E.J.
    Corey, Effects of leukotriene E on pulmonary mechanics in
    the guinea pig, Am. Rev. Respir. Dis. 125:290 (1982).
13. A.G. Leitch, E.J. Corey, K.F. Austen, and J.M. Drazen, Indo-
    methacin potentiates the pulmonary response to aerosol
    leukotriene C_4 in the guinea pig, Amer. Rev. Respir. Dis.
    128:639 (1983).
14. G. Smedegård, P. Hedqvist, S.-E. Dahlén, B. Revenäs, S.
    Hammarström, and B. Samuelsson, Leukotriene C_4 affects
    pulmonary and cardiovascular dynamics in monkey, Nature.
    295:327 (1982).

15. J.M. Drazen and K.F. Austen, Effects of intravenous administration of slow reacting substance of anaphylaxis, histamine, bradykinin, and prostaglandin $F_{2\alpha}$ on pulmonary mechanics in the guinea pig, J. Clin. Invest. 53:1679 (1974).

16. J.M. Drazen, R.A. Lewis, K.F. Austen, and E.J. Corey, Pulmonary pharmacology of the SRS-A leukotrienes, in: "Leukotrienes and Prostacyclin," F. Berti, G. Folco, and G Velo, eds., Plenum Press, New York (1983).

17. M.C. Holroyde, R.E.C. Altounyan, M. Cole, M. Dixon, and E.V. Elliot, Bronchoconstriction produced in man by leukotriene C and D, Lancet. 2:17 (1981).

18. J.W. Weiss, J.M. Drazen, N. Coles, E.R. McFadden, Jr., P.F. Weller, E.J. Corey, R.A. Lewis, and K.F. Austen, Bronchoconstrictor effects of leukotriene C in humans, Science. 216:196 (1982).

19. J.W. Weiss, J.M. Drazen, E.R. McFadden, Jr., P.F. Weller, E.J. Corey, R.A. Lewis, and K.F. Austen, Airway constriction in normal humans produced by inhalation of leukotriene D. Potency, time course, and effect of aspirin therapy, J. Amer. Med Assoc. 249:2814 (1983).

20. Z. Marom, J.H. Shelhamer, M.K. Bach, D.R. Morton, and M. Kaliner, Slow-reacting substances, leukotrienes C_4 and D_4, increase the release of mucus from human airways in vitro, Am. Rev. Respir. Dis. 126:449 (1982).

21. S.J. Coles, K.H. Neill, L.M. Reid, K.F. Austen, Y. Nii, E.J. Corey, and R.A. Lewis, Effects of leukotrienes C_4 and D_4 on glycoprotein and lysozyme secretion by human bronchial mucosa, Prostaglandins. 25:155 (1983).

22. S.-E. Dahlén, J. Bjork, P. Hedqvist, K.-E. Årfors, S. Hammarström, J.-Å. Lindgren, and B. Samuelsson, Leukotrienes promote plasma leakage and leukocyte adhesion in postcapillary venules: in vivo effects with relevance to the acute inflammatory response, Proc. Natl. Acad. Sci. USA. 78:3887 (1981).

23. N.A. Soter, R.A. Lewis, E.J. Corey, and K.F. Austen, Local effects of synthetic leukotrienes (LTC_4, LTD_4, LTE_4, and LTB_4) in human skin, J. Invest. Derm. 80:115 (1983).

24. F. Michelassi, L. Landa, R.D. Hill, E. Lowenstein, W.D. Watkins, A.J. Petkau, and W.M. Zapol, Leukotriene D_4: a potent coronary artery vasoconstrictor associated with impaired ventricular contraction, Science. 217:841 (1982).

25. M.A. Pfeffer, J.M. Pfeffer, R.A. Lewis, E. Braunwald, E.J. Corey, and K.F. Austen, Systemic hemodynamic effects of leukotrienes C_4 and D_4 in the rat, Am. J. Physiol. 244:H628 (1983).

26. J. Bittl, M.A. Pfeffer, R.A. Lewis, J.M. Pfeffer, J.S. Ingwall, and K.F. Austen, Mechanism of the negative ionotropic action of leukotrienes C_4 and D_4 on the isolated rat heart, J. Amer. College Cardiol. 3:503 (1984).

27. K.F. Badr, C. Baylis, J.M. Pfeffer, M.A. Pfeffer, R.J. Soberman, R.A. Lewis, K.F. Austen, E.J. Corey, and B.M. Brenner, Renal and systemic hemodynamic responses to intravenous infusion of leukotriene C_4 in the rat, Circ. Res. 54:492 (1984).

28. P. Sirois, S. Roy, and P. Borgeat, The lung parenchymal strip as a sensitive assay for leukotriene B_4, Prostaglandins Med. 6:153 (1981).

29. E.J. Goetzl and W.C. Pickett, The human polymorphonuclear leukocyte chemotactic activity of complex hydroxy-eicosatetraenoic acids (HETEs), J. Immunol. 125:1789 (1980).

30. R.A. Lewis, J.M. Drazen, E.J. Corey, and K.F. Austen, Structural and functional characteristics of the leukotriene components of slow reacting substance of anaphylaxis (SRS-A), in: "SRS-A and the Leukotrienes," P.J. Piper, ed., John Wiley and Sons, London (1981).

31. R.L. Hoover, M.L. Karnovsky, K.F. Austen, E.J. Corey, and R.A. Lewis, Leukotriene B_4 action on endothelium mediates augmented neutrophil/endothelial adhesion, Proc. Natl. Acad. Sci. USA. 81:2191 (1984).

32. D. Atluru and J.S. Goodwin, Control of polyclonal immunoglobulin production from human lymphocytes by leukotrienes; LTB_4 induces an OKT8(+), radiosensitive suppressor cell from resting human OKT8(-) T cells, J. Clin. Invest. (in press).

33. D.G. Payan and E.J. Goetzl, Specific suppression of human T lymphocyte function by leukotriene B_4, J. Immunol. 131:551 (1983).

34. M.P. Rola-Plezczynski, P. Borgeat, and P. Sirois, Leukotriene B_4 induces human suppressor lymphocytes, Biochem. Biophys. Res. Commun. 198:1531 (1982).

35. R.A. Lewis, J.M. Drazen, K.F. Austen, M. Toda, F. Brion, A. Marfat, and E.J. Corey, Contractile activities of structural analogs of leukotrienes C and D: role of the polar substituents, Proc. Natl. Acad. Sci. USA. 78:4579 (1981).

36. S. Krilis, R.A. Lewis, E.J. Corey, and K.F. Austen, Specific binding of leukotriene C_4 on a smooth muscle cell line, J. Clin. Invest. 72:1516 (1983).

37. S. Krilis, R.A. Lewis, E.J. Corey, and K.F. Austen, Specific binding of leukotriene C_4 to ileal segments and subcellular fractions of ileal smooth muscle, Proc. Natl. Acad. Sci. USA. 81:4529 (1984).

38. S.S. Pong, R.N. DeHaven, F.A. Kuehl, Jr., R.W. Egan, Leukotriene C_4 binding to rat lung membranes, J. Biol. Chem. 258:9616 (1983).

39. G.K. Hogaboom, S. Mong, H.-L. Wu, and S. Crooke, Peptidoleukotrienes: distinct receptors for leukotrienes C_4 and D_4 in the guinea pig lung, Biochem. Biophys. Res. Commun. 116:1136 (1983).

40. R.F. Bruns, W.J. Thomsen, and T.A. Pugsley, Binding of leuko-
    trienes C_4 and D_4 to membranes from guinea pig lung:
    regulation by ions and guanine nucleotides, Life Sci.
    33:645 (1983).

41. S.S. Pong and R.N. DeHaven, Characterization of a leukotriene
    D_4 receptor in guinea pig lung, Proc. Natl. Acad. Sci.
    USA. 80:7415 (1983).

42. S. Krilis, R.A. Lewis, and K.F. Austen, Classes of receptors
    for the sulfidopeptide leukotrienes, in: "Icosanoids and
    Ion Transport," P. Braquet and B. Samuelsson, eds., Raven
    Press, New York (in press).

43. B.J. Ballermann, R.A. Lewis, E.J. Corey, K.F. Austen, and
    B.M. Brenner, Identification of leukotriene C_4 (LTC_4)
    receptors in isolated rat renal glomeruli, Clin. Res.
    32:440A (1984).

44. E.J. Goetzl and W.C. Pickett, Novel structural determinants of
    the human neutrophil chemotactic activity of leukotriene B,
    J. Exp. Med. 153:482 (1981).

45. R.A. Lewis, E.J. Goetzl, J.M. Drazen, N.A. Soter, K.F. Austen,
    and E.J. Corey, Functional characterization of synthetic
    leukotriene B and its stereochemical isomers, J. Exp. Med.
    154:1243 (1981).

46. A.W. Ford-Hutchinson, M.A. Bray, F.M. Cunningham, E.M.
    Davidson, and M.J.H. Smith, Isomers of LTB_4 posess differ-
    ent biological potencies, Prostaglandins 21:143 (1981).

47. D.W. Goldman and E.J. Goetzl, Specific binding of leukotriene
    B_4 to receptors on human polymorphonuclear leukocytes, J.
    Immunol. 129:1600 (1982).

48. D.W. Goldman and E.J. Goetzl, Selective transduction of human
    polymorphonuclear leukocyte functions by subsets of recep-
    tors for leukotriene B_4, J. Allergy Clin. Immunol. (in
    press).

49. P.F. Weller, C.W. Lee, D.W. Foster, E.J. Corey, K.F. Austen,
    and R.A. Lewis, Generation and metabolism of 5-lipoxygen-
    ase pathway leukotrienes by human eosinophils: predominant
    production of leukotriene C_4, Proc. Natl. Acad. Sci. USA.
    80:7626 (1983).

50. C.W. Lee, R.A. Lewis, A.I. Tauber, M. Mehrotra, E.J. Corey,
    and K.F. Austen, The myeloperoxidase-dependent metabolism of
    leukotrienes C_4, D_4, and E_4 to 6-trans-leukotriene B_4 dia-
    stereoisomers and the subclass-specific S-diastereoisomeric
    sulfoxides, J. Biol. Chem. 258:15004 (1983).

51. A.O. Fels, N.A. Pawlowski, E.B. Cramer, T.K.C. King, Z.A.
    Cohn, and W.A. Scott, Human alveolar macrophages produce
    leukotriene B_4, Proc. Natl. Acad. Sci. USA. 79:7866
    (1982).

52. T.R. Martin, L.C. Altman, R.K. Albert, and W.R. Henderson,
    Leukotriene B_4 production by the human alveolar macro-
    phage: a potential mechanism for amplifying inflammation
    in the lung, Amer. Rev. Respir. Dis. 125:106 (1984).

53. P. Godard, M. Damon, F.B. Michel, E.J. Corey, K.F. Austen, and R.A. Lewis, Leukotriene B$_4$ production from human alveolar macrophages, Clin. Res. 31:548A (1983).

54. J.D. Williams, J.K Czop, and K.F. Austen, Release of leukotrienes by human monocytes on stimultion of their phagocytic receptor for particulate activators, J. Immunol. 132:3034 (1984).

55. D.W. MacGlashan, R. Schleimer, S.P. Peters, E.S. Schulman, G.K. Adams, H.H. Newball, and L.M. Lichtenstein, Generation of leukotrienes by purified human lung mast cells, J. Clin. Invest. 70:747 (1982).

56. S.P. Peters, D.W. MacGlashan, E.S. Schulman, R.P. Schleimer, E.C. Hayes, J. Rokach, N.F. Adkinson and L.M. Lichtenstein, Arachidonic acid metabolism in purified human lung mast cells, J. Immunol. 132:1972 (1984).

57. T. Shimizu, O. Rådmark, and B. Samuelsson, Enzyme with dual lipoxygenase activities catalyzes leukotriene A$_4$ synthesis from arachidonic acid, Proc. Natl. Acad. Sci. USA. 81:689 (1984).

58. O. Rådmark, C. Malmsten, B. Samuelssson, G. Goto, A. Marfat, and E.J. Corey, Leukotriene A: isolation from human polymorphonuclear leukocytes, J. Biol. Chem. 255:11828 (1980).

59. A.L. Maycock, M.S. Anderson, D.M. DeSousa, and F.A. Kuehl, Jr., Leukotriene A$_4$: preparation and enzymatic conversion in a cell-free system to leukotriene B$_4$, J. Biol. Chem. 257:13911 (1982).

60. M.K. Bach, J.R. Brashler, and D.R. Morton, Jr., Solubilization and characterization of the leukotriene C$_4$ synthetase of rat basophil leukemia cells: a novel, particulate glutathione-S-transferase, Arch. Biochem. Biophys. 230:455 (1984).

61. R.A. Lewis and K.F. Austen, The biologically active leukotrienes: biosynthesis, metabolism, receptors, functions, and pharmacology, J. Clin. Invest. 73:889 (1984).

62. E.J. Corey, H. Park, A. Barton, and Y. Nii, Synthesis of three potential inhibitors of the biosynthesis of leukotrienes A-E, Tetrahedron Lett. 21:4243 (1980).

63. E. Razin, L.C. Romeo, S. Krilis, F.-T. Liu, R.A.Lewis, E.J. Corey, and K.F. Austen, An analysis of the relationship between 5-lipoxygenase product generation and the secretion of preformed mediators from mouse bone marrow-derived mast cells, J. Immunol. 133:938 (1984).

64. M.K. Bach, J.R. Brashler, H.W. Smith, F.A. Fitzpatrick, F.F. Sun, and J.C. Maguire, 6,9-deepoxy-6,9-(phenylimino)-$\Delta^{6,8}$-prostaglandin I$_1$ (U-60,257), a new inhibitor of leukotriene C and D synthesis: in vitro studies, Prostaglandins 23:759 (1982).

65. B.M. Weichman, M.A. Wasserman, D.A. Holden, R.R. Osborn, D.F. Woodward, T.W. Ku, and J.G. Gleason, Antagonism of the pulmonary effects of the peptidoleukotrienes by a leukotriene D_4 analog, J. Pharmacol. Exp. Ther. 227:700 (1983).

66. R.C. Murphy, W.C. Pickett, B.R. Culp, and W.E.M. Lands, Tetraene and pentaene leukotrienes: selective production from murine mastocytoma cells after dietary manipulation, Prostaglandins. 22:613 (1981).

67. J.D. Prickett, D.R. Robinson, and A.D. Steinberg, Dietary enrichment with the polyunsaturated fatty acid eicosapentaenoic acid prevents proteinuria and prolongs survival in NZB x NZW F_1 mice, J. Clin. Invest. 68:556 (1981).

68. J.D. Prickett, D.W. Trentham, and D.R. Robinson, Dietary fish oil augments the induction of arthritis in rats immunized with type II collagen, J. Immunol. 132:725 (1984).

69. E.J. Corey, C. Shih, and J.R. Cashman, Docosahexaenoic acid is a strong inhibitor of prostaglandin but not leukotriene biosynthesis, Proc. Natl. Acad. Sci. USA 80:3581 (1983).

70. R.P.Orange, M.D. Valentine, and K.F. Austen, Antigen-induced release of slow reacting substance of anaphylaxis (SRS-A^{rat}) in rats prepared with homologous antibody, J. Exp. Med. 127:767 (1968).

71. A.G. Leitch, T.H. Lee, E.W. Ringel, J.D Prickett, D.R. Robinson, S.G. Pyne, E.J. Corey, J.M. Drazen, K.F. Austen, and R.A. Lewis, Immunologically-induced generation of tetraene and pentaene leukotrienes in the peritoneal cavities of menhaden-fed rats, J. Immunol. 132:2559 (1984).

72. T.H. Lee, J.-M. Mencia-Huerta, C. Shih, E.J. Corey, R.A. Lewis, and K.F. Austen, Characterization and biologic properties of 5,12-dihydroxy derivatives of eicosapentaenoic acid, including leukotriene B_5 and the double lipoxygenase product, J. Biol. Chem. 259:2383 (1984).

73. S. Hammarström, Conversion of ^{14}C-labeled eicosapentaenoic acid (N-3) to leukotriene C_5, Biochim. Biophys. Acta. 663:575 (1981).

74. S.-E. Dahlén, P. Hedqvist, and S. Hammarström, Contractile activities of several cysteine-containing leukotrienes in the guinea pig lung strip, Eur. J. Pharmacol. 86:207 (1982).

75. T.H. Lee, R.A. Lewis, D.R. Robinson, J.M. Drazen, and K.F. Austen, The effects of a diet enriched in menhaden fish oil on the pulmonary response to antigen challenge, J. Allergy Clin. Immunol. 73:150 (1984).

76. E.A. Ham, D.D. Soderman, M.E. Zanetti, H.W. Dougherty, E. McCauley, and F.A. Kuehl, Jr., Inhibition by prostaglandins of leukotriene B_4 release from activated neutrophil, Proc. Natl. Acad. Sci. USA. 80:4349 (1983).

77. L. Levine, R. Morgan, R.A. Lewis, K.F. Austen, D.A. Clark, A. Marfat, and E.J. Corey, Radioimmunoassay of the leukotrienes of slow reacting substance of anaphylaxis (SRS-A), Proc. Natl. Acad. Sci. USA. 78:7692 (1981).

78. E.C. Hayes, D.L. Lombardo, Y. Girard, A.L. Maycock, J. Rokach A.S. Rosenthal, R.M. Young, R.W. Egan, and H.J. Zweerink, Measuring leukotrienes of slow reacting substance of anaphylaxis: development of specific radioimmunoassay, J. Immunol. 131:429 (1983).

79. K. Ochi, T. Yoshimoto, S. Yamamoto, K. Taniguchi, and T. Miyamoto, Arachidonate 5-lipoxygenase of guinea pig peritoneal polymorphonuclear leukocytes, J. Biol. Chem. 258:5754 (1983).

80. R.J. Soberman, R.A. Lewis, E.J. Corey, and K.F. Austen, The characterization of two lipoxygenases from the human PMN, Fed. Proc. 43:1879 (1984).

81. T.H. Lee, J.-M. Mencia-Huerta, C. Shih, E.J. Corey, R.A. Lewis, and K.F. Austen, Effects of exogenous arachidonic, eicosapentaenoic, and docosahexaenoic acids on the generation of 5-lipoxygenase pathway products by ionophore-activated human neutrophils, J. Clin. Invest. (in press).

82. S. Fischer, C.V. Schacky, W. Siess, T. Strasser, and P.C. Weber, Uptake, release and metabolism of docosahexaenoic acid in human platelets and neutrophils, Biochem. Biophys. Res. Commun. 120:907 (1984).

83. H.O. Bang, and J. Dyerberg, Lipid metabolism and ischemic heart disease in Greenland Eskimoes, Adv. Lipid Res. 3:1 (1980).

84. H. Herxheimer and O. Shaefer, Asthma in Canadian Eskimoes, N. Engl. J. Med. (correspondence) 291:1419 (1974).

85. J. Dyerberg, H.O. Bang, G. Stoffersen, S. Moncada, and J.R. Vane, Eicosapentaenoic acid and prevention of thrombosis and atherosclerosis, Lancet. 1:117 (1978).

86. P. Needleman, A. Raz, N.S. Minkes, A. Ferendelli, and H. Sprecher, Triene prostaglandins: prostacyclin and thromboxane biosynthesis and unique biological properties, Proc. Natl. Acad. Sci. USA. 76:944 (1979).

87. G.H.R. Rai, E. Radha, and J.G. White, Effect of docosahexaenoic acid (DHA) on arachidonic acid metabolism and platelet function, Biochem. Biophys. Res. Commun. 117:5498 (1983).

STUDIES WITH INHIBITORS OF LEUKOTRIENE BIOSYNTHESIS WITH SPECIAL REFERENCE TO PIRIPROST (U-60,257)

Michael K. Bach

Department of Hypersensitivity Diseases Research
The Upjohn Company
Kalamazoo, MI

INTRODUCTION

The underlying and motivating force behind the search for inhibitors of the formation of the leukotrienes is the hypothesis that these substances play an important if not an etiologic role in the elicitation of the symptoms of inflammation in general and of asthma in particular. An essential element in the final "proof" of this assumption is the demonstration that the selective inhibition of the formation or action of these substances can result in meaningful improvement in the condition of patients suffering from these disorders. Thus, even though relatively non-selective inhibitors may have their place, and even though in certain circumstances it may actually be desirable to combine the specific inhibition of certain pathways in one and the same molecule, the goal of the studies to be reported here is the development of selective inhibitors of the formation of the leukotrienes in the hope that these agents might then be useful in providing the remaining needed element of proof for the role of the leukotrienes in disease.

This paper will describe the in vitro experiments which led to the identification of piriprost (U-60,257) as a selective inhibitor of leukotriene synthesis. It will also review the evidence from in vivo experiments which indicates that this compound can inhibit leukotriene-induced manifestations of anaphylactic reactions in living animals. It will then consider the evidence that piriprost is a selective inhibitor of the 5-lipoxygenase and that, in terms of leukotriene biosynthesis, it does not appear to have other sites of action. Finally, and deriving from this conclusion, it will present some more recent results which demonstrate that this compound can profoundly synergize the action of another inhibitor of leukotriene synthesis whose site of action is elsewhere in the biosynthetic pathway to the sulfidopeptide leukotrienes.

DISCOVERY OF PIRIPROST

With the discovery almost ten years ago, that the challenge of resident or induced rat peritoneal cells, or the mononuclear cell fraction derived from these, with the calcium ionophore, A23187, could result in the production of large amounts of slow reacting substance, it became possible for the first time to design meaningful biochemical studies with potential inhibitors and modulators of the synthesis of this material. It became apparent early on that the production of these mediators under ionophore stimulation was independent of regulation via the adenylate cyclase system so that one could extrapolate, at least for the first level of simplification, that inhibitors of the formation of slow reacting substance in this system were actually inhibiting the enzymatic steps involved in the synthesis of these substances rather than pharmacologically modulating the controls on this synthesis. Our studies then led us to the conclusion that slow reacting substance was derived from arachidonate[1] even though it did not seem to fit into the pattern of compounds whose biosynthesis could be inhibited by low doses of indomethacin. At the same time, we knew that the cells which we were using also produced products of the cyclooxygenase pathway of arachidonate metabolism under the same challenge conditions. Thus, even before we knew the structures of the slow reacting substances, we postulated that compounds that had been found to have marginal activity on the eicosanoid pathways which were then being monitored, might be good candidates for testing for their ability to inhibit this new pathway. If any of these compounds should prove to be active, then the already known low or absent activity on the other pathways would automaticaly impart to the new inhibitor a level of selectivity.

Piriprost (U-60,257) which is 6,9-deepoxy-6,9-(phenylimino)-$\Delta^{6,8}$ prostaglandin I_1 (Fig. 1) had been prepared by Dr. Herman Smith and his colleagues as part of a program of defining the structure activity characteristics within the prostacyclin family. It had virtually no activity in the cyclooxygenase screen and thus became a candidate for us. We found that piriprost, and especially its methyl ester, were potent inhibitors of leukotriene biosynthesis in our mononuclear cells while, at the same time the formation of thromboxane was moderately enhanced in the same cells (Fig. 2)[2]. We also found that these compounds could inhibit the formation of leukotrienes in anaphylactically-challenged human lung fragments while, at the same time, the release of preformed mediators was unaffected. We further showed that the activity of

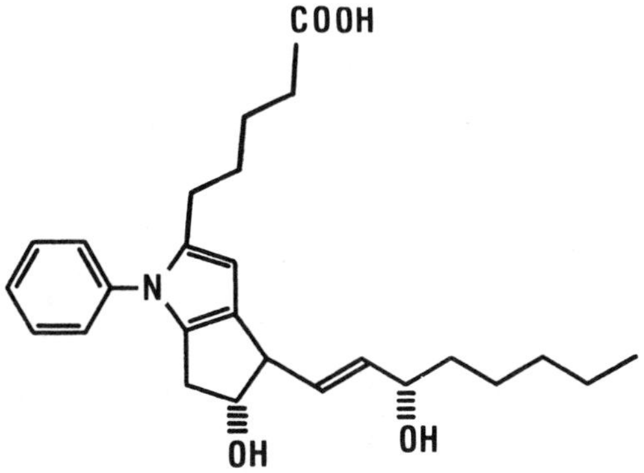

Fig. 1. The structure of piriprost.

piriprost was not a general property of the prostacyclins since neither PGI$_2$ nor 6-β-PGI$_1$ inhibited leukotriene synthesis in our mononuclear cell preparations. Finally, and to further distinguish this new activity from the activities of compounds which inhibit the release of preformed mediators during anaphylactic challenge (e.g. sodium cromoglycate), we showed that there was no need to preincubate cells with piriprost in order to demonstrate full inhibition, that the inhibition persisted as long as the cells remained in contact with the inhibitor, that the inhibition was readily reversible upon removal of the inhibitor, and that the inhibition could be reinstituted upon readdition of the inhibitor. Despite the increased potency of the methyl ester in vitro, piriprost, which has a free carboxylic acid, was selected for further development because its solubility in buffers markedly facilitated the in vivo studies.

IN VIVO ACTIONS OF PIRIPROST

Though it is well recognized by now that the leukotrienes contribute to the anaphylactic responses which can be elicited in animal models, it is a bit more difficult to devise situations in which the contribution of the leukotrienes to the total response is of sufficient magnitude that their selective inhibition results in a marked inhibition of the total response. A number of methods for achieving this in the egg albumin-sensitized, anaphylactically-challenged guinea pig have been described and we adopted one of these methods for our studies[3]. In this model, guinea pigs are pretreated with an antihistamine, a nonsteroidal

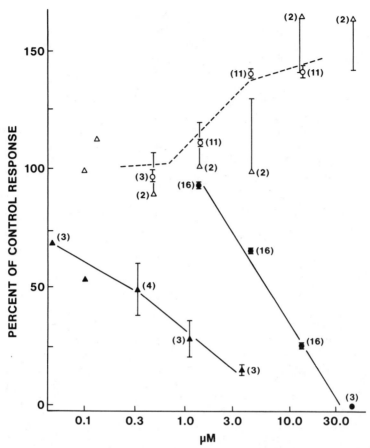

Fig. 2. Dose-dependent inhibition by piriprost of leukotriene
formation in ionophore A23187-challenged rat peritoneal
mononuclear cells, and dose-dependent stimulation of
thromboxane formation in the same cells. (Reproduced
from ref. 9) Open symbols, thromboxane; closed symbols,
leukotriene formation; circles, piriprost; triangles,
piriprost and methyl ester.

anti-inflammatory compound and atropine and are then given a bolus
injection of arachidonate, iv, immediately before intravenous
challenge with antigen. Under these conditions, the bronchoconstriction which is inhibited by approximately 50% by the antihistamine, is increased to a level which approximately equals that
in untreated control animals. This enhanced bronchoconstriction
was readily inhibitable by a selective end-organ antagonist of
the leukotrienes, FPL 55712, at low concentrations. Piriprost
also inhibited the enhanced bronchoconstriction in this model at
doses in the 1 to 10 mg/kg range (iv). The potency of piriprost
was increased by several orders of magnitude when the compound

was administered to the animals by the aerosol route. Under these conditions we found that letting the animals breath the aerosol generated from a 0.01% solution for 180 seconds was sufficient to completely inhibit the response. Duration of action studies then showed that this dose was sufficient to protect the animals for 90 min while exposure to a 1% solution protected for as long as 6 h (Fig. 3).

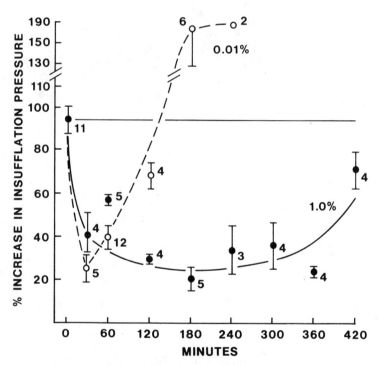

Fig. 3.   Duration of action of piriprost in the anaphylactically challenged guinea pig. Conscious guinea pigs were exposed to an aerosol of 1% solution of piriprost (closed circles, solid line) or 0.01% solution (open circles, dashed line) for 180 seconds and were then dosed and challenged with antigen after the elapsed times noted in the figure. Results are expressed relative to the insufflation pressure prior to challenge with antigen.

There was no change in the capacity of a 0.01% solution to afford protection after the animals had been exposed to this dose daily for 7 days[4] (Fig. 4).

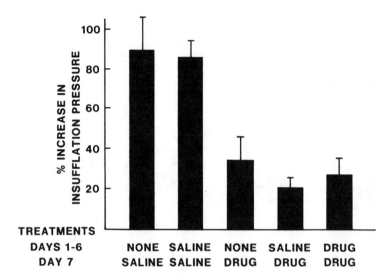

Fig. 4.   Effect of repeated dosing with piriprost on the capacity to inhibit increases in insufflation pressure upon challenge with antigen. Animals were randomly assigned to the different treatment groups and, within treatment groups, to specific days for initiation of treatment and for challenge. All treatment exposures were for 180 seconds to a tham solution in saline. Drug concentration, where employed was 0.01%. Results are the means of 7 animals per group.

Another model of anaphylaxis which has been studied extensively is the bronchospasm which can be induced in spontaneously Ascaris-sensitive monkeys upon aerosol exposure to Ascaris antigen. We have at our laboratories a small colony of Ascaris responder monkeys which have been studied in detail over many years. Thus the response of each animal to antigen challenge in the presence of various drug treatments can be compared to the historic control responses in the same animal. It was found[5] that pretreatment of the monkeys with piriprost, either intravenously or by aerosol, afforded a dose-dependent protection from both the decreases in dynamic lung compliance (a measure of changes in the peripheral airways) and the increases in lung resistance (a measure of constriction of the central airways) which occur when these animals are challenged with antigen. The doses at which this protection was achieved were comparable to those which had been found to be protective in the guinea pigs. Even more interestingly, when a combination of a low dose of piriprost (0.01 mg/kg, iv) and a low dose of an H_1 antihistamine was used, such that neither agent caused significant protection by itself, virtually complete inhibition of both the changes in compliance and resistance could be shown. This synergism suggests that, rather than merely acting independently, the different mediators which are released or produced during an anaphylactic challenge may well potentiate the response of one another.

In addition to bronchospasm, the excessive production of mucus, the inappropriate viscosity of the mucus and the slowing of mucus transport velocity are other serious aspects of the asthmatic syndrome. Dr. H. G. Johnson at our laboratories has been studying a model in the dog, in which mucus production can be quantitated on the longitudinally sectioned upper portion of the trachea by counting the number of "hillocks" of mucus which form on the tracheal surface after the tissue has been dusted with tantalum powder to prevent the mucus droplets from coalescing. In this model, the exogenous administration of leukotrienes into the cranial thyroid artery which feeds the trachea, resulted in a marked increase in mucus secretion[6] suggesting that the leukotrienes may play a role in these aspects of the asthmatic syndrome as well. This is further stressed by the findings[7] that FPL 55712 can markedly increase mucus transport velocity and, furthermore, can inhibit the decrease in this parameter which is ordinarily demonstrable upon anaphylactic challenge. The administration of piriprost into the cranial thyroid artery, or its aerosolization into the lung in Dr. Johnson's dog model resulted in an inhibition of the spontaneous production of mucus as well as in the elicited increased production which accompanies hypoxia or the exogenous administration of arachidonate in this model[8].

MODE OF ACTION STUDIES

Initial observations suggested that low concentrations of piriprost actually increased the production of 5-HETE and LTB in ionophore-challenged human polymorphonuclear cells (PMN's)[9]. At the same time, it was found that the conversion of LTA to LTC by crude rat liver cytosolic glutathione S-transferase preparations was inhibited in dose-dependent manner by this compound[2] and this led to the suggestion that piriprost was an inhibitor of the terminal step in sulfidopeptide leukotriene synthesis, the LTA: glutathione S-transferase (LTC synthetase). This conclusion was inconsistent with the observation by R. J. Smith et al[10] that piriprost was a potent inhibitor of the formation of LTB from endogenous substrates in human PMN's.

Subsequent studies proved the original conclusion wrong on two counts. First it was found that the particulate LTC synthetases of RBL cells, rat mononuclear cells, and human lung, which appear to be responsible for the synthesis of sulfidopeptide leukotrienes in these tissues[11] were not sensitive to inhibition by piriprost while the ability of piriprost to inhibit purified fractions of liver glutathione S-transferase was readily confirmed. Second, it was found that the apparent enhanced formation of 5-lipoxygenase products in the presence of piriprost was a peculiarity of the high concentrations of exogenous arachidonate which had been used in the initial studies. When the arachidonate concentration was reduced to the trace level, the formation of products of the 5-lipoxygenase pathway was inhibited by piriprost in a dose-dependent fashion[12].

At this point, piriprost has been studied in a large number of settings by a considerable number of investigators. Many of their results are in various stages of publication and it would not be appropriate, nor does time permit me to review them here. However, all the results are consistent with the conclusion that piriprost is a selective inhibitor of the 5-lipoxygenase.

Piriprost is presently undergoing clinical trials as a potential therapeutic for the treatment of asthma. While it is too early to tell what its fate will be, both the toxicologic studies and the early studies in man suggest that the drug is well tolerated.

INHIBITORS OF THE LTC SYNTHETASE AND SYNERGISM WITH PIRIPROST

Our initial studies with the LTC synthetase of RBL cells[11] revealed that the profile of inhibition of this enzyme by a variety of known inhibitors of glutathione S-transferase was distinctly different from those of the cytosolic rat liver or RBL cell glutathione S-transferases. Compounds which are good inhibitors of the liver enzyme turned out to be nearly inactive in the LTC synthetase system. This suggested that a selective inhibitor of the LTC synthetase, if it could be found, might be a relatively non-toxic inhibitor of sulfidopeptide leukotriene synthesis[13].

We have been interested in two compounds which have been known for some time to inhibit the formation of the leukotrienes. One of these is sulfasalazine which, at the admittedly high concentrations which might be found in bowel contents of patients being medicated with this drug, can inhibit the formation of both 5-HETE and LTB[14], and the other is diethylcarbamazine which has been known to be an inhibitor of SRS-A formation for over 16 years[15]. While sulfasalazine turned out to be a potent inhibitor of rat liver cytosolic glutathione S-transferases (K_i in the micromolar range), diethylcarbamazine was virtually inactive on these enzymes. On the other hand, both of these compounds inhibited the LTC synthetase at concentrations which were comparable to those which were required to demonstrate the inhibition of sulfidopeptide leukotriene synthesis in intact RBL cells (Fig.5).

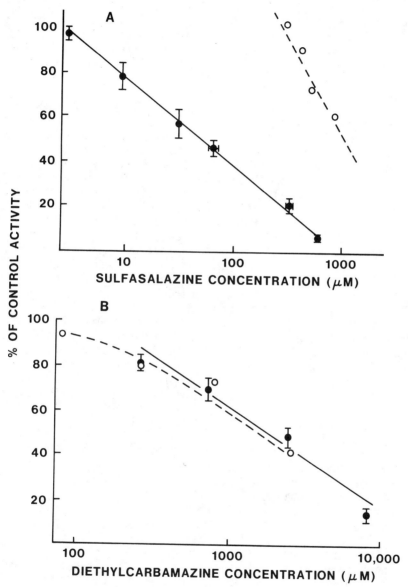

Fig. 5.   Dose-response curves for the inhibition of leukotriene production by intact RBL cells (solid circles and lines) and by the solubilized LTC synthetase (broken lines, open circles). A. Sulfasalazine; B Diethylcarbamazine

Kinetic studies have shown that sulfasalazine is a competitive inhibitor for glutathione, both with the liver enzymes and with the RBL-derived, solubilized LTC synthetase. While both 5-aminosalicylic acid and N'-2-pyridylsulfanilamide, the two breakdown products of sulfasalazine, were weak inhibitors of these enzymes, the kinetics of inhibition were not consistent with competitive inhibition with glutathione for either of these compounds. These results do not explain the action of sulfasalazine in inhibiting LTB formation[14], but rather, they indicate that these molecules which are known to possess a large and seemingly diverse series of activities, possess in addition, yet another action which had not been appreciated thus far.

Kinetic studies on the inhibition of LTC synthetase by diethylcarbamazine are consistent with the inhibition being competitive with LTA_4 although the limited supplies of LTA_4 at our disposal have not permitted a detailed analysis of this inhibition. If piriprost is indeed an inhibitor of the 5-lipoxygenase, its effect on leukotriene formation will be to limit the available supply of LTA_4 in the cells. Under such conditions, a second inhibitor, which is kinetically a competitor for LTA_4 in the LTC synthetase reaction, might then be expected to become markedly more active in the presence of low concentrations of piriprost. Thus we asked whether synergism between piriprost and diethylcarbamazine in the synthesis of sulfidopeptide leukotrienes by RBL cells could be demonstrated. As seen in Fig. 6, this was indeed the case. Concentrations of piriprost which, by themselves, had no inhibitory activity on leukotriene formation (0.2 and 0.7 M), in combination with concentrations of diethylcarbamazine which were also without significant effect (26 to 260 M), caused a profound inhibition of leukotriene formation. Indeed, in the presence of these non-inhibitory concentrations of piriprost, a plot of the log of the EC_{50} concentration of diethylcarbamazine against the piriprost concentration was linear; a doubling of the piriprost concentration (0.12 to 0.23 M) caused a 2.9-fold decrease in the EC_{50} value for diethylcarbamazine.

Since both sulfasalazine and diethylcarbamazine inhibit the LTC synthetase but differ in their kinetics, we expected that synergistic inhibition of leukotriene synthesis might be demonstrable with this combination of inhibitors as well. This was in fact the case. However, the magnitude of the synergism was considerably smaller than the one we had observed between piriprost and diethylcarbamazine. We were able to show (Fig. 7) that increasing concentrations of diethylcarbamazine increased the apparent inhibitory potency of sulfasalazine. Even though the data are plotted as a log-log plot in the figure, it should be stressed that the fit of the data to the curve does not permit us to discriminate between this method of presentation and plots of

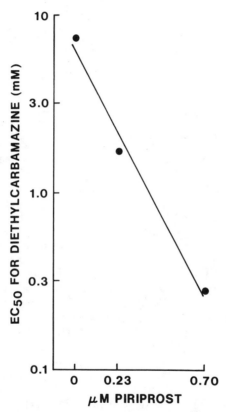

Fig. 6.   Synergism in the inhibition of leukotriene formation in RBL cells by combinations of piriprost and diethyl-carbamazine. At these concentrations, piriprost by itself did not inhibit leukotriene production.

a linear relationship or the relationship between diethylcarbamazine concentration and the log of the fold increase in potency of sulfasalazine.

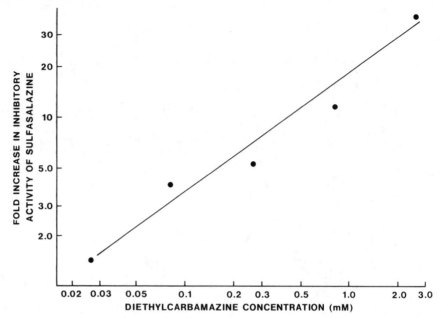

Fig. 7.   Synergism in the inhibition of leukotriene formation in RBL cells by combinations of diethylcarbamazine and sulfasalazine. For each diethylcarbamazine concentration, a dose response curve for sulfaslazine was constructed taking the activity in the absence of sulfasalazine as 100%. These curves were compared to the dose-response curve for sulfasalazine in the absence of diethylcarbamazine. It was found that increasing concentrations of diethylcarbamazine caused a parallel shift to the right in the dose-response curves for sulfasalazine. The magnitude of this shift, for a given diethylcarbamazine concentration, could be equated to a "fold increase in the inhibitory activity of sulfasalazine, as read from the log dose vs. response plot for sulfasalazine in the absence of diethylcarbamazine. The log of the "fold increase inhibitory activity" was plotted against the log of the diethylcarbamazine concentration.

These recent results highlight the power which can be derived from the judicious application of combinations of inhibitors having different sites of action on the same biochemical pathway. At the same time, one can envision that the use of such combinations might minimize the toxicity which might be encountered other than that which is due to intended action(s) of the combinations since, under ideal conditions, neither drug in the combination would be present at a concentration which is sufficient to elicit any of the undesired responses which higher concentrations of the same drug might elicit. We hope that, with a judicious educational program, it will become possible to consider the use of such combinations in the rational design of better therapeutics.

ACKNOWLEDGEMENTS

The studies which were reviewed here were conducted by a large number of investigators at our Company and, wherever possible, their original papers have been cited. The studies which were carried out in my own laboratory involved, in addition to John R. Brashler, the assistance of Dr. Mark A. Johnson for biostatistical evaluations, Dr. Douglas G. Morton for the preparation of LTA_4, Dr. Ivan M. Richards and Mr. Robert L. Griffin for the studies in guinea pigs, and Rebecca E. Peck and John O'Brien for assistance with the bioassays for leukotrienes.

REFERENCES

1.   M. K. Bach, J. R. Brashler, and R. R. Gorman, On the structure of slow reacting substance of anaphylaxis: Evidence of biosynthesis from arachidonic acid, Prostaglandins 14:21 (1977).
2.   M. K. Bach, J. R. Brashler, H. W. Smith, F. A. Fitzpatrick, F. F. Sun, and J. C. McGuire, 6,9-deepoxy-6,9(phenylimino)$-_\Delta{}^{6,8}$-prostaglandin I_1, (U-60,257), a new inhibitor of leukotriene C and D synthesis: In vitro studies. Prostaglandins 23:759 (1982).
3.   D. M. Ritchie, J. N. Sierchio, R. J. Capetola, and M. E. Rosenthale, SRS-A-mediated bronchospasm by pharmacologic modification of lung anaphylaxis in vivo, Agents Actions 11:396 (1981).
4.   M. K. Bach, R. L. Griffin, and I. M. Richards, Inhibition of the presumably leukotriene-dependent component of the antigen-induced bronchoconstriction in the guinea pig by piriprost (U-60,257), to be presented at the 15 Symposium of the Collegium Internationale Allergologicum, Puerto Vallarata, Mexico, September 1984.
5.   H. G. Johnson, M. L. McNee, M. K. Bach, and H. W. Smith, The activity of a new, novel inhibitor of leukotriene synthesis in Rhesus monkey Ascaris reactors, Int. Archs Allergy Appl. Immunol. 70:169 (1983).
6.   H. G. Johnson and M. L. McNee, Secretagogue responses of leukotrienes C_4 and D_4: A comparison of potency in canine trachea in vivo, Prostaglandins 25:237 (1983).

7. T. Ahmed, D. W. Greenblatt, S. Birch, B. Marchette, and A. Wanner, Abnormal mucocilliary transport in allergic patients with antigen-induced bronchospasm: Role of slow reacting substance of anaphylaxis. Am. Rev. Resp. Dis. 124:110 (1981).

8. H. G. Jonson and M. L. McNee, Regulation of canine mucus secretion by a novel leukotriene synthesis inhibitor (U-60,257), In Press.

9. M. K. Bach, J. R. Brashler, F. A. Fitzpatrick, R. L. Griffin, S. S. Iden, H. G. Johnson, M. L. McNee, J. C. McGuire, H. W. Smith, R. J. Smith, F. F. Sun, and M. A. Wasserman, In vivo and in vitro actions of a new selective inhibitor of leukotriene C and D synthesis. Adv. Prostaglandin Thromboxane Leukotriene Research 11:39 (1983).

10. R. J. Smith, F. F. Sun, B. J. Bowman, S. S. Iden, H. W. Smith and J. C. McGuire, Effect of 6,9-deepoxy-6,9(phenylimino) $-_\Delta^{6,8}$ prostaglandin I_1, (U-60,257), an inhibitor of leuko-triene synthesis, on human neutrophil function, Biochem. Biophys. Res. Commun. 109:943 (1982).

11. M. K. Bach, J. R. Brashler and D. R. Morton, Jr., Solubilization and characterization of the leukotriene C_4 synthetase of rat basophil leukemia cells: A novel, particulate glutathione S-transferase, Archs Biochem. Biophys. 230:455 (1984).

12. F. F. Sun and J. C. McGuire, Inhibition of human neutrophil arachidonate 5-lipoxygenase by 6,9-deepoxy-6,9(phenylimino) $-_\Delta^{6,8}$ prostaglandin I_1 (U-60,257), Prostaglandins 26:211 (1983).

13. M. K. Bach, Prospects for the inhibition of leukotriene synthesis, Biochem. Parmacol. 33:515 (1984)

14. W. F. Stenson and E. Lobos, Sulfasalazine inhibits the synthesis of chemotactic lipids by neutrophils, J. Clin. Invest., 69:494 (1982).

15. R. P. Orange, M. D. Valentine, and K. F. Austen, Inhibition of release of slow reacting substance of anaphylaxis in the rat with diethylcarbamazine, Proc. Soc. Expt. Biol. Med. 127:127 (1968).

PULMONARY AND VASCULAR EFFECTS OF LEUKOTRIENES: INVOLEMENT IN

ASTHMA AND INFLATION

Per Hedqvist and Sven-Erik Dahlén

The National Institute of Environmental Medicine and
Department of Physiology, Karolinska Institutet
S-104 01 Stockholm, Sweden

INTRODUCTION

The prostaglandins, thromboxanes and leukotrienes comprise a
complex system of bioregulators, synthesized on demand in almost
every tissue, and demonstrating a broad range of activities. They
all derive from some closely related polyunsaturated fatty acids,
particularly arachidonic acid, which may be oxidized and further
transformed in reactions initiated either by a fatty acid cyclooxygenase or, alternatively by a number of lipoxygenases. Prostaglandins, prostacyclin (PGI_2) and thromboxane A_2 (TXA_2) are formed
via the cyclooxygenase pathway, whereas leukotrienes, lipoxins, and
related monohydroxy acids are generated by specific lypoxygenases.
Most of the products thus formed either contract of relax vascular
and nonvascular smooth muscle, and several of them have been implicated a mediator role in various inflammatory and hypersensitivity
reactions. The antiflogistic effect of aspirin and related non-
steroidal antiinflammatory drug (NSAID:s) is well established, and
apparently correlates with the capacity to inhibit the formation of
cyclooxygenase products, notably PGE_2, PGD_2, and PGI_2. Although
these three substances are considered proinflammatory and potently
enhance the response to other stimuli, they do not themselves elicit
significant edema, and their pain producing capacity is at best moderate (cf. Kuehl and Egan, 1980; Goetzl, 1981). The same prostaglandins seem to have no effect per se on activation or migration
of leukocytes, although they have been reported to enhance chemokinesis (Goetzl et al., 1979) and to inhibit the release of lysosomal enzymes induced by other stimuli (Weissman et al., 1980). In
the pulmonary system, PGD_2, $PGF_{2\alpha}$, and TXA_2 are potent broncho-

constrictors, and most asthmatic patients are remarkable hyper-
reactive to inhalation of $PGF_{2\alpha}$ (Mathé et al., 1973; Pasarglikian
et al., 1977). Moreover, asthmatic patients provoked by inhalation of specific allergen demonstrate increased plasma levels of
15-keto-13,14-dehydro-$PGF_{2\alpha}$, major metabolite of $PGF_{2\alpha}$ and PGD_2,
in correlation with the severety of the asthmatic attack (Green et
al., 1974). However, cyclooxygenase inhibitors do not significantly alleviate the symptoms of asthma, and sometimes they even precipitate a life-threatening reaction, the so called aspirin asthma.

The lipoxygenase-derived metabolites of arachidonic acid form
another heterogenous group of biologically active substances. However, some of them, the leukotrienes, differ conspicuously from the
cyclooxygenase products inasmuch they have the capacity themselves
to mimic most, if not all, of the events in hypersensitivity and
inflammatory states. The responses elicited include bronchoconstriction, hypersecretion of mucus into the airways, formation of
mucosal and interstitial edema, and finally, but not the least,
migration and activation of leukocytes. The purpose of this chapter
is to briefly review the pulmonary and microvascular effects of the
leukotrienes, and the possible role of these substances as mediators
in acute inflammation and immediate hypersensitivity.

BIOCHEMICAL BACKGROUND

The biosynthesis of the leukotrienes (cf. Samuelsson, 1983) is
initiated by a lipoxygenase which catalyzes the introduction of
molecular oxygen at C-5, leading to the formation of 5-hydroper-
oxyeicosatetraenoic acid (5-HPETE), and subsequent enzymatic de-
hydration yields 5,6-oxido-7,9,11,14-eicosatetraenoic acid (LTA_4).
The epoxide, being highly unstable, is rapidly transformed into a
number of hydroxy acids, including 5(S), 12(R)-dihydroxy-6,8,10,
14-eicosatetraenoic acid (LTB_4), or by conjugation with glutathione
into 5(R)-hydroxy 6(S)-glutationyl-7,9,11,14-eicosatetraenoic acid
(LTC_4). Enzymatic elimination of glutamic acid from LTC_4 by γ-
glutamyl transpeptidase forms LTD_4, and subsequent hydrolysis of
the remaining peptide bond by a dipeptidase gives rise to LTE_4.
Although LTD_4 and LTE_4 are metabolites of LTC_4, they have the same
or occasionally an even higher biological potency. Together, the
three substances comprise SRS-A, and they have been identified in
a number of biological systems, but the relative proportions apparently vary with tissue and experimental conditions. At present,
the metabolic fate of the cysteinyl-containing leukotrienes is
largely unknown, although it has been shown that LTE_4 can function
as an acceptor of γ-glutamic acid forming a γ-glutamyl, cysteinyl
derivative, designated LTF_4 (Bernström and Hammarström, 1982). As
regards LTB_4, it is metabolized to trihydroxy LTB_4, and subsequently
to dicarboxy LTB_4 which seems to have lower biological potency than

the parent substance and hence may be regarded as initial step of bioinactivation (Hansson et al., 1981).

Leukotrienes may be formed also in lipoxygenase reactions starting with oxygenation at C-12 and C-15 rather than at C-5 (Jubiz et al., 1981, Maas et al., 1981). The biological significance of these substances has not been clarified, but it is of potential interest that 15-HPETE, precurser of the 14,15-leukotrienes,is a major lipoxygenase product formed in human lung (Hamberg et al., 1980, Dahlén et al., 1983a). It is also worth noting that 15-HPETE is the precursor of a number of trihydroxytetraenes, named lipoxines (Serhan et al., 1984a,b). These substances stimulate degranulation and superoxide generation in polymorphonuclear leukocytes (Serhan et al., 1984b), and they cause constriction of pulmonary tissue (Dahlén et al., 1984).

PULMONARY EFFECTS OF LEUKOTRIENES

In the 40 years between the discovery of SRS (Kellaway and Trethewie, 1940) and its chemical identification as a mixture of LTC_4, LTD_4 and LTE_4 (cf. Samuelsson,1983) a great deal of evidence was produced suggesting that SRS is released during allergic reactions and also mediates some of the manifestations. In particular, attention was paid to the possibility that SRS triggered attacks of bronchial asthma. As distinct from other presumed mediators, and in keeping with the fact that contraction of both larger and smaller passages contribute to the breathing difficulties of asthmatic patients, SRS proved very effective on all types of airways, and especially on the peripheral ones (Drazen and Austen, 1974). Careful analysis, over the past few years, of the pulmonary effects of the cysteinyl-containing leukotrienes has revealed that they are by far the most potent natural bronchoconstrictors, being 100-1000 times or more potent than histamine when given as aerosols to guinea pig, monkey and man (Hedqvist et al., 1980; Smedegård et al., 1982; Weiss et al., 1982). Like SRS they differ from histamine also in other respects. Thus, the bronchoconstriction induced by the leukotrienes is considerably slower in onset and of much longer duration (Hedqvist et al., 1980). Furthermore, they are particularly prone to act on terminal airways, as indicated by a decrease of pulmonary dynamic compliance rather than an increase in airways resistance (Drazen et al., 1980; Smedegård et al., 1982; Weiss et al., 1982). The contractile responses to the cysteinyl-containing leukotrienes in isolated airway preparations from guinea pig and man exhibit the same slow onset and long duration as under in vivo conditions (Dahlén et al., 1980; Drazen et al., 1980; Hedqvist et al., 1980). Likewise, the leukotrienes are particularly inclined to affect peripheral airways, but central airways are also very sensitive. Furthermore, noncumulative dose-response curves for LTC_4 and LTD_4 in human bronchi (diameter 2-4 mm), and for LTC_4, LTD_4 and LTE_4 in

guinea pig parenchymal lung strips, evidently show that these substances are virtually equiactive contractile agonists, and that
their potency, on a molar basis, exceeds that of histamine by at
least three orders of magnitude (Dahlén et al., 1980, 1983b; Jones
et al., 1982). The very same pattern, both regards contractile
potency and duration of the response, apparently applies to the 11-
trans isomers of LTC_4 and LTE_4, and cysteinyl-containing leukotrienes belonging to the 3 and 5 series, e.g. LTC_3 and LTC_5 (Dahlén et al., 1983b). Leukotriene B_4, on the other hand, is much
less potent than its cysteinyl-containing congeners on human bronchi and guinea pig lung strips (Sirois et al., 1981; Dahlén et al.,
1983c). In addition, the response to LTB_4 develops and vanishes
more rapidly, and has the apparent requirement of secondarily released cyclooxygenase products, particularly TXA_2 (Dahlén et al.,
1983c). Also the intermediate in leukotrien formation, $LTA4$,
elicits relatively short-lived contractile responses in human
bronchi and guinea pig lung strips, and demonstrates dose-response
relations comparable to LTB_4 (Dahlén et al., 1983c).

The typical slow onset of the bronchoconstrictive response to
LTC_4, LTD_4, and LTE_4 implies that these substances act by releasing
other smooth muscle stimulants. However, neither in vivo nor in
vitro is there any indication that acetylcholine, noradrenaline,
serotonin, or histamine are directly involved in the process (Dahlén
et al., 1980; Dahlén, 1983). On the other hand, there is more than
circumstantial evidence that cyclooxygenase products may contribute
to the response. Thus, LTC_4 causes the release of TXA_2 from guinea
pig lung, both in vitro and in vivo, and inhibitors of prostaglandin
cyclooxygenase or tromboxane synthetase may attenuate the bronchoconstrictive response to LTC_4 (Folco et al., 1982; Hamel et al.,
1982; Weichman et al., 1982; Dahlén, 1983; Dahlén et al., 1983c).
However, the potential of the inhibitors is highly dependent upon
route of leukotriene administration, and the experimental design.
In the guinea pig, indomethacin pretreatment shifts the dose-response
curve for intravenously injected LTC_4 by one order of magnitude to
the right (Dahlén 1983). Actually, this means that responses to
low doses of LTC_4 are markedly attenuated, whereas high doses still
may attain full agonist activity. Responses to LTC_4 given as an
aerosol were not at all inhibited, but rather enhanced by indomethacin. Removal of the bronchorelaxant PGE_2, known to be released by LTC_4 from guinea pig trachea (Piper and Tippins, 1982),
might offer an explanation of this enhancement.

Even though LTC_4 provokes the release of substantial amounts
of TXA_2 from the guinea pig lung strip, the contractile response to
LTC_4 in this preparation is generally quite resistant to indomethacin, presumably because of lower contractile potency of TXA_2
relative to LTC_4 (Dahlén et al., 1983c). However, if the preparation is superfused at high rate and LTC_4 is given as a bolus, a

situation less favourable to the tardy LTC_4, then the contractile response becomes inhibitable by indomethacin, suggesting that under these conditions the rapidly acting TXA_2 plays a significant role in the pharmacological activity of LTC_4 in isolated guinea pig tissue (Piper and Samhoun, 1982; Dahlén et al., 1983c). Together, all these findings indicate that cysteinyl-containing leukotrienes are potent bronchoconstrictors by themselves, and that secondarily released cyclooxygenase products contribute, or play a major role, only if the time of exposure is kept short, as when a superfusion technique is used in vitro, or when the leukotrienes are given by the intravenous route. Finally, neither in vitro (Jones et al., 1982; Dahlén et al., 1983a) nor in vivo (Barnes, personal commumications) is the bronchoconstrictive action of LTC_4 in humans affected by NSAID:s.

CARDIOVASCULAR EFFECTS OF LEUKOTRIENES

The cysteinyl-containing leukotrienes have been shown to greatly affect a number of important cardiovascular parameters. Thus, they cause vasoconstriction in many vascular beds (Dahlén et al., 1981; Peck et al., 1981; Terashita et al., 1981; Yokochi et al., 1982), and they may provoke a decrease of cardiac performance (Letts and Piper, 1982; Smedegård et al., 1982). When injected intravenously or intraatrially into guinea pig and monkey, the leukotrienes evoke biphasic changes of blood pressure in both circulations; initial increase followed by sustained hypotension (Smedegård et al., 1982; Dahlén, 1983). In the monkey (Smedegård et al., 1982) the hypotension was accounted for by decreased cardiac performance rather than vasodilatation. Thus, stroke volume and cardiac output fell markedly, whereas total peripheral resistance, if anything, was elevated. In addition, there was an increase in hematocrit indicating loss of plasma from the circulation. Decreased stroke volume and an increase of hematocrit has been noted after injection of LTC_4 also in man (Kaijser et al., 1984). Recently, it was reported that inhibitors of leukotriene biosynthesis and action block hypoxic vasoconstriction in the isolated perfused rat lung (Morganrothe et al., 1984). While this is an observation of interest, it remains to be established whether leukotrienes are involved in the regional control of ventilation-perfusion ratio in the lung.

In line with previous observations with SRS, intradermal injections of cystenyl-containing leukotrienes induce local extravasation of plasma to a variable extent in several species, including man (Drazen et al., 1980; Hedqvist et al., 1980; Peck et al., 1981; Lewis et al., 1982; Soter et al., 1983). When given systemically, the leukotrienes may evoke generalized leakage of plasma (Smedegård et al., 1982; Hua et al., 1984; Kaijser et al., 1984). In the guinea pig, LTC_4 and LTD_4 were virtually equiactive and provoked plasma exudation in most tissues throughout the body, with the respiratory and urinary tracts being particuarly sensitive. Furthermore, the extent of plasma exudation induced by a single bolus of LTC_4(1 nmol x kg^{-1}) was impressive, as indicated by 20% hemoconcentration, occurring within 5 min and lasting for 30 min, or more.

The mechanism for the edema-promoting action of leukotrienes has been studied in some detail by means of intravital microscopy of the terminal vascular bed of the hamster cheek pouch (Dahlén et al., 1981; Björk et al., 1982a; Björk et al., 1983). In this in vivo model, LTC_4, LTD_4, and LTE_4 elicited constriction of terminal arterioles and leakage of plasma from the venules. The two effects were not interrelated, inasmuch low concentrations of the leukotrienes evoked substantial extravasation in the absence of visible arteriolar constriction. The three leukotrienes proved to be very effective in causing macromolecular leakage; on a molar basis they were at least 1000 times more potent than histamine. Furthermore, the effect was specifically oriented towards postcapillary venules (leakage from larger venules was not observed), and apparently uninfluenced by depletion of circulating polymorphonuclear leukocytes, or administration of mepyramine and indomethacin. Leukotriene B_4 was also found to promote plasma leakage in the hamster cheek pouch, but it was considerably less potent than the cysteinyl-containing leukotrienes. As distinct from the cysteinyl-containing leukotrienes, LTB_4 caused extravasation from both postcapillary and larger venules, and the reaction occurred with some latency, and apparently required adhesion of leukocytes to the endothelial lining. In the rat and rabbit, LTB_4 has been reported to cause little leakage, unless given together with a vasodilator prostaglandin (Bray et al., 1981; Wedmore and Williams, 1981).

There is considerable in vitro evidence indicating that LTB_4 is chemokinetic and chemotactic for leukocytes; i.e. it increases random and directional migration of the cells (Ford-Hutchinson et al., 1980; Goetzl and Pickett, 1980; Malmsten et al., 1980; Palmer et al., 1980). The chemotactic effect of LTB_4 was equivalent to that of complement-derived C5a and the synthetic peptide fMLP, and it showed stereochemical selectivity, inasmuch a number of other lipoxygenase products, including cysteinyl-containing leukotrienes and non-enzymatic isomers of LTB_4, were considerably less active or virtually inactive. In addition, LTB_4 has been reported to stimulate cAMP formation in leukocytes (Claesson, 1982), and to cause aggregation, degranulation, superoxide generation, and mobilization of membrane-associated calcium in these cells (Serhan et al., 1983).

Apparently, LTB_4 is leukotactic also in vivo. Thus, intradermal injection of LTB_4 is associated with local accumulation of leukocytes in several species, including man (Bray et al., 1981; Lewis et al., 1981, 1982; Soter et al., 1983), and polymorphonuclear leukocytes and macrophages, in large numbers, may be harvestered after intraperitoneal injection of LTB_4 (Smith et al., 1980). When given systemically to rabbit or monkey, LTB_4 causes a reversible drop in circulating leukocytes (Bray et al., 1981; Smedegård et al., 1982). Intravital microscopy of the terminal vascular bed in hamster cheek pouch and rabbit teniussimus muscle (Dahlén et al.,1981; Björk et al., 1982b; Lindbom et al., 1982) has disclosed that LTB_4 causes dramatic changes in the behaviour of circulating leukocytes. Upon topical administration of LTB_4 to either of the two in vivo models, marginating leukocytes began to roll slower in spite of unchanged flow rate of the blood, and to in adhere, in increasing numbers, to the endothelial lining of postcapillary and larger venules. The adhesion of leukocytes, present after one minute, was followed after some time lag (usually 10 min) by massive diapedesis and further migration of the cells in the interstitium surrounding the vessels. Electronmicroscopic follow-up of the events in the tenuissimus muscle (Thureson-Klein et al., 1984a,b) showed adhesion of leukocytes in venules and small veins, but never in transverse or terminal arterioles. All types of leukocytes adhered, but with exposure to LTB_4 for 30 min, neutrophils and monocytes were the only ones to pass the vessel wall. Diapedesis always occurred through junctions between interdigitating endothelial cells, but junctional gaps were not formed. Degranulation of leukocytes was sparse and clearly seen only in a few basophils, but even in the vicinity of degranulated cells there was no evidence of local injury to the endothelial cells. Extravasation of macromolecules was localized to the sites of adhering leukocytes, and apparently occurred through the junctions in the wake of leukocyte diapedesis.

It seems justified to conclude that chemoattraction of leukocytes, particularly neutrophils, is the prime and specific microvascular effect of LTB_4, and that plasma exudation, generally requiring higher concentrations and occurring with some time lag, is a secondary phenomenon caused by massive recruitment of leukocytes. The cysteinyl-containing leukotrienes, on the other hand, apparently have little capacity to attract and/or activate leukocytes, although they may cause a reversible drop in the number of circulating leukocytes when injected intravenously. Rather, they cause extravasation on plasma, in surprisingly low concentrations, and, specifically from postcapillary venules. It is an intriguing corollary that LTB_4 and any of the cysteinyl-containing leukotrienes produce accumulation of leukocytes, and edema, cardinal signs of acute inflammation. Whether the leukotrienes actually are significant mediators of this important reaction must await further experimentation, however.

LEUKOTRIENES AS MEDIATORS OF ALLERGIC ASTHMA

Allergic astham is characterized by episodes of airway obstruction, and an exaggerated bronchoconstrictor response to a variety of stimuli. As a consequence of a specific interaction of allergen and IgE antibody on the surface of tissue mast cells, mediators are released from these cells, and possibly also from interstitial cells, to bring about obstruction in three concurrent ways; smooth muscle contraction, mucosal edema, and hypersecretion of mucus. In addition, the tissue may be invaded by phagocytes recruited from the circulation.

When the leukotrienes entered the scene a few years ago they brought with them the information that their alter ego, SRS-A, is released from lung tissue by immunological challenge, and that it is a potent bronchoconstrictor, also capable of inducing tissue edema (Brocklehurst, 1960). Indeed the cysteinyl-containing leukotrienes have proved to be bronchoconstrictors and inducers of tissue edema of hitherto unsurpassed potency. In addition, they do evoke hypersecretion into the airways (Johnsson et al., 1982; Marom et al., 1982; Peatfield et al., 1982), and, as already pointed out, the related LTB_4 is the most potent natural leukotactic factor identified to date. While much of our current information about the leukotrienes is from animal experiments, all the aforementioned effects have been documented in man, at least in vitro. In addition, the equisite bronchoconstrictor potency of LTC_4 in healthy subjects, is exaggerated in asthmatics (Barnes, personal communications),and inhalation of LTC_4 or LTD_4 is associated with a long-lived reduction in expiratory flow rate that is reminiscent of the effect of allergen challenge (Weiss et al., 1982; Griffin et al., 1983; Barnes et al., 1984).

A question of great concern is whether leukotrienes are released in sufficient amounts to account for the symptoms of asthma when the host is invaded by specific allergen. For methodological reasons, no chemical method is at present available to accurately quantitate overflow of leukotrienes to the blood after immunological challenge of the lung. However, it has been shown that immunological challenge causes the release of cysteinyl-containing leukotrienes from passively sensitized human lung fragments (Lewis et al., 1980), and mast cells from human lung apparently release LTC_4 and LTD_4 via an IgE-dependent mechanism (McGlashan et al., 1982). More direct evidence for leukotrienes as mediators of allergen-induced bronchoobstruction has recently been obtained in experiments with lung tissue from two asthmatic patients, both of which were sensitive to birch pollen (Dahlén et al., 1983a). Brief incubations of lung tissue with birch pollen provoked the release of LTC_4, LTD_4 and LTE_4. In fact, the amounts released were estimated to be large enough to give rise to maximal bronchial contraction, as indicated by the reactivity of bronchi isolated from the very same patients. When challenged with specific allergen, the bronchi contracted with the same time course as after administration of LTC_4, and independently of whether mepyramine and indomethacin were present or not. Further in proof of leukotrienes mediating the reaction, a selective inhibitor of the 5-lipoxygenase, U-60257 (Bach et al., 1982), severely depressed both the release of leukotrienes and the bronchial contraction induced with birch pollen.

It is of some interest that similar observations have been made with lung tissue from actively sensitized guinea pigs (Hedqvist et al., 1984). Thus, allergen challenge elicited dose-related contractions of parenchymal strips, which were uninfluenced by mepyramine, enhanced by indomethacin, and depressed by U-60257. Also when given as an aerosol to anesthetized guinea pigs the allergen elicited dose-dependent bronchoconstriction, which, interestingly, was further enhanced by indomethacin. As distinguished from the in vitro situation, mepyramine attenuated the response, and shifted the dose-response curve approximately one order of magnitude to the right. In the presence of both indomethacin and mepyramine, U-60257 offered substantial protection and left but a residual response to the highest antigen dose. By contrast, U-60257 alone had little effect on allergen-induced bronchoconstriction.

It is apparent that the mediator mechanisms involved in allergic bronchoconstriction are rather complex, and, moreover, the relative importance of any one putative mediator may vary between species, and, perhaps, even with the method employed for allergen challenge. In addition, as inferred from e.g. IgE-triggered cutaneous reactions (cf. Gleich, 1982), there is good reason to believe that acute responses and late phase reactions differ as regards contributing mediators. Nevertheless, as evident from the data presented in this chapter, the cysteinyl-containing leukotrienes must at present be considered as major mediator-candidates of the acute bronchial response to allergen in man. Furthermore, distinct leukotriene-dependent airway reactions may be identified both in vivo and in vitro in the guinea pig as well. The animal model may be of use to identify leukotriene antagonists or synthesis inhibitors with potential applicability in the human provocation studies that are necessary to test the "leukotriene-hypothesis". As mentioned above, further biochemical developments are required to obtain reliable methods for quantitation of leukotrienes under in vivo conditions in humans. In that context, it should be observed that measurements of LTB_4 by no means can be assumed to reflect release of its congener LTC_4. In fact, in human lung tissue (Dahlén et al., 1983a; Folco et al., this volume), allergen challenge appears to selectively trigger the release of the cysteinyl-containing leukotrienes, whereas the ionophore A 23187 induces formation of both LTB_4 and LTC_4.

It is well established that steroids with antiinflammatory activity alleviate the symptoms of bronchial asthma, and that NSAID:s do not. The members of either group affect the biosynthesis of arachidonic acid derivatives, but they differ inasmuch steroids inhibit the liberation of arachidonic acid, and, hence, may block the formation of both lipoxygenase and cyclooxygenase products, whereas NSAID:s have only the cyclooxygenase as a target. While this again stresses the potential impact of the leukotrienes, it remains to explain the functional role of the various cyclooxygenase products released in relatively large measure by allergen challenge. The failure of the leukotriene synthesis inhibitor, U-60257, to block aerosol-induced airway responses to allergen in the guinea pig, unless indomethacin is present, may indicate an interaction between leukotrienes and cyclooxygenase products. One current view is that blockade of the cyclooxygenase makes more arachidonic acid available for synthesis of lipoxygenase products. However, studies with radioactive tracer indicate that different pools of arachidonic acid are involved in the synthesis of leukotrienes and cyclooxygenase products in the lung (Dahlén et al., 1983a). Mechanisms other than shunting of substrate, might therefore be responsible for the as yet unexplained enhanced bronchoconstrictor response to allergen challenge in guinea pigs after treatment with indomethacin, and the aspirin asthma in man.

ACKNOWLEDGEMENTS

Supported by grants from the Swedish Medical Research Council, projects 14X-4342 and 03P-6949, from the National Association against Heart and Chest Diseases, from Karolinska Institutet, and from the National Institute of Environmental Medicine.

REFERENCES

Bach, M.K., Brashler, J.R., Smith, H.W., Fitzpatrick, F.A., Sun, F.F., and McGuire, J.C., 1982, 6,9-deepoxy-6,9-(phenylimino)-Δ6,8 -prostaglandin I$_1$, (U-60,257), a new inhibitor of leukotriene C and D synthesis: in vitro studies. Prostaglandins, 23:759-771.

Barnes, N.C., Piper, P.J., and Costello, J.F., 1984, Comparative effects of inhaled leukotriene C$_4$, leukotriene D$_4$, and histamine in normal human subjects. Thorax, 39:500-504.

Bernström, K., and Hammarström, S., 1982, A novel leukotriene formed by transpeptidation of leukotriene E. Biochem.Biophys. Res.Commun., 109:800-804.

Björk, J., Hedqvist, P., and Arfors, K.-E., 1982a, Increase in vascular permeability induced by leukotriene B$_4$ and the role of polymorphonuclear leukocytes. Inflammation, 6:189-200.

Björk, J., Arfors, K.-E., Hedqvist, P., Dahlén, S.-E., and Lindgren, J.Å., 1982b, Leukotriene B$_4$ causes leukocyte migration in vivo. Microcirculation, 2:271-281.

Björk, J., Dahlèn, S.-E., Hedqvist, P., and Arfors, K.-E., 1983, Leukotrienes B_4 and C_4 have distinct microcirculatory actions in vivo, in: "Advances in Prostaglandin, Thromboxane and Leukotriene Research", B. Samuelsson, R. Paoletti and P. Ramwell, eds, Vol. 12, Ch. 81, pp.1-6, Raven Press, New York.

Bray, M.A., Cunningham, F.M., Ford-Hutchinson, A.W., and Smith, M.J.H., 1981, Leukotriene B_4: a medator of vascular permeability. Br. J.Pharmacol., 72:483-486.

Brocklehurst, W.E., 1960, The release of histamine and formation of a slow-reacting substance (SRS-A) during anaphylactic shock. J Physiol (Lond) 151:416-435.

Claesson, H.-E., 1982, Leukotreiens A_4 and B_4 stimulate the formation of cyclic AMP in human leukocytes. FEBS Lett., 139: 305-308.

Dahlèn, S.-E., 1983, The significance of liberated cyclooxygenase products for the pulmonary and cardiovascular actions of leukotriene C_4 in the guinea pig depends upon the route of administration. Acta Physiol Scand, 118:415-421.

Dahlèn, S.-E., Hedqvist, P., Hammarström, S., and Samuelsson, B., 1980, Leukotrienes are potent constrictors of human bronchi. Nature, 288:484-486.

Dahlèn, S.-E., Björk, J., Hedqvist, P., Arfors, K.-E., Hammarström, S., Lindgren, J.A., and Samuelsson, B., 1981, Leukotrienes promote plasma leakage and leukocyte adhesion in postcapillary venules: In vivo effects with relevance to the acute inflammatory response. Proc.Natl.Acad.Sci.USA, 78:3887-3891.

Dahlèn, S.-E., Hansson, G., Hedqvist, P., Björck, T., Granström, E., and Dahlèn, B., 1983a, Allergen challenge of lung tissue from asthmatics elicits bronchial contraction that correlates with the release of leukotrienes C_4, D_4 and E_4. Proc.Natl.Acad. Sci.USA, 80:1712-1716.

Dahlèn, S.-E., Hedqvist, P., and Hammarström, S., 1983b, Contractile activities of several cysteine-containing leukotrienes in the guinea pig lung strip. Eur J Pharmacol, 86:207-215.

Dahlèn, S.-E., Hedqvist, P., Westlund, P., Granström, E., Hammarström, S., Lindgren, J.A., and Rådmark, O., 1983c, Mechanisms for leukotriene-induced contractions of guinea pig airways: Leukotriene C_4 has a potent direct action whereas leukotriene B_4 acts indirectly. Acta Physiol Scand, 118:393-403.

Dahlèn, S.-E., Serhan, C.N., and Samuelsson, B., 1984, Spasmogenic activity of lipoxin A in isolated guinea pig tissues. FEBS Lett, In press.

Drazen, J.M., and Austen, K.F., 1974, Effects of intravenous administration of slow-reacting substance of anaphylaxis, histamine, bradikinin, and prostaglandin $F_{2\alpha}$ on pulmonary mechanics in the guinea pig. J.Clin.Invest, 53:1679-1685.

Drazen, J.M., Austeen, K.F., Lewis, R.A., Clark, D.A., Goto, G., Marfat, A., and Corey, E.J., 1980, Comparative airway and vascular activities of leukotrienes C-1 and D in vivo and in vitro. Proc.Natl.Acad.Sci.USA, 77:4354-4358.

Folco,G.C., Omini, C., Viganò,T., Brunelli, G., Rossoni, G., and Berti, F., 1982, Biological activity of leukotriene C_4 in guinea pigs: in vitro and in vivo studies, in:"Leukotrienes and Other Lipoxygenase Products", B. Samuelsson and R.Paoletti, eds, pp.153-167, Raven Press, New York.

Ford-Hutchinson, A.W., Bray, M.A., Doig, M.V., Shipley,M.E., and Smith, M.J.H., 1980, Leukotriene B, a potent chemokinetic and aggregating substance released from polymorphonuclear leukocytes. Nature, 286:264-265.

Gleich, G.J., 1982, The late phase of the immunoglobin E-mediated reaction: a link between anaphylaxis and common allergic disease. Clin. Immun., 70:160-169.

Goetzl, E.J., 1981, Oxygenation products of arachidonic acid as mediators of hypersensitivity and inflammation. Med.Clin. North Am., 65:809-828.

Goetzl, E.J., and Pickett, W.C., 1980, The human PMN leukocyte chemotactic activity of complex hydroxy-eicosatetraenoic acids (HETEs). J. Immunol., 125:1789-1791.

Goetzl, E.J., Weller, P.F., and Valone, F.H., 1979, Biochemical and functional bases of the regulatory and protective roles of the human eosinophil, in:" Advances in Inflammation Research", G. Weissman, B. Samuelsson and R. Paoletti, eds, Vol. 14, pp. 157-167, Raven Press, New York.

Greén, K., Hedqvist, P., and Svanborg, N., 1974, Increased plasma levels of 15-keto-13,14-dihydro-prostaglandin $F_{2\alpha}$ after allergen-provoked asthma in man. Lancet, II:1419-1421.

Griffin, M., Weiss, J., Leitch,A.G., McFadden, E.R., Corey, E.J., Austen, K.F., and Drazen, J.M., 1983, Effects of leukotriene D on the airways in asthma. N.Engl.J.Med., 308:436-439.

Hamberg, M., Hedqvist, P., and Rådegren, K., 1980, Identification of 15-hydroxy-5,8,11,13-eicosatetraenoic acid (15-HETE) as the major metabolite of arachidonic acid in human lung. Acta Physiol Scand, 110:219-221.

Hamel, R., Masson, P., Ford-Hutchinson, A.W., Jones, T.R., Brunet, G., and Piechuta, H., 1982, Differing mechanisms for leukotriene D_4-induced bronchoconstriction in guinea pigs following intravenous and aerosol administration. Prostaglandins,24: 419-432.

Hansson, G., Lindgren, J.Å., Dahlèn,S.-E., Hedqvist, P., and Samuelsson, B., 1981, Identification and biological activity of novel ω-oxidized metabolites of leukotriene B_4 from human leukocytes. FEBS Lett., 130:107-112.

Hedqvist, P., Dahlèn,S.-E., Gustafsson, L., Hammarström, S., and Samuelsson, B., 1980, Biolgical profile of leukotrienes C_4 and D_4. Acta Physiol Scand, 110:331-333.

Hedqvist, P., Dahlèn, S.-E., and Palmertz, U., 1984, Leukotriene-dependent airway anaphylaxis in guinea pigs. Prostaglandins, in press.

Hua, X.-Y., Dahlèn,S.-E., Hammarström, S., and Hedqvist, P., 1984, Leukotrienes C_4, D_4 and E_4 cause extensive plasma extravasation in the guinea pig. Naunyn-Schmiedebergs Arch Pharmacol., in press.

Johnson, H.G., Chinn, R.A., McNee, M.L., Miller, M.D., and Nadel,J.A., 1982, Studies in the in vivo canine trachea: pharmacological blockage of leukotriene enhanced mucus secretion. Int. J. Immunopharm. 4:348 (A52).

Jones, T.R., Davis, C., and Daniel, E.E., 1982, Pharmacological study of the contractile activity of leukotriene C_4 and D_4 on isolated human airway smooth muscle. Can.J.Physiol.Pharmacol., 60:638-643.

Jubiz, W., Rådmark, O., Lindgren, J.A., Malmsten, C., and Samuelsson, B., 1981, Novel leukotrienes: products formed by initial oxygenation at C-15. Biochem.Biophys.Res.Commun., 99:976-986.

Kaijser, L., Dahlèn,S.-E., Hansson, G., Kumlin,M., Hedqvist, P., and Samuelsson, B., 1984, Cardiovascular effects of leukotriene C_4 in man. Prostaglandins, in press.

Kellaway, C.H., and Trethewie,E.R., 1940, The libration of a slow reacting smooth muscle-stimulating substance in anaphylaxis. Quart.J.Exp.Physiol., 30:121-145.

Kuehl, F.A., and Egan,R.,1980, Prostaglandins, arachidonic acid, and inflammation. Science, 210:978-984.

Letts, L.G., and Piper, P.J., 1982, The actions of leukotrienes C_4 and D_4 on guinea pig isolated hearts. Br.J.Pharmacol. 76:169-176.

Lewis, R.A., Austen, K.F., Drazen, J.M., Clark, D.A., Marfat, A., and Corey, E.J., 1980, Slow reacting substances of anaphylaxis: Identification of leukotrienes C-1 and D from human and rat sources. Proc.Natl.Acad.Sci.USA, 77:3710-3714.

Lewis, R.A., Austen, K.F., Drazen, J.M., Soter, N.A., Figueiredo, J.C., and Corey, E.J., 1982, Structure, function and metabolites of leukotriene constituents of SRS-A, in:"Leukotrienes and Other Lipoxygenase Products, Samuelsson,B. and Paoletti, R., eds, pp.137-151, Raven Press, New York.

Lindbom, L., Hedqvist, P., Dahlèn,S.-E., Lindgren, J.A., and Arfors, K.-E., 1982, Leukotriene B_4 induces extravasation and migration of polymorphonuclear leukocytes in vivo. Acta Physiol Scand, 116:105-108.

MacGlashan, D.W., Schleimer, R.P., Peters, S.P., Schulman, E.D., Adams, G.A., Newball, H.N. & Lichtenstein, L.M., 1982, Generation of leukotrienes by purified human lung mast cells. J.Clin.Invest., 70:747-751.

Maas, R.L., Brash, A.R., and Oates, J.A., 1981, A second pathway of leukotriene biosynthesis in porcine leukocytes. Proc. Natl.Acad.Sci.USA, 78:5523-5527.

Malmsten, C.L., Palmblad, J., Udén, A.-M., Rådmark, O., Engstedt,L., and Samuelsson, B., 1980, Leukotriene B_4: A highly potent and stereospecific factor stimulating migration of polymorphonuclar leukocytes. Acta Physiol Scand, 110:449-451.

Marom, Z., Shelhamer, J.H., Bach, M.K.,Morton,D.R., and Kaliner,M., 1982, Slow reacting substances, leukotrienes C_4 and D_4, increase the release of mucus from human airways in vitro. Am. Rev.Resp.Dis., 126:449-451.

Mathé, A.A., Hedqvist, P., Holmgren, A., and Svanborg, N., 1973, Bronchial hyperreactivity to prostaglandin F_2 and histamine in patients with asthma. Brit.Med.J., 1:193-196.

Morganroth,M.L., Reeves, J.T., Murphy, R.C., and Voelkel, N.F., 1984, Leukotriene synthesis and receptor blockers block hypoxic pulmonary vasoconstriction. J. Appl. Physiol., 56:1340-1346.

Palmer,R.M.J., Stephney,R.J., Higgs, G.A., and Eakins, K.-E., 1980, Chemokinetic activity of arachidonic acid lipoxygenase products on leukocytes of different species. Prostaglandins, 20:411-418.

Pasarglikian, M., Bianco, S., Allegra, L., Moavaro, N.E., Petrigrini, G., Robuschi, A., and Grugni, A., 1977, Aspects of bronchial reactivity to prostaglandins and aspirin in asthmatic patients. Respiration, 34:79-91.

Peatfield, A.C., Piper,P.J., and Richardson, P.S., 1982, The effect of leukotriene C_4 on mucin release into the cat trachea in vivo and in vitro. Br.J.Pharmacol., 77:391-393.

Peck, M.J., Piper, P.J., and Williams, T.J., 1981, The effect of leukotrienes C_4 and D_4 on the microvasculature of guinea pig skin. Prostaglandins, 21:315-321.

Piper, P.J., and Samhoun, M., 1982, Stimulation of arachidonic acid metabolism and generation of thromboxane A_2 by leukotrienes B_4, C_4, and D_4 in guinea-pig lung in vitro. Br. J. Pharmacol., 77:267-275.

Piper, P.J., and Tippins. J.R., 1982, Interaction of leukotrienes with cyclo-oxygenase products in guinea pig isolated trachea. in:"Advances in Prostaglandin, Thromboxane and Leukotriene Research", B. Samuelsson and R. Paoletti,eds, Vol. 9, pp.183-185, Raven Press, New York.

Samuelsson, B., 1983, Leukotrienes: mediators of immediate hypersensitivity reactions and inflammation. Science, 220:568-575.

Serhan, C.N., Hamberg, M., and Samuelsson, B., 1984a, Trihydroxytetraenes: a novel series of compounds formed from arachidonic acid in human leukocytes. Biochem.Biophys.Res.Commun., 118: 934-949.

Serhan,N.C., Hamberg, M., and Samuelsson, B., 1984b, Lipoxins: a novel series of biologically active compounds formed from arachidonic acid in human leukocytes. Proc.Natl.Acad.Sci.USA 81: in press.

Serhan, C.N., Radin,A., Smolen, J.E., Korchak, H., Samuelsson,B., and Weissmannn, G., 1983, Leukotriene B_4 is a complete secretagogue in human neutrophils. Biochem.Biophys.Res.Commun. 107:1006-1012.

Sirois, P., Borgeat, P., and Jeanson, A., 1981, Comparative effects of leukotriene B_4, prostaglandins I_2 and E_2,6-keto-PGF$_{1\alpha}$, tromboxane B_2 and histamine on selected smooth muscle preparations. J.Pharm.Pharmacol., 33:466-468.

Smedegård, G., Hedqvist,P., Dahlën,S.-E., Revenäs, B., Hammarström, S., and Samuelsson, B., 1982, Leukotrienes C_4 affects pulmonary and cardiovascular dynamics in monkey. Nature, 295: 327-329.

Smith, M.J.H., Ford-Hutchinson,A.W., and Bray, M.A., 1980, Leukotriene B: a potent mediator of inflammation. J.Pharm.Pharmacol., 32:517-518.

Soter, N.A., Lewis, R.A., Corey, E.J., and Austen, K.F., 1983, Local effects of synthetic leukotrienes (LTC$_4$, LTD$_4$, LTE$_4$, and LTB$_4$) in human skin. J.Invest.Dermatol., 80:115-119.

Terashita, Z.I., Fukui, H., Hirata, M., Terao,S., Ohkawa,S., Nishikawa, K., and Kikuchi,S., 1981, Coronary vasoconstriction and PGI$_2$ release by leukotrienes in isolated guinea pig hearts. Eur.J.Pharmacol., 73:357-361.

Thureson-Klein,Å., Hedqvist, P., and Lindbom, L., 1984a, Ultrastructure of polymorphonuclear leukocytes in postcapillary venules after exposure to leukotriene B_4 in vivo. Acta Physiol Scand 122:221-224.

Thureson-Klein,Å, Hedqvist, P., and Lindbom, L., 1984b, Ultrastructural effects of LTB$_4$ on leukocytes and blood vessels. Prostaglandins, in press.

Weichman, B.M., Muccitelli,R.M., Osborn,R.R., Holden, D.A., Gleason, J.G., and Wasserman, M.A., 1982, In vitro and in vivo mechanisms of leukotriene-mediated bronchoconstriction in the guinea pig. J.Pharm.Exp.Ther., 222:202-208.

Wedmore, C.V., and Williams, T.J., 1981, Control of vascular permeability by polymorphonuclear leukocytes in inflammation. Nature, 289:646-650.

Weiss, J.W., Drazen, J.M., Coles, N., McFadden, E.R., Weller, P.W., Corey, E.J., Lewis, R.A, and Austen, K.F., 1982, Bronchoconstrictor effects of leukotriene C in humans. Science, 216:196-198.

Weissmann, G., Smolen, J.E., and Korchak, H., 1980, Prostaglandins and inflammation: Receptor/cyclase coupling as an explanation of why PGEs and PGI$_2$ inhibit functions of inflammatory cells. in:"Advances in Prostaglandin and Thromboxane Research", Samuelsson,B., Ramwell, P.W. and Paoletti,R., eds, Vol. 8, pp.1637-1646, Raven Press, New York.

Yokochi,K.,Olley,P.M.,Sideris,E.,Hamilton,F.,Huhtanene,D,and Coceani,F., 1982, Leukotriene D$_4$: A potent vasoconstrictor of the pulmonary and systemic circulations in the newborn lamb, in: "Advances in Prostaglandin, Thromboxane and Leukotriene Research, Samuelsson,B.and Paoletti,R., eds, Vol. 9, pp.211-214, Raven Press, New York.

MODULATION OF THE RELEASE OF LEUKOTRIENES AND PROSTAGLANDINS AND OF THEIR FUNCTIONAL EFFECTS IN HUMAN AND GUINEA-PIG LUNG PARENCHYMA

G.C. Folco, L. Sautebin, G. Rossoni, T. Viganò
M.T. Crivellari, G. Galli, F. Berti and M. Messetti*

Institute of Pharmacology and Pharmacognosy, University of Milan, Via A. Del Sarto 21, 20129 Milano and *IV Clinic of Thoracic surgery, Policlinico di Milano Via F. Sforza, 20122 Milano, Italy

INTRODUCTION

The elucidation of the structure of SRS-A (slow reacting substance of anaphylaxis) has led to the discovery of Leukotrienes (LTs), a family of arachidonate metabolites produced by the enzyme 5-lipoxygenase [1] [2]. A stereospecific synthesis brings about formation of two classes of LTs, one major class composed of the sulfidopeptide leukotrienes, LTC_4, LTD_4 and LTE_4, and another class represented solely by LTB_4. A variety of stimuli, cleaving arachidonate from membrane phospholipids, provide the necessary substrate for the synthesis of prostaglandins (PGs), thromboxanes (TX) and LTs [3]. PGs and to a minor extent TX are formed ubiquitarily, whereas the synthesis of LTs seems to require a considerable cellular specificity [4] [5]: all of them are formed by normal and asthmatic human lung where they may play a role as potent bronchoconstrictors as well as primary mediators of airway hyperreactivity [6].

PGs, TX and LTs do not represent the final product of distinct and independent biosynthetic pathways but a tight network of interrelationships exists among these bioactive lipids. In fact in a number of preparations [7] [8] LTs stimulate further metabolism of arachidonic acid (AA) and mediate complex, indirect airway smooth muscle actions. Further involvement of eicosanoids in the etiology of asthma can be inferred from the observation that LTC_4 and LTD_4 increase the release of mucus from human airways in vitro [9]: however this effect seems to be independent on a specific structure (10) and it is therefore not possible at the present status of our knowledge to attribute to a specific sulfidopeptide leukotriene a selective biologic effect on mucous secreting cells.

In the present chapter we would like to present evidence on the fate of LTs and of some cyclo-oxygenase products in human and guinea-pig lung, and ways to control pharmacotherapeutically their biosynthesis and/or functional effects.

HUMAN STUDIES

Macroscopically normal human lung tissue obtained following resection for cancer or bronchiectasis was dissected free of pleura and visible blood vessels. Tissue fragments of approximately 100 mg each were washed extensively in Tyrode's buffer and incubated overnight at 25°C: the following day replicates of lung fragments were washed again and resuspended in Tyrode's solution (1g/10 ml, w/v) according to different experimental protocols. Passive sensitization was accomplished by incubation of the tissue overnight with an idiopathic hyper-IgE serum (1500 ng/ml of IgE) kindly provided by Prof. Staffan Ahlstedt, Pharmacia AB, Uppsala, Sweden, who also provided the necessary anti-human IgE antibody necessary for the immunological challenge.

At the end of the incubation the supernatant solutions from all the replicates of lungs were immediately assayed biologically for SRS-A-like activity using a longitudinal strip of guinea-pig ileum smooth muscle, superfused with Tyrode's solution (0.2 ml/min), containing a mixture of receptor antagonists and indomethacin (1.5×10^{-5} M) (11), according to the laminar flow technique described by Ferreira (12). Concomitantly the remaining incubation media were divided into aliquots for subsequent determination of PGs, TXB_2 and LTs.

Leukotrienes were identified and measured quantitatively hy high pressure liquid chromatography (HPLC) as described by Sautebin et al. (13). Briefly the leukotriene containing fraction was evaporated to dryness under nitrogen and the residue resuspended with the HPLC mobil phase (methanol/water, 70: 30; v/o, added with tetrabutylammonium phosphate (PIC-A), 0.005 M, and adjusted to pH 5.7 with acetic acid): flow rate was 1 ml/min, detector 280 nm. The retention times of the compounds were the following: PGB_2 11 min, LTC_4 15 min 4 sec, LTD_4 18 min 4 sec, LTB_4 20 min 3 sec and LTE_4 22 min 2 sec.

A calibration curve was prepared by adding a fixed amount (500 ng) of PGB_2 and increasing amounts of LTB_4, LTC_4, LTD_4 and LTE_4 to blank samples. Each sample was then processed and analyzed as reported for the biological specimens. For each leukotriene a linearity curve was obtained by plotting the ratio of peak intensities of leukotrienes and PGB_2 (y) against the concentration of the added leukotriene (x). The regression coefficient was 0.99 for all the leukotrienes. The amounts of leukotrienes in the biological samples were calculated from the peak ratios on the basis of the slope of the linearity curve. The detection limits ranged between 5 and 10 ng for each leukotriene tested, except LTE_4 which is detectable from 50-80 ng. The recovery for each leukotriene ranged between 50 and 70%.

Assay of cyclo-oxygenase products was carried on by radioimmunoassay (14) (15). The antisera vs. $6-K-PGF_{1\alpha}$ and PGD_2 were kindly supplied by Dr. Jacques Maclouf, Hospital Lariboisiere, Paris.

When human lung parenchymal fragments were stimulated by the Ca^{++}-Ionophore A23187 (10 μM), formation of LTD_4, LTE_4 and LTB_4 occurred following different patterns. Maximal net cumulative mediator release for LTD_4 was 1.33 ± 0.16 nmoles/g fresh tissue at 45', which then declined to 0.76 ± 0.07 two hours after A23187. Levels of LTE_4 continued to accumulate even of 120' where they averaged 4.95 ± 0.35 nmoles/g fresh tissue. The release kinetic of LTB_4 reached a plateau at 45', 0.89 ± 0.25 nmoles/g fresh tissue and was comparable to that of the cyclo-oxygenase products measured in these experiments, i.e. TXB_2, $6-K-PGF_{1\alpha}$ and PGE_2 (16). LTC_4 was mostly undetectable, to indicate the effectiveness of the interconversion LTC_4 LTD_4 brought about by the enzyme -glutamyl transpeptidase. This finding was confirmed in separate experiments where exogenous LTC_4 (1.2 nmoles/g fresh tissue) was incubated with unstimulated human lung parenchymal fragments.

The half life of LTC_4 was 8-10 min in these experimental conditions and complete conversion to LTD_4 and LTE_4 took place at longer incubation times (30 - 45 min). In these experiments no secondary formation of cyclo-oxygenase products followed the addition of LTC_4 to parenchymal fragments: in this respect human lung differs markedly from guinea-pig where LTC_4 causes modifications of airway tone and caliber which are partly or totally TXA_2-mediated (17) (18). Pretreatment of the tissue with Piriprost (U-60257, see M.K. Bach, this volume) potently inhibited LTs biosynthesis without an apparent shift of AA metabolism towards the cyclo-oxygenase products (Fig. 1).

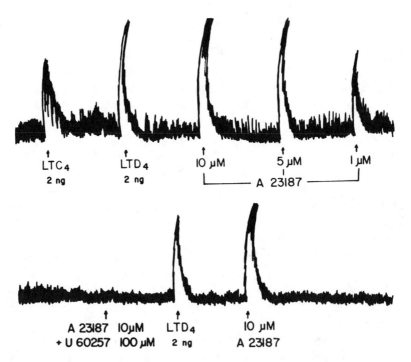

Fig. 1 - Bioassay of SRS-A activity on a longitudinal strip of guinea-pig ileum.

In a similar manner other compounds such as the flavonoid quercetin (19) were investigated for their potential activity as 5-lipoxygenase inhibitors in human lung parenchymal fragments.

This compound when preincubated for 15' at 100 μM is able to block completely, or at least reduce below the limit of our detection, formation of LTD_4, LTE_4 and LTB_4 evoked by A23187 2.5 μM (Tab. 1).

Table 1 – Effect of Quercetin (100 μM) on the formation of Leukotrienes and TXB_2 in human lung parenchymal fragments stimulated with the Ca^{++}-Ionophore A-23187 (2.5 – 10 μM).

Stimulus	LTB_4	LRD_4	LTE_4	TXB_2
A-23187 2.5 μM	0.36	0.53	0.68	0.40
A-23187 10 μM	0.54	0.76	1.42	–
Quercetin 100 μM + A-23187 2.5 μM	N.D.	N.D.	0.08	0.68

Net release, nmoles/g fresch tissue.

Suppression of 5-lipoxygenase activity was not accompanied by inhibition of cyclooxygenase activity: in fact net TXB_2 increase after A23187 challenge was 0.40 nmoles/g fresh tissue and 0.68 nmoles/g fresh tissue in presence of 100 μM Quercetin. These results speak in favour of a certain degree of specificity of Quercetin as a 5-lipoxygenase inhibitor: however there are profound differences among various flavonoids in their actions on the enzymes involved in arachidonate metabolism. Inhibition of 5-, 12- as well as 15-lipoxygenase has been reported for quercetin and other flavonoids (20) while their effects on cyclo-oxygenase were reported to be either stimulatory or inhibitory (21). The therapeutic applications of quercetin and more generally of flavonoids are certainly of great interest as potentially useful for the treatment of asthma: unfortunately carefully controlled clinical trials have not been reported so far, nevertheless they remain important prototypes of drugs which are both mediator release inhibitors (like disodiumchromoglycate) and inhibitors of leukotriene biosynthesis (19).

The inhibition of leukotriene synthesis is certainly a desirable feature for drugs which are aimed at alleviating the symptoms of asthma. However since this disease is likely to be the final result of a complex combination of different factors (airway hyperreactivity, increased production of mediators together with their positive feed-back interactions, genetic predisposition etc.) drugs which are able to interact with multiple targets might have a better therapeutic utility.

β_2-adrenoceptor stimulants are commonly employed for the treatment of reversible airway obstruction and relax human bronchial smooth muscle precontracted with LTC_4 (22). In addition this class of compounds prevents anaphylactic release of spasmogens such as histamine and SRS-A from human lung fragments (23). Certainly the autonomic nervous system provides, via the β_2-adrenergic stimulation an efficient way to control airway smooth muscle tone and caliber, since allergic subjects were shown to possess reduced β-adrenergic responsiveness: furthermore blockade of β_2-adrenergic receptors has been reported to cause bronchospasm in asthmatic as well as in normal subjects and potentiate very strongly LTC_4-induced bronchoconstriction in the guinea-pig (24). Previous studies carried on in this laboratory have shown that stimulation of β_1 and β_2 adrenoceptors in isolated guinea-pig lungs can reduce the release of TXA_2 triggered by histamine and SRS-A (25). It was therefore of interest to investigate the effects of fenoterol, a highly broncho selective β_2-agonist (26), on the release from human lung of sulfido- and non sulfidopeptide leukotrienes as well as of PGD_2, a potent bronchoactive eicosanoid (27), induced by antigen challenge and by the Ca^{++}-ionophore A23187.

Normal human lung parenchyma, obtained at thoracotomy for lung cancer, was cut into fragments of approximately 100 mg each, extensively washed using Tyrode's buffer and passive sensitization performed as described above. Replicates of the lung fragments (1g/10 ml, w:v) were suspended in Tyrode's solution at 37° for 5' with or without fenoterol 10^{-6}M and subsequently challenged with anti human IgE for 15'.

Leukotriene and PGD_2 release was also induced by the Ca^{++}-Ionophore A23187 (10 uM). Lung parenchymal fragments were preincubated for 15' at 25°C with or without fenoterol 10^{-6}M and subsequently stimulated with the Ionophore for 45'. Aliquots (100-200 µl) of the supernatant solution from all the replicates of lungs were immediately assayed for SRS-A like activity using a longitudinal strip of guinea-pig ileum.

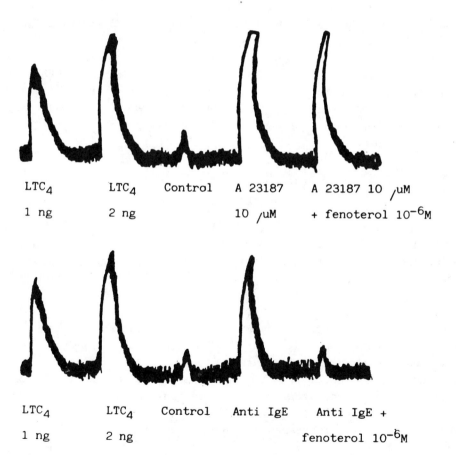

LTC$_4$	LTC$_4$	Control	A 23187	A 23187 10 µM
1 ng	2 ng		10 µM	+ fenoterol 10^{-6}M

LTC$_4$	LTC$_4$	Control	Anti IgE	Anti IgE +
1 ng	2 ng			fenoterol 10^{-6}M

Fig. 2 - Bioassay of SRS-A activity induced by antigen challenge and by the calcium ionophore A-23187: effect of fenoterol.

Aliquots for HPLC Leukotriene assay (6-8 ml) and for PGD_2 radioimmunoassay (200-400 μl) were processed as described (13) (15).

Antigen challenge of passively sensitized human lung parenchymal fragments is followed by a marked release of leukotrienes. LTD_4, LTE_4 and minute amounts of LTB_4 were detected in the incubation medium and their relative proportions varied according to the lenght of the incubations.. Spontaneous release (nmoles/g fresh tissue) was 0.025 ± 0.001 for LTD_4, 0.05 ± 0.001 for LTB_4 and 0.126 ± 0.02 for LTE_4 and net release following stimulus was 0.39 ± 0.08 for LTD_4, 0.48 ± 0.05 for LTE_4 and 0.06 ± 0.02 for LTB_4.

Prostaglandin D_2 (PGD_2) was the cyclo-oxygenase metabolite that was synthetized in higher amounts: its spontaneous release was 0.16 nmoles/g fresh tissue and increase to 1.28 nmoles/g fresh tissue following immunological stimulus and to 1.22 nmoles/g fresh tissue after A23187. Fenoterol (10^{-6} M) totally prevented the antigen-induced release of leukotrienes (Fig. 2) and PGD_2 but caused a modest inhibition of A23187 induced leukotriene formation and reduced PGD_2 output by 50%. The quantitation of leukotriene release by HPLC was confirmed by SRS-A bioassay using a superfused guinea-pig ileum.

GUINEA PIG STUDIES

Since the discovery of SRS-A the guinea pig has been a preferential experimental animal for studies involving immediate hypersensitivity reactions of the respiratory tract. This occurred mostly because of its exquisite sensitivity to a variety of agonists including histamine, bradykinin, SRS-A, PGD_2 etc. (28) (29). A secondary generation of TXA_2 can play an important role in the bronchoconstrictor action of different mediators provided that these are administered i.v. In fact as shown in fig 3, and more thoroughly investigated by Rossoni et al. (28), histamine-induced bronchoconstriction is only slightly dependent an TXA_2 formation, acetylcholine- is completely independent an a synthesis of TXA_2 or other cyclo-oxygenase products whereas bradykinin and LTC_4 are able to trigger an increased airway tone that is largely dependent on TXA_2 (28).

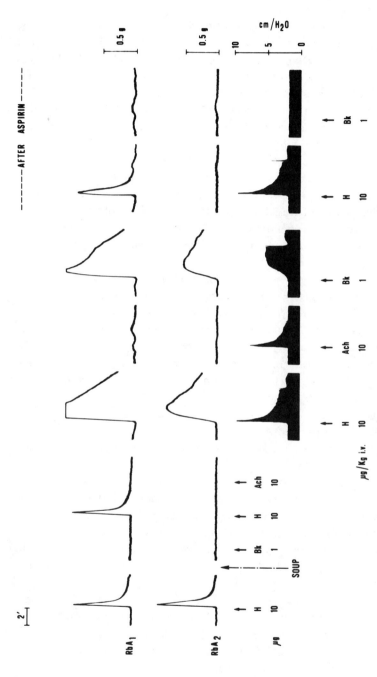

Fig. 3 – Bronchoconstriction caused by i.v. injection of different agonists in the anaesthetized guinea-pig, prepared according to Konzett and Rössler. Arterial blood in extracorporeal circulation superfuses to helical strips of rabbit aorta to monitor TXA_2-like activity. RbA_2 is treated with a mixture of receptor anatagonists (soup) to increase its specificity (11).

111

The guinea-pig is undoubtedly a rather unique model since different experimental conditions can provide a different picture as far as the relative incidence of "per se" bronchocostrictive effects compared to those in which primary mediators require a bioamplification via cyclo-oxygenase products. It seemed therefore of interest to investigate the therapeutic potential of β_2-adrenoceptor stimulants which are commonly utilized for the treatment of reversible airway obstruction, are powerful broncho-dilators and inhibit TXA_2 and SRS-A synthesis from the guinea-pig isolated lung parenchymal strip (25). One of the most promising of this family of compounds is procaterol: in 1976 Yoshizaki et al. (30) reported the synthesis of a new serie of sympathomimetic amines with a carbostyril nucleus: a member of this serie is procaterol, or 5-(1-hydroxy-2 isopropylaminobutyl)-8-hydroxy-carbostyril hydrochloride hemihydrate, a powerful and selective bronchodilator The selectivity of procaterol for $beta_2$-adrenocep-tors vs $beta_1$-adrenoceptors in animals has been described in detail by Yabuuchi et al. (31).

Guinea-pigs were anaesthetized with ethyl-urethane (1.2 g/kg, i.p.) and prepared for recording of arterial blood pressure and respiratory mechanics, according to Drazen et al. (32). Dynamic compliance (C_{Dyn}), lung resistance (R_L), transpulmonary pressure (TPP), tidal volume (V) and respiratory air flow (V) were registered using Hewlett-Packard instruments. The animals were also prepared for extracorporeal circulation according to the blood bathed organ technique of Rossoni et al. (28) in order to monitor TXA_2-like activity in the blood. Helical strips of rabbit aorta (RbA), superfused overnight with a mixture of receptor antagonist and indomethacin were used in cascade as bioassay tissues.

Following the procedure described by Davies and Johnston (33), passively sensitized guinea-pigs anaesthetized with sodium-pentobarbitone (70 mg/kg i.p.) were prepared in order to monitor bronchoconstriction and appearance of TXA_2-like activity during the anaphylactic reaction. Anaphylactic challenge was induced in control guinea-pigs and in groups of animals treated with different doses of procaterol (0.3-1-3 µg/kg i.v.) and salbutamol (5 µg/kg i.v.) 1 min before the antigen (Ovalbumin 5 mg/kg i.v.). Bronchospasm severity was evaluated according to Davies and Johnston (33) and the protecting activity of the ß-adrenergic compounds was expressed as percent of the bronchoconstriction observed in control guinea-pigs.

Blood was collected for radioimmunoassay of plasma TXB_2 before and after antigen injection in control and Procaterol-treated animals.

Intravenous administration of LTC_4 (0.8-1.6 nmoles/kg) causes a bronchoconstriction which involves primarily peripheral airways (Fig. 4).

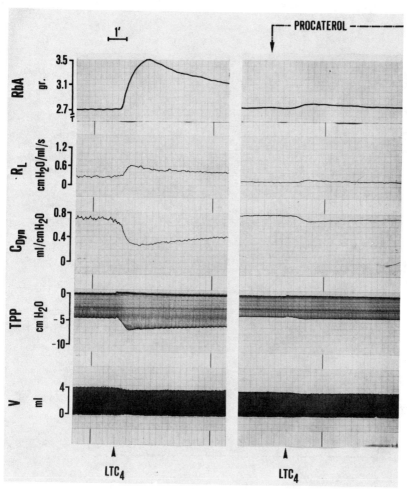

Fig. 4 - Effect of LTC_4 (1 ug/kg i.v.) on lung resistance (R_L), dynamic compliance (C_{Dyn}), transpulmonary pressure (TPP) and respiratory volume (V) in anaesthetized guinea-pig. Blood (extracorporeal circulation) superfuses a strip of rabbit aorta (RbA) in order to detect TXA_2-like activity. Procaterol (3 ug/kg i.v.).

TXA$_2$ is also released in the circulating blood, a phenomenon which is reduced by procaterol as well as the modifications of respiratory mechanics. In this respect it must be noted that the effectiveness of procaterol is higher against histamine that LTC$_4$ (Not shown).

Procaterol displays a dose-dependent protecting activity in passively sensitized guinea-pigs during anaphylactic shock (Fig. 5).

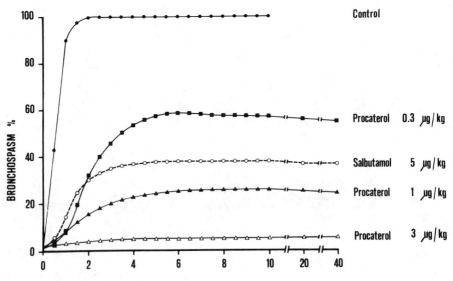

Fig. 5 - Procaterol and Salbutamol protect anaesthetized guinea-pigs against anaphylactic bronchoconstriction. Control animals died in 10 minutes. Time after injection of antigen is reported in minutes.

114

In fact the severe bronchoconstriction which is lethal in control animals, is efficiently controlled by procaterol at the dose of 0.3 µg/kg i.v., and completely antagonized at 3 µg/kg. Salbutamol, a well known β_2-adrenoceptor agonist, even at the dose of 5 µg/kg i.v., shows a significantly weaker protecting activity. In these experiments a substantial release of TXB_2 in the blood takes place during antigen-antibody interaction, and procaterol prevents this phenomenon and the associated bronchoconstriction (Fig. 6).

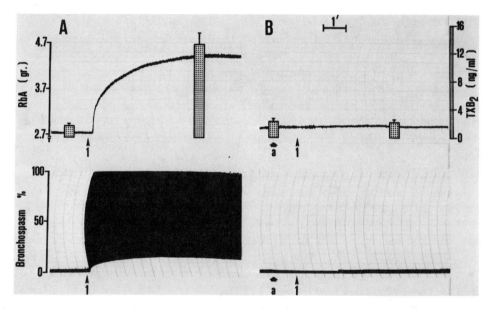

Fig. 6 - A, anaphylactic bronchoconstriction in anaesthetized guinea-pigs prepared according to Konzett and Rössler. TXA_2-like activity in the circulating blood is monitored by contraction of blood bathed rabbit aorta (RbA). At 1 injection of antigen (ovalbumin 5 mg/kg i.v.).
B, the guinea-pig prepared as in A, but pretreated 1 minute before ovalbumin with procaterol (3 µg/kg i.v. in a).

These "in vivo" observations demonstrate quite clearly that procaterol, and more generally β_2-adrenoceptor agonists, antagonize not only the direct effect of the mediators which are thought to be responsible for anaphylactic bronchoconstriction but also their capacity to stimulate formation of arachidonate metabolites.

These observations would imply that procaterol controls lung-parenchymal phospholipase-A_2 (PLA$_2$) and subsequent formation of prostaglandins and TXA$_2$. Procaterol behaves similarly to other β-adrenoceptor stimulants such as salbutamol, fenoterol, and clenbuterol (34) and the mechanism of action of these compounds is likely related to their ability to activate adenylate-cyclase and to increase formation of cyclic adenosine- 3'-5'-monophosphate (cyclic-AMP) in guinea-pig lungs (unpublished data). In this respect Lapetina et al. (35) have already demonstrated that cyclic-AMP inhibits arachidonic acid cleavage from membrane phospholipids in platelets.

The results obtained with passively sensitized guinea-pigs indicate that after ovalbumin challenge, the massive bronchoconstriction is accompanied by an increased concentration of circulating TXA$_2$. This ephemeral eicosanoid is one of the most powerful bronchoconstrictors and, together with other mediators of anaphylaxis such as histamine and leukotrienes, participates to the sudden and sustained changes of airway caliber. The observed protecting activity of procaterol could be attributed to its adenylate-cyclase stimulating property (36). This compound, in fact, besides its bronchodilating activity, may modulate the release of mediators from passively sensitized lungs following immunological reaction (37). In conclusion, with the same mechanism (intracellular increase of cyclic AMP) several sites of action may be proposed to explain the antiasthmatic activity of procaterol: on the bronchomotor tone through its regulation by β_2-adrenoceptor activation, on mast cells and basophils through an inhibition of their mediator's release and finally through an impairment of primary mediators of anaphylaxis to amplify their signals via release of bronchoconstrictive eicosanoids.

REFERENCES

1. R. C. Murphy, S. Hammarström and B. Samuelsson, Leucotriene C: a slow reacting substance from murine mastocytoma cells, Proc. Natl. Acad. Sci. U.S.A. 76: 4275 (1979).

2. P. Borgeat and B. Samuelsson, Transformation of arachidonic acid by polymorphonuclear leukocytes, J. Biol. Chem. 254: 7865 (1979).

3. P. Borgeat, B. Fruteau de Laclos and J. Maclouf, New concepts in the modulation of leukotriene synthesis, Biochem. Pharmacol. 32: 381 (1983).

4. R. A. Lewis and K.F. Austen, The biologically active leukotrienes: biosynthesis, metabolism, receptors, functions and pharmacology, J. Clin. Invest. 73: 889 (1984).

5. A. O. S. Fels, N.A. Pawlowski, E.B. Cramer, T.K.C. King, Z.A. Cohn and W.A. Scott, Human alveolar macrophages produce leukotriene B_4, Proc. Natl. Acad. Sci. U.S.A. 79: 7866 (1982).

6. J. W. Weiss, J.M. Drazen, N. Coles, E.R. McFadden, P.F. Weller, E.J. Corey, R.A. Lewis and K.F. Austen, Bronchoconstrictor effects of leukotriene C in humans, Science 216: 196 (1982).

7. G. C. Folco, G. Hansson and E. Granström, Leukotriene C_4 stimulates TXA_2 formation in isolated sensitized guinea-pig lungs, Biochem. Pharmacol. 30: 2491 (1981).

8. P. J. Piper and M.N. Samhoun, Stimulation of arachidonic acid metabolism and generation of thromboxane A_2 by leukotrienes B_4, C_4 and D_4 in guinea-pig lung in vitro, Br. J. Pharmacol. 77: 267 (1982).

9. Z. Marom, J.H. Shelhamer, M.K. Bach, D.R. Morton and M. Kaliner, Slow-reacting substances, leukotrienes C_4 and D_4, increase the release of mucus from human airways in vitro, Am. Rev. Respir. Dis. 126: 449 (1982).

10. S. J. Coles, K.H. Neill, L.M. Reid, K.F. Austen, Y. Nii, E.J. Corey and R.A. Lewis, Effects of LTC_4 and D_4 on glycoprotein and lysozime secretion by human bronchial mucosa, Prostaglandins 25: 155 (1983).

11. N. Gilmore, J.R. Vane, J.H. Willie, Prostaglandins released by the spleen, Nature 218: 1135 (1968).

12. S. H. Ferreira and F.S. Costa, A laminar flow technique with much increased sensitivity for the detection of smooth

muscle stimulating substances, <u>Europ. J. Pharmac.</u> 39: 379 (1976).

13. L. Sautebin, D. Caruso and G. Galli, Analysis of cyclo-oxyge-
    nase and lipoxygenase products in incubation media,
    <u>Prostaglandins</u> 27: 361 (1984).

14. E. Granström and H. Kindahl, Radioimmunoassay of prostaglan-
    dins and thromboxanes, <u>in</u>: "Advances in Prostaglandins and
    Thromboxane Research", J.C. Frolich, ed., Raven Press, N.Y.
    (1978).

15. J. Maclouf, E. Corvazier and Z. Wang, Development of a
    radioimmunoassay for PGD_2 using an antiserum against
    9-methoxime PGD_2. Submitted to <u>Analytical Biochemistry</u>
    (1984).

16. L. Sautebin, R. Viganò, E. Grassi, M.T. Crivellari, G. Galli,
    F. Berti, M. Mezzetti and G.C. Folco, Release of leukotrie-
    nes induced by the Ca^{++}-ionophore A23187, from human lung
    parenchyma in vitro, <u>J. Pharmacol. Exp. Therap.</u>, submitted
    (1984).

17. B. B. Vargaftig, J. Lefort and R.C. Murphy, Inhibition by
    aspirin of bronchoconstriction due to leukotrienes C_4
    and D_4 in the guinea-pig, <u>Europ. J. Pharmac.</u> 72: 417
    (1981).

18. F. Berti, G.C. Folco and C. Omini, An outline of the pharma-
    cological control of the formation and release of thrombo-
    xane A_2 and 12-HETE in the lung, <u>in</u> "Atherosclerosis
    Reviews: Prostaglandins and Cardiovascular Disease", R.J.
    Hegyeli, ed., Raven Press, N.Y. (1981).

19. W. C. Hope, A.F. Welton, C.F. Nagy, C.B. Bernardo, J.W.
    Coffey, In vitro inhibition of the biosynthesis of SRS-A
    and lipoxygenase activity by quercetin, <u>Biochem. Pharmacol.</u>
    32(2): 367 (1983).

20. R. J. Gryglewski, J. Robak and J. Swies, Flavonoids-lipoxyge-
    nase-Platelet aggregation. <u>This volume.</u>

21. K. Sekiya and H. Okuda, Selective inhibition of platelet
    lipoxygenase by baicalein, <u>Biophys. Biochim. Res. Commun.</u>
    105: 1090 (1982).

22. S. E. Dahlen, P. Hedqvist, S. Hammarström and B. Samuelsson,
    Leukotrienes are potent constrictors of human bronchi,
    <u>Nature</u> 288: 484 (1980).

23. J. M. Hughes, J.P. Seale, D.M. Temple, Effect of fenoterol on
    immunological release of leukotrienes and histamine from
    human lung in vitro: selective antagonism by ß-adrenoceptor
    antagonists, <u>Eur. J. Pharmacol.</u> 95: 239 (1983).

24. S. Bongrani, G.C. Folco, R. Razzetti and P. Schiantarelli, ß-adrenoceptor blockade is the basis of guinea-pig bronchial hyperresponsiveness to LTC_4 and other agonists, Br. J. Pharmacol. 79: 839 (1983).

25. G. C. Folco, C. Omini, T. Viganò, G. Brunelli, G. Rossoni and F. Berti, Biological activity of LTC_4 in guinea pigs: in vitro and in vivo studies, in: "Leukotrienes and other lipoxygenase productions", B. Samuelsson and R. Paoletti, eds., Raven Press, N.Y. (1982).

26. S. O'Donnell, A selective ß-adrenoceptor stimulant (Th 1165 a) related to orciprenaline, Europ. J. Pharmac. 12: 34 (1970).

27. M. Hamberg, P. Hedqvist, K. Strandberg, J. Svensson and B. Samuelsson, Prostaglandin endoperoxides. IV Effects on smooth muscle, Life Sci. 16: 451 (1975).

28. G. Rossoni, C. Omini, T. Viganò, V. Mandelli, G.C. Folco and F. Berti, Bronchoconstriction by histamine and bradykinin in guinea-pig: relationship to thromboxane A_2 generation and effect of aspirin, Prostaglandins 20: 547 (1980)

29. J. M. Drazen and K.F. Austen, Effect of intravenous administration of SRS-A, histamine, bradykinin and PGF_2 on pulmonary mechanichs in the guinea-pigs, J. Clin. Invest. 53: 1679 (1974).

30. S. Yoshizaki, K. Tanimura, S. Tamada, Y. Yabuuchi and K. Nakagawa, Sympathomimetic amines having a carbostyryl nucleus, J. Med. Chem. 19: 1138 (1976).

31. Y. Yabuuchi, S. Yamashita and S. Tei, Pharmacological studies of OPC-2009 a newly synthetized selective ß-adrenoceptor stimulant, J. Pharmacol. Exp. Therap. 202: 326 (1977).

32. J. M. Drazen, M.W. Schneider and C.S. Venugopalan, Bronchodilator activity of dimaprit in the guinea-pig in vitro and in vivo, Europ. J. Pharmacol. 55: 233 (1979).

33. G. E. Davies and T.P. Johnston, Quantitative study on anaphylaxis in guinea-pig passively sensitized with homologous antibody, Int. Arch. Allergy 41: 648 (1971).

34. R. T. Brittain, C.M. Dean and D. Jack, Sympathomimetic bronchodilator drugs, in: "Respiratory Pharmacology", J.G. Widdicombe, ed., Pergamon Press, Oxford (1981).

35. E. G. Lapetina, C.J. Schmitges, K. Chandrabose and P. Cuatrecasas, Regulation of phospholipase activity in platelets, in: "Advances in Prostaglandin and Thromboxane Res., Vol. 3", C. Galli, G. Galli and G. Porcellati, eds., Raven Press, N.Y. (1978).

36. Y. Saitoh, T. Hosokawa, T. Igawa and Y. Irie, Effect of a selective β_2-adrenoceptor agonist, procaterol, on tissue cyclic AMP level, <u>Biochem. Pharmacol.</u>, 28: 1319 (1979).

37. G. C. Folco, E. Passoni, T. Viganò, L. Daffonchio, G. Rossoni, G. Brunelli and F. Berti, New pharmacological aspects of the bronchodilating activity of procaterol, <u>Pharm. Res. Commun.</u> 15: 909 (1983).

COMPARATIVE EFFECTS OF LEUKOTRIENES IN RESPIRATORY TISSUE

OF VARIOUS SPECIES

Marwa N. Samhoun, Priscilla J. Piper and Neil C. Barnes*

Department of Pharmacology
Royal College of Surgeons of England
London WC2A 3PN, U.K.
*Chest Unit King's College Hospital Medical School
London SE5, U.K.

INTRODUCTION

It is now recognised that leukotrienes (LTs) C_4, D_4 and their probable metabolite E_4, which contain a sulphur linkage and amino acid side chain at C-6, collectively account for the biological activity of slow-reacting substance of anaphylaxis (SRS-A) obtained from various sources which, for many years, has been proposed as an important mediator of bronchoconstriction in man. These LTs display pronounced spasmogenic and vasoactive properties in various preparations and possess unprecedented potencies in respiratory smooth muscle in particular[1].

In this chapter we describe the actions of these LTs in isolated lung preparations of guinea pig, rat, rabbit and man, used in a superfusion cascade system, as well as their effects in human volunteers, following their administration by inhalation. In addition studies investigating the biological effects of the dihydroxyacid, LTB_4 and of LTF_4[2], the most recently described peptidolipid LT, in guinea-pig lung in vitro will also be included for comparative purposes.

RESULTS AND DISCUSSION

I. STUDIES IN ISOLATED LUNG PREPARATIONS

1) Guinea-pig tissues: LTC_4 and LTD_4 were equiactive and approximately 1,000 times more active than histamine in

contracting isolated strips of guinea-pig trachea (GPT) and guinea-pig lung parenchyma (GPP), in vitro preparations of large and small airways respectively[3,4].

a) Isolated perfused lungs:
When injected into isolated perfused lungs LTC_4 and LTD_4 (1-10 pmol) were equiactive and approximately 10 times more active than LTE_4 (10-100 pmol) in inducing the release of thromboxane A_2 (TXA_2) and prostaglandin (PG)-like materials, as shown by contractions of isolated strips of rabbit aorta and rat stomach respectively[4,5,6]. This action of LTs was antagonised by FPL 55712 (1.9 μM), the SRS-A/LT antagonist, and inhibited by indomethacin (2.8 μM) and imidazole (2.9 μM)[4,5,6], inhibitors of cyclo-oxygenase and Tx synthetase respectively. Thus, LTs displayed a similar pharmacological profile to that previously described for SRS-A[7]. Mepacrine (200 μM), a phospholipase inhibitor, inhibited generation of TXA_2 and PG-like materials induced by LTD_4 but not that due to exogenous arachidonic acid (AA)(15-80 nmol), strongly suggesting that LTD_4 exerts its action via stimulation of phospholipase with subsequent release of endogenous AA and generation of cyclo-oxygenase products[5].

b) Parenchymal strips:
Leukotrienes were very active contracting agents of GPP. There was a marked similarity, with respect to potency and profile of responses induced, between LTC_4 and LTD_4 on one hand and LTE_4 and LTF_4 on the other[5,6,8]. Thus, as in the perfused lung model, LTC_4 and LTD_4 (1-30 pmol) were equiactive and, in terms of threshold dose and height of response, about ten times more active than LTE_4 in inducing dose-related contractions of GPP. This similarity between LTC_4 and LTD_4 may be attributed to the presence of high levels of γ-glutamyltranspeptidase, in guinea-pig lung tissue, which are sufficient to convert tens of nmol/min of LTC_4 into LTD_4 and suggests that part of the biological acitivity of LTC_4 may be due to its conversion to LTD_4[9].

LTE_4 and LTF_4 (10-1000 pmol) were approximately equiactive and induced contractions which were easily differentiated from those due to LTC_4 and LTD_4 by being more protracted and lasting up to four times as long[6,8]. This long duration of action of LTE_4 and LTF_4 suggests that these LTs are less readily metabolised or bind more firmly to receptors than the other LTs in GPP. In the event of the direct involvement of LTs in respiratory disorders LTF_4, if present in man in vivo[2], and LTE_4, which may be present as a degradation product of LTC_4 and LTD_4, may prolong bronchoconstriction initiated by LTC_4 and LTD_4 by contributing to the long-lasting narrowing of the airways which occurs in asthma.

LTB_4 was equiactive with LTC_4 and LTD_4 in GPP and produced contractions which were very similar to those elicited by these peptidolipid LTs[5]. In contrast to cysteinyl-containing LTs, when administered successively, LTB_4 induced tachyphylaxis in GPP. Tachyphylaxis was not observed however when doses of LTB_4 were alternated with doses of other agonists[5].

FPL 55712 (1.9 μM) effectively antagonised contractions induced by LTC_4, LTD_4, LTE_4 and LTF_4 but not those due to LTB_4[4,5,6,8]. Resistance of the response induced by LTB_4 to FPL 55712 emphasizes requirement of the amino acid functional group in the LT molecule for antagonism by FPL 55712 and, together with occurrence of tachyphylaxis, strongly suggests the presence of a specific LTB_4 receptor population in GPP[5].

Although differences were observed between the various LTs in GPP, they all appear to share the same mechanism of action in this airway preparation. Indomethacin (2.8 μM) inhibited actions caused by all LTs[4,6,8] and imidazole (2.9 μM), carboxyheptylimidazole (24 μM) and mepacrine (200 μM) greatly reduced contractions of GPP induced by LTB_4, LTC_4, LTD_4[5] and LTE_4[6]. These findings indicate that, at the low doses used, LTs stimulate endogenous AA metabolism via cyclo-oxygenase in guinea-pig lung in vitro, leading to generation of TxA_2, which will in turn amplify the direct bronchoconstrictor effect of the LTs. This illustrates a type of "additive" interaction between products of cyclo-oxygenase and lipoxygenase pathways[10] and is in contrast to results obtained in GPT where actions of LTD_4 were markedly enhanced in the presence of indomethacin (2.8 μM)[11]. This could be attributed to redirection of AA metabolism via lipoxygenase, leading to formation of a bronchoconstrictor lipoxygenase product, or may be due to inhibition of synthesis of bronchodilator cyclo-oxygenase products (PGE_2, PGI_2), which may be acting as physiological antagonists to the contractile actions of LTs[11]. The above results are in agreement with previous work in the guinea pig describing synthesis of Txs mainly in the parenchyma whereas that of PGs occurs predominantly in the trachea[12], which would provide an explanation for the lower sensitivity of GPT to LTs, compared with GPP.

c) The combined use of superfused strips of guinea-pig lung parenchyma and ileum as a sensitive and selective bioassay for LTB_4:

Of all the LTs, only LTB_4 has little spasmogenic activity. It is a potent chemotactic, chemokinetic and aggregating agent for polymorphonuclear leucocytes (PMNs) and is usually assayed in terms of one or more of these properties[13,14]. As described above LTB_4 contracts the GPP but, in contrast to LTC_4, LTD_4, LTE_4 and LTF_4, is inactive on isolated strips of guinea-pig ileum smooth muscle (GPISM) even when administered at high doses (up to 1nmol), suggesting that the cysteinyl-substituent at C-6 in the LT molecule is a prerequisite for contracting this tissue[5]. This has given rise to the use of the combination of GPP and GPISM, suspended in series in a cascade superfusion system, as a simple and selective bioassay for LTB_4-like materials generated in biological fluids[15]. Comparative studies with other substances showed that LTB_4 was more active than bradykinin and angiotensin II by a 100 fold and by at least 3-4 orders of magnitude than PGD_2, $PGF_{2\alpha}$ and PGI_2 in contracting the GPP. PGE_1 and PGE_2 were about 1,000 - 10,000 times less active than LTB_4 but, in contrast to all other agonists used, relaxed the GPP. More significantly however, with the exception of 6-oxo-$PGF_{1\alpha}$ and 5-hydroxyeicosatetraenoic acid which lacked activity on both GPP and GPISM, only LTB_4 was inactive on GPISM whereas the cysteinyl-containing LTs and other substances investigated induced stable contractions of GPISM at doses which caused myotropic effects on GPP[15].

These results demonstrate that this assay is particularly selective for LTB_4. Thus any material which contracts GPP but not GPISM, causing tachyphylaxis in the former when given in succession, and induces contractions of the lung strip which are resistant to FPL 55712 but reduced by inhibitors of cyclo-oxygenase and Tx synthetase, is highly likely to be LTB_4. This method has been successfully used to initially detect[16] and later confirm and assay LTB_4[17], generated by rat basophilic leukaemia cells and, more recently, by porcine blood vessels[18].

2)   Rat tissues: LTC_4 and LTD_4 displayed very little activity on strips of rat lung parenchyma and caused only small contractions at doses ranging between 0.5 - 50 nmol[4].

3)   Rabbit tissues: LTC_4 and LTD_4 (50 pmol - 25 nmol) were equiactive on strips of rabbit parenchyma (RbP) and contractions produced were not reduced in the presence of indomethacin (2.8 μM)[4]. In contrast to results obtained in GPP, FPL 55712 (1.9 μM) did not antagonise the effect of LTs in RbP[4].

4)   Human tissues: LTC_4 and LTD_4 were about 3 orders of magnitude more active in contracting human tissues than histamine.

a)   Parenchymal strips:
      LTC_4 and LTD_4 (50 - 200 nmol) exhibited comparable activity on strips of human lung parenchyma (HP) and induced contractions which were resistant to indomethacin (2.8 μM). FPL 55712 antagonised responses induced by these LTs when superfused over the HPs at 19 μM but not at the lower concentrations of 1.9 μM and 10 μM.

      LTE_4 was 2 - 3 orders of magnitude less active than either LTC_4 or LTD_4[19].

b)   Bronchial strips:
      LTC_4 and LTD_4 (3 - 300 pmol) were equiactive and considerably more active in inducing dose-related contractions of strips of human bronchus (HB) than of HP. LTE_4 was at least one hundred times less active than LTC_4 or LTD_4, in terms of threshold dose and height of response, but induced contractions which were much more sustained as in GPP[19]. Indomethacin (2.8 μM) did not inhibit contractions caused by LTs which were antagonised by FPL 55712 (0.19 - 1.9 μM)[19].

Lack of inhibition of LT-induced contractions of the RbP, HP and HB by indomethacin indicates that LTs exert direct actions which are independent of a cyclo-oxygenase mechanism.

II. STUDIES IN NORMAL HUMAN SUBJECTS

The initial study of inhaled LTC_4 and LTD_4 in man[20] showed these LTs to be potent bronchoconstrictors and because of their marked effect on the flow at 1.5 litres above residual volume (approximately equivalent to the flow at 30% of vital capacity above residual volume - $\dot{V}max_{30}$), and smaller effect on the forced expiratory volume in one second (FEV_1), it was suggested that inhaled LTs had a preferential action on peripheral airways in man. Two further studies of inhaled LTC_4[21] and LTD_4[22] showed that LTC_4 and LTD_4 are respectively 3,900 and 5,900 times more potent than inhaled histamine in causing a fall in the $\dot{V}max_{30}$; this led to the suggestion that LTs have a preferential action on peripheral airways. Owing to the actions of LTs on human bronchial and parenchymal strips in vitro (see above), we have studied the actions of LTC_4 and LTD_4, following administration by inhalation, in six normal, non-asthmatic subjects[23]. We have measured the $\dot{V}max_{30}$ and the specific airways conductance (sGaw), a measurement of comparable sensitivity to $\dot{V}max_{30}$ but mainly dependent on large airway function.

1) _Actions of LTC_4 and LTD_4_: LTC_4 and LTD_4 were approximately 1000 times as potent as histamine and caused a longer-lasting bronchoconstriction than histamine. There were equal percentage falls in the sGaw and $\dot{V}max_{30}$ after inhalation of histamine, LTC_4 and LTD_4, indicating that inhaled LTC_4 and LTD_4 affect both large and small airways, with no evidence for a selective action on small airways, which is also in agreement with another study[24].

Approximately half of the biological activity of LTC_4 and LTD_4, as assayed on guinea-pig ileum smooth muscle (GPISM), was lost during nebulisation; thus the activity of the inhaled LTs is probably underestimated by at least 50%. Following inhalation of LTC_4 and LTD_4 there was neither cough nor throat irritation but wheezing was observed in subjects who bronchoconstricted sufficiently.

2) _Action of LTE_4_: In another study LTE_4, administered by inhalation to five normal subjects, was 88 times as potent as histamine but 13 times less potent than LTD_4[25]. Further, the bronchoconstriction induced by LTE_4 lasted about twice as long as that due to LTD_4. In contrast to results obtained using LTC_4 and LTD_4, LTE_4, as assayed on GPISM, was stable during nebulisation.

CONCLUSION

The studies described in this chapter show that LTC_4, LTD_4 and LTE_4 are potent bronchoconstrictor agents in guinea-pig and human isolated pulmonary tissues. Although the mechanism of action of LTs differs in these species, there were marked similarities in effects of LTs, with respect to potency and responses elicited , in GPP and HB. In the event of limitations of experimental work in human lung, these results strongly suggest that guinea-pig lung treated with indomethacin, may represent a suitable _in vitro_ model for further studies on LTs.

It is of interest that the results obtained in humans _in vivo_ are in close agreement with those obtained on human tissues _in vitro_, suggesting a possible role for these LTs in the long-lasting bronchoconstriction which occurs in asthma.

ACKNOWLEDGEMENTS

We wish to thank the Frances and Augustus Newman Foundation, the Asthma Research Council and King's College joint research committee for financial support, as well as Dr J. Rokach, Merck Frosst Laboratories, Canada, for leukotrienes.

REFERENCES

1. Piper, P.J. (1983) Pharmacology of leukotrienes. Br.med.Bull. 39: 255-259.

2. Anderson, M.E., R.D. Allison and Meister, A. (1982) Interconversion of leukotrienes catalyzed by purified γ-glutamyltranspeptidase: concomitant formation of leukotriene D_4 and γ-glutamyl amino acids. Proc.Natl.Acad.Sci.USA 79: 1088-1091.

3. Piper, P.J., Samhoun, M.N., Tippins, J.R., Williams, T.J., Palmer, M.A. and Peck, M.J. (1981) Pharmacological studies on pure SRS-A and synthetic leukotrienes C_4 and D_4. In: SRS-A and Leukotrienes, ed. Piper, P.J., Research Studies Press, John Wiley, Chichester, New York, Brisbane, Toronto, pp.81-89.

4. Piper, P.J. and Samhoun, M.N. (1981) The mechanism of action of leukotrienes C_4 and D_4 in guinea pig isolated perfused lung and parenchymal strips of guinea pig, rabbit and rat. Prostaglandins 21: 793-803.

5. Piper, P.J. and Samhoun, M.N. (1982) Stimulation of arachidonic acid metabolism and generation of thromboxane A_2 by leukotrienes B_4, C_4 and D_4 in guinea-pig lung _in vitro_. Br.J.Pharmac. 77: 267-275.

6. Piper, P.J. and Samhoun, M.N. (1983) Comparison of the actions of leukotriene E_4 with those of leukotrienes B_4, C_4 and D_4 on guinea-pig lung and ileal smooth muscle _in vitro_. In: Advances in Prostaglandin, Thromboxane and Leukotriene Research, ed. Samuelsson, B., Paoletti, R. and Ramwell, P., Raven Press, New York, vol. 12, pp. 127-131.

7. Engineer, D.M., Morris, H.R., Piper, P.J. and Sirois, P. (1978) The release of prostaglandins and thromboxanes from guinea-pig lung by slow reacting substance of anaphylaxis, and its inhibition. Br.J.Pharmac. 64: 211-218.

8. Samhoun, M.N. and Piper, P.J. (1984) Leukotriene (LT) F_4: comparison of its pharmacological profile with that of other cysteinyl-containing LTs. In: Proceedings of IUPHAR 9th International Congress of Pharmacology (in press).

9. Morris, H.R., Taylor, G.W., Jones, C.M., Piper, P.J., Samhoun, M.N. and Tippins, J.R. (1982) Slow reacting substances (leukotrienes): enzymes involved in their biosynthesis. Proc.Natl.Acad.Sci.USA 79: 4838-4842.

10. Samhoun, M.N. and Piper, P.J. (1984) Actions and interaction of lipoxygenase and cyclo-oxygenase products in respiratory and vascular tissues. Prostaglandins, Leukotrienes Med. 13: 79-87.

11. Piper, P.J. and Tippins, J.R. (1982) Interaction of leukotriene with cyclo-oxygenase products in guinea-pig isolated trachea. In: Leukotrienes and Other Lipoxygenase Products, ed. Samuelsson, B. and Paoletti, R., Raven Press, New York, pp. 183-185.

12. Gryglewski, R.J., Dembinska-Kiec, Grodzinska, L. and Panczenko, B. (1976) Differential generation of substances with prostaglandin-like and thromboxane-like activities by guinea pig trachea and lung strips. In: Lung Cells and Diseases, ed. Bouhuys, A., Elsevier/North Holland Biomedical Press, Amsterdam, New York, Oxford, pp. 289-307.

13. Goetzl, E.J. and Pickett, W.C. (1980) The human PMN leukocyte chemotactic activity of complex hydroxy-eicosatetraenoic acids (HETEs). J.Immunol. 125 1789-1791.

14. Ford-Hutchinson, A.W., Bray, M.A. Doig, M.V., Shipley, M.E. and Smith, M.J.H. (1980) Leukotriene B_4: a potent chemokinetic and aggregating substance released from polymorphonuclear leucocytes. Nature 286: 264-265.

15. Samhoun, M.N. and Piper, P.J. (1984) The combined use of isolated strips of guinea-pig lung parenchyma and ileum as a sensitive and selective bioassay for leukotriene B_4. Prostaglandins 27: 711-724.

16. Morris, H.R., Piper, P.J., Samhoun, M.N. and Taylor, G.W. (1981) Generation of a leukotriene (LT)B$_4$-like material from rat basophilic leukaemia (RBL-1) cells, and its actions in guinea-pig lung in vitro. Br.J.Pharmac. 74: 922-923P.

17. Ford-Hutchinson, A.W., Piper, P.J. and Samhoun, M.N. (1982) Generation of leukotriene B$_4$, its all trans isomers and 5-hydroxyeicosatetraenoic acid by rat basophilic leukaemia cells. Br.J.Pharmac. 76: 215-220.

18. Piper, P.J., Stanton, A.W.B., McLeod, L.J., Galton, S.A. and Letts, L.G. (1984) Actions of leukotrienes in the circulation. In: Proceedings of IUPHAR 9th International Congress of Pharmacology (in press).

19. Samhoun, M.N. and Piper, P.J. (1983) Comparative actions of leukotrienes in lung from various species. In: Leukotrienes and Other Lipoxygenase Products, ed. Piper, P.J., Research Studies Press, John Wiley, pp. 161-177.

20. Holroyde, M.C., Altounyan, R.E.C., Cole, M., Dixon, M. and Elliott, E.V. (1981) Bronchoconstriction produced in man by leukotrienes C and D. Lancet 2: 17-18.

21. Weiss, J.W., Drazen, J.M., McFadden, E.R. Weller, P., Corey, E.J., Lewis, R.A. and Austen, K.F. (1983) Airway constriction in normal humans produced by inhalation of leukotriene D. JAMA 249: 2814-2817.

22. Weiss, J.W., Drazen, J.M., Coles, N., McFadden, E.R., Weller, P., Corey, E.J., Lewis, R.A. and Austen, K.F. (1982) Bronchoconstrictor effects of leukotriene C in humans. Science 216: 196-198.

23. Barnes, N.C., Piper, P.J. and Costello, J.F. (1984) Comparative effects of inhaled leukotriene C$_4$, leukotriene D$_4$ and histamine in normal human subjects. Thorax 39: 500-504.

24. Smith, L.J., Patterson, R., Greenberger, P., Krell, R. and Bernstein, P. (1984) Airway response to inhaled leukotriene D$_4$ in man. Am.Rev.Respir.Dis. 129: 4 Part 2: A1 (abstract).

25. Barnes, N.C., Piper, P.J. and Costello, J.F. (1984) Bronchoconstrictor effect of leukotriene E$_4$ in normal humans. In: Leukotrienes and prostaglandins, Washington Symposium, Abstract Book, ed. Bailey, J.M.

THE EFFECTS OF LOW-DOSE ASPIRIN AND SELECTIVE INHIBITORS OF THROMBOXANE-SYNTHASE ON EICOSANOID PRODUCTION IN MAN

Carlo Patrono, Paola Filabozzi and Paola Patrignani

Department of Pharmacology and Centro di Studio per la
Fisiopatologia dello Shock C.N.R., Catholic University
School of Medicine, Rome, Italy

INTRODUCTION

The appreciation that two cyclooxygenase products, i.e.
prostacyclin (PGI$_2$) and thromboxane (TX) A$_2$ have potent and con-
trasting effects on platelet function and vascular tone (see ref.
1 for a review) has prompted attempts to develop selective pharmacologic tools affecting their production with the aim of understanding their pathophysiologic role and possibly treating human
disease states. Two different approaches have been followed: 1)
differential inhibition of platelet vs vascular cyclooxygenase by
low-dose aspirin [2,3,4] and 2) selective inhibition of TX-synthase
by a variety of imidazole derivatives, such as dazoxiben[5,6], UK-
38,485[7], CGS 13080[8] and OKY-046[9]. The former has a clear advanta-
ge in achieving a profound and long-lasting suppression of platelet
TXA$_2$ production with a high safety margin and low cost. The latter
approach has theoretically two distinct advantages over low-dose
aspirin, i.e. it can result in enhanced PGI$_2$ production by virtue
of platelet-derived prostaglandin (PG) endoperoxides, and it can
be expected to inhibit TXA$_2$ production in all TXA$_2$-producing cells.

The purpose of this paper is to review the available information on biochemical selectivity and platelet inhibitory effects of
both therapeutic strategies in human health and disease.

ANALYSIS OF TXA$_2$ AND PGI$_2$ BIOSYNTHESIS IN MAN

The methodologic and conceptual problems inherent to the
assessment of vascular and platelet eicosanoid production in man
have been reviewed by FitzGerald et al.[10]. Currently used ex vivo
and in vivo indices of TXA$_2$ and PGI$_2$ production are detailed in

Tables 1 and 2. Both eicosanoids are not measurable as such in human biological fluids because of chemical instability. Detection of their biological activity in plasma in unrealistic because of very low levels and limited sensitivity of bioassay techniques. Thus, all the relevant measurements are largely confined to chemically stable hydration products or enzymatically formed metabolites. Both TXB_2 and 6-keto-$PGF_{1\alpha}$ can be detected in peripheral venous plasma by either radioimmunoassay (RIA) or gas chromatography/mass spectrometry (GC/MS). However, their very low levels (in the low picogram range), short half-life and ease of artefactual formation by blood cells during and after sampling make such measurements highly questionable. One method of circumventing problems of sampling-induced artifact and ex vivo eicosanoid formation is by measurement of plasma metabolites that have an extended half-life. Although the 13,14-dihydro-6,15-diketo-$PGF_{1\alpha}$ metabolite of PGI_2 has a longer half-life than 6-keto-$PGF_{1\alpha}$ and has been identified by RIA in human plasma after PGI_2 infusion[11], experience with other PGs has shown that the metabolites initially formed from the hydration products are rapidly replaced by more polar products as the major derivatives in plasma. Quantitative assays for stable oxidative metabolites of TXA_2 and PGI_2 in plasma are currently being developed.

The urinary excretion of TXB_2 and 6-keto-$PGF_{1\alpha}$ is largely a reflection of renal TXA_2 and PGI_2 production, respectively, both in health[12,13] and disease [14,15]. The dinor metabolites of TXB_2 and 6-keto-$PGF_{1\alpha}$ are the most abundant products of systemically administered TXB_2 and PGI_2, respectively, in man[10]. Although these measurements represent the only noninvasive method of quantifying systemic (largely extrarenal) generation of TXA_2 and PGI_2, they are not specific to the tissue of origin of these compounds. Thus, the relative contribution of platelet and extra-platelet sources to urinary 2,3-dinor-TXB_2 remains to be determined in pathophysiologic conditions. The finding that daily dosing with 20 mg aspirin can reduce urinary 2,3-dinor-TXB_2 excretion by 67% in healhty subjects[3] suggests that it may represent primarily platelet TXB_2 production under physiologic conditions.

More specific indices have been studied ex vivo, such as TXB_2 production in whole blood[16] or in stimulated platelet-rich plasma [3], or 6-keto-$PGF_{1\alpha}$ formation by biopsies of vascular tissue[5,17] or in whole blood[6]. These methods clearly assess the capacity of platelets, vascular tissue or white blood cells to synthesize TXB_2 or 6-keto-$PGF_{1\alpha}$ in response to native or exogenously added stimuli and by no means reflect the actual production rate of these substances in vivo[10]. Such tissue-specific indices can be used appropriately in pharmacologic studies where drug-induced changes of cyclooxygenase or TX-synthase are being investigated. In our studies, we have used serum TXB_2 determinations as a reflection of thrombin-induced platelet TXA_2 production during whole blood clotting[2,16]. Serum levels of this eicosanoid averaged 300±108 ng/ml (Mean±SD) in a

Table 1. Ex vivo and in vivo indices of TXA_2 biosynthesis

Eicosanoid measured	Biological fluid	Analytical technique
TXB_2	plasma urine incubates of tissue fragments serum	RIA, GC/MS
2,3-dinor-TXB_2	urine	GC/MS, RIA

Table 2. Ex vivo and in vivo indices of PGI_2 biosynthesis

Eicosanoid measured	Biological fluid	Analytical technique
6-keto-$PGF_{1\alpha}$	plasma urine gastric juice incubates of tissue fragments serum	RIA, GC/MS GC/MS
13,14-DH-6,15-DK-$PGF_{1\alpha}$	plasma	RIA
2,3-dinor-6-keto-$PGF_{1\alpha}$	urine	GC/MS

group of 177 healthy subjects, with no statistically significant difference between men and women[18]. Consistent results have been reported from different laboratories, measuring serum TXB_2 by RIA[4,5,7] or GC/MS[19].

SELECTIVE INHIBITION OF PLATELET CYCLOOXYGENASE

Aspirin selectively acetylates the hydroxyl group of a single serine residue within the polypeptide chain of cyclooxygenase (PGH_2-synthase), thereby inactivating the enzyme[20,21]. As a consequence of this acetylation, the cyclooxygenase activity (Arachidonate $\rightarrow$ PGG_2) of the enzyme is lost, while the peroxidase activity (PGG_2 $\rightarrow$ PGH_2) results unaffected. The stoichiometry of this reaction is 1:1, one acetyl group transferred per enzyme monomer[20,21]. At low concentrations, aspirin acetylates PGH_2-synthase rapidly (within minutes) and selectively. At high concentrations, over longer time periods, aspirin will also acetylate nonspecifically a variety of proteins and nucleic acids. When given orally to healthy subjects, aspirin acetylates circulating platelet cyclooxygenase[22] and inhibits TXB_2 production[2] in a dose- and time-dependent fashion. A linear inhibition of platelet cyclooxygenase activity was found in the range of 0.1 to 2 mg/kg, after a single dosing[2]. Moreover, such a dose-response relationship is substantially identical in healthy subjects[2] and in atherosclerotic patients[4], when assessed with the same technique i.e. ex vivo TXB_2 production in whole blood. No sex-related difference in aspirin effect was noted in these studies.

Because of irreversible enzyme inactivation and lack of de novo enzyme synthesis in platelets, acetylation of platelet cyclooxygenase and consequent inhibition of TXA_2 production by low-dose (20-40 mg) aspirin is cumulative on repeated dosing[2,22]. We have recently characterized the variables affecting the rate and maximal degree of cumulative inhibition of platelet cyclooxygenase activity in healthy subjects undergoing chronic dosing with oral aspirin in the range of 5 to 40 mg per day[23]. Our findings suggest that the fractional dose of aspirin necessary for achieving a given level of acetylation by virtue of cumulative effects approximately equals the fractional daily platelet turnover[23]. In view of these findings and of recent studies of Pedersen and FitzGerald[24] demonstrating unchanged systemic bioavailability of aspirin in the range 20-1300 mg and presystemic acetylation of platelet cyclooxygenase by low-doses of the drug, it appears likely that platelet life-span represents a major variable affecting cumulative inhibition, within this particular dose range. For a given dose, both the rate at which cumulative acetylation occurs and its maximal extent would essentially depend upon the rate of platelet turnover.

Although the long-lasting suppression of TXA_2-related platelet function by aspirin has been disputed on the basis of studies employing pairs of aggregating agents[25], the likely occurrence of this phenomenon in vivo is suggested by the positive results (i.e. > 50% reduction in thrombotic events) of 3 clinical trials using single daily dosing of the drug: 160 mg in patients on hemodialysis[26], 324 mg in men with unstable angina[27] and 100 mg in patients with aortocoronary bypass[28]. These results are consistent with the hypothesis that the antithrombotic effect of aspirin is largely or entirely related to irreversible inactivation of platelet cyclooxygenase and consequent suppression of TXA_2-related platelet function. That suppression of platelet rather than vascular actions of TXA_2 is involved in aspirin effects is suggested by Harter's study[26] and by the finding of the VA Cooperative study of unchanged incidence and severity of angina in aspirin-treated patients[29]. Further support to this contention derives from recent studies of Steele et al.[30] demonstrating that low-dose aspirin (1 mg/kg/day) is equally effective to high-dose aspirin (20 mg/kg/day) combined with dipyridamole in preventing platelet deposition and mural thrombus formation following arterial balloon angioplasty in pigs. Although mechanisms other than acetylation of platelet cyclooxygenase may be operative at aspirin dosage of 10-20 mg/kg, the likelihood of this occurring at doses 10-20 times lower is limited by the stoichiometry of the acetylation reaction and its dose-dependence[2,22].

Dissociation of vascular from platelet effects of aspirin has been attempted on the assumption that intact PGI_2 production might enhance the antithrombotic efficacy of the drug. Though probably not serving the role of a circulating antiplatelet hormone, as originally proposed, PGI_2 may still be important in the local modulation of platelet-endothelial interactions, particularly in patients with severe atherosclerosis and platelet activation[31]. Complete separation of platelet from vascular effects of aspirin can not be demonstrated after single dosing[4,17]. However, continuous administration of aspirin in low doses (20 to 40 mg/day) has no statistically significant effects on the urinary excretion of either 6-keto-$PGF_{1\alpha}$[2] or 2,3-dinor-6-keto-$PGF_{1\alpha}$[3]. Inasmuch as the cumulative nature of aspirin-induced inhibition of cyclooxygenase activity is a function of the different rates of daily acetylation and turnover of the enzyme (cell turnover or de novo synthesis), careful consideration should be given to the possibility of variable effects of the drug when pathologic processes affect platelet and/or endothelial behaviour. Thus, enhanced platelet turnover and/or endothelial damage might decrease effectiveness and/or biochemical selectivity of low-dose aspirin. De Caterina et al.[32] have reported that in patients recovering from myocardial infarction, low-dose aspirin (0.4 mg/kg/day) persistently inhibits platelet cyclooxygenase activity and TXA_2-dependent platelet function during one month of therapy, without significantly reducing urinary 6-keto-$PGF_{1\alpha}$ excretion. In contrast, Weksler et al.[33] have reported evidence for a significant cumulative inhibition of vascular PGI_2 synthesis in patients with atherosclerotic cardiovascular disease given 20 mg aspirin daily for 7 days. Whether the severity of atherosclerotic involvement and/or the _ex vivo_ rather than the _in vivo_ type of assessment can account for the apparent discrepancy remains to be determined. Similar studies reporting a profound antiplatelet effect of low-dose aspirin in patients with cerebrovascular disease have recently appeared[34,35]. However, no measurements of PGI_2 production were included in these studies. Inasmuch as PGI_2 biosynthesis is enhanced in patients with severe atherosclerotic lesions, possibly as a result of platelet interactions with endothelium or other vascular insults[31], preservation of the capacity of the vessel wall to produce this natural platelet inhibitory compound would then be desirable in the setting of platelet activation _in vivo_. Whether such a selective sparing of PGI_2 production will result in increased antithrombotic efficacy, fewer toxic reactions or both remains to be established in prospective clinical trials of low-dose aspirin.

SELECTIVE INHIBITION OF PLATELET TX-SYNTHASE

The development of selective inhibitors of TX-synthase as potential antithrombotic agents was predicated on two assumptions i.e. 1) that inhibition of platelet TXA_2 production could not be obtained by aspirin-like drugs without also suppressing vascular PGI_2 synthesis, and 2) that accumulation of platelet-derived PG-endoperoxides consequent to TX-synthase blockade might lead to enhanced vascular PGI_2 production by virtue of an endothelial "steal" mechanism. That the first assumption was rather dogmatic has been clearly shown by the above studies of low-dose aspirin. That the second assumption was only partially correct and rather optimistic has been demonstrated by several recent studies of TX-synthase inhibitors in man. These studies have reported a variable increase in the urinary excretion of 2,3-dinor-6-keto-$PGF_{1\alpha}$ following the oral administration of dazoxiben[5] and CGS 13080[8] and no change after UK-38,485[7], with no apparent relation to the biological half-life and potency of the drug. Moreover, it should be pointed out that a 2-fold increase in the urinary excretion of 2,3-dinor-6-keto-$PGF_{1\alpha}$ (presumably reflecting a doubling of vascular PGI_2 production) is well within the capacity of the vessel wall to respond to mechanical[36] or pathologic[31] insults in the absence of any endoperoxide "steal" mechanism. Moreover, no functional correlate of such drug-induced enhancement of PGI_2 production became apparent in the above cited studies. Given the low rate of endogenous PGI_2 secretion (0.1 ng/kg/min as a maximal estimate[37]), a 2-3 fold increase over the basal rate would still be insufficient to cause any systemic effects. Studies with exogenous PGI_2 suggest that infusion rates of 2-4 ng/kg/min are required to achieve the threshold for either inhibition of platelet function _ex vivo_[38] or systemic hemodynamic effects in man[13]. Peripheral plasma measurements of 6-keto-$PGF_{1\alpha}$ after dazoxiben have failed to detect significant increases into the biologically relevant range of PGI2 concentrations[6]. Furthermore, the predominant redirection of platelet PG-endoperoxide metabolism toward proaggregatory PGE2, as detected ex vivo after dazoxiben[6] or OKY-046[9], may account for limited antiplatelet effect of these drugs and its unmasking by low concentrations of aspirin[39]. White blood cell PGI2-synthase, a possible source of PGI2 production in whole blood, only utilized a minor fraction of platelet-derived PG-endoperoxides after exposure to dazoxiben, as judged by either in vitro[19,40] or ex vivo[6] studies. Thus, it appears more plausible that the local hemostatic consequences of inhibited platelet TX-synthase represent a complex reflection of changes in PG-endoperoxide metabolism by platelets, endothelial cells and leukocytes, rather than simply resulting from an altered "TXA2/PGI2 balance". The clinical significance of such metabolic changes remains to be determined.

ACKNOWLEDGEMENTS

The Authors gratefully acknowledge the expert editorial assistance of Ms Angelamaria Zampini. The studies of the Authors were supported by grants from Consiglio Nazionale delle Ricerche (82.00389.96 and 83.02535.04) and Ministero della Pubblica Istruzione (60/82, 60/83).

REFERENCES

1. P.W. Majerus, Arachidonate metabolism in vascular disorders, J.Clin. Invest. 72:1521 (1983).
2. P. Patrignani, P. Filabozzi and C. Patrono, Selective cumulative inhibition of platelt thromboxane production by low-dose aspirin in healthy subjects, J.Clin. Invest. 69:1366 (1982).
3. G.A. FitzGerald, J.A. Oates, J. Hawiger, R.L. Maas, L.J. Roberts II, J.A. Lawson and A.R. Brash, Endogenous biosynthesis of prostacyclin and thromboxane and platelet function during chronic administration of aspirin in man, J. Clin. Invest. 71:676 (1983).
4. B.B. Weksler, S.B. Pett, D. Alonso, R.C. Richter, P. Stelzer, V. Subramanian, K. Tack-Goldman, and W.A. Gay, Differential inhibition by aspirin of vascular and platelet prostaglandin synthesis in atherosclerotic patients, N. Engl. J. Med. 308:800 (1983).
5. G.A. FitzGerald, A.R. Brash, J.A. Oates and A.K. Pedersen, Endogenous prostacyclin biosynthesis and platelet function during selective inhibition of thromboxane synthase in man, J. Clin. Invest. 71:1336 (1983).
6. P. Patrignani, P. Filabozzi, F. Catella, F. Pugliese and C. Patrono, Differential effects of dazoxiben, a selective thromboxane-synthase inhibitor, on platelet and renal prostaglandin-endoperoxide metabolism, J. Pharmacol. Exp. Ther. 228:472 (1984).

7. S. Fisher, M. Struppler, B. Böhlig, C. Bernutz, W. Wober, and P.C. Weber, The influence of selective thromboxane synthetase inhibition with a novel imidazole derivative, UK-38,485, on prostanoid formation in man, Circulation 68:821 (1983).
8. G.A. FitzGerald and J.A. Oates, Selective and nonselective inhibition of thromboxane formation, Clin. Pharmacol. Ther. 35:633 (1984).
9. P. Patrignani, F. Catella, P. Filabozzi, F. Pugliese, A. Pierucci, B.M. Simonetti, L. Forni, M. Segni and C. Patrono, Differential effects of OKY-046, a selective thromboxane-synthase inhibitor, on platelet and renal prostaglandin endoperoxide metabolism, Clin. Res. 32:246A, (abstract) (1984)
10. G.A. FitzGerald, A.K. Pedersen and C. Patrono, Analysis of prostacyclin and thromboxane biosynthesis in cardiovascular disease, Circulation 67:1174 (1983).
11. C. Patrono, G. Ciabattoni, B.M. Peskar, F. Pugliese, and B.A. Peskar, Is plasma 6-keto-PGF$_{1\alpha}$ a reliable index of circulating Prostacyclin ? Clin. Res. 29:276A (abstract) (1981).
12. G. Ciabattoni, F. Pugliese, G.A. Cinotti, G. Stirati, R.Ronci, G. Castrucci, A. Pierucci and C. Patrono, Characterization of furosemide induced activation of the renal Prostaglandin system, Eur. J. Pharmacol. 60:181 (1979).
13. C. Patrono, F. Pugliese, G. Ciabattoni, P. Patrignani, A. Maseri, S. Chierchia, G.A. Cinotti, B.M. Simonetti, Pierucci A. and B.A. Peskar, Evidence for a direct stimulatory effect of prostacyclin on renin release in man, J. Clin. Invest. 69: 231 (1982).
14. G. Ciabattoni, G.A. Cinotti, A. Pierucci, B.M. Simonetti, M. Manzi, F. Pugliese, P. Barsotti, G. Pecci, F. Taggi and C. Patrono, Effects of sulindac and ibuprofen in patients with chronic glomerular disease. Evidence for the dependence of renal function on prostacyclin, N. Engl. J. Med. 310:279 (1984)
15. C. Patrono, G. Ciabattoni, P. Patrignani, P. Filabozzi, E. Pinca, M.A. Satta, D. Van Dorne, G.A. Cinotti, F. Pugliese, A. Pierucci and B.M. Simonetti, Evidence for a renal origin of urinary thromboxane B$_2$ in health and disease, Adv. Prostaglandin, Thromboxane and Leukotriene Res. 11:493 (1983).
16. C. Patrono, G. Ciabattoni, E. Pinca, F. Pugliese, G. Castrucci, A. De Salvo, M.A. Satta and B.A. Peskar, Low-dose aspirin and inhibition of thromboxane B$_2$ production in healthy subjects, Thromb. Res. 17:317 (1980).
17. F.E. Preston, S. Whipps, C.A. Jackson, A.J. French, P.J. Wyld and C. J. Stoddard, Inhibition of prostacyclin and platelet thromboxane A$_2$ after low-dose aspirin, N. Engl. J. Med. 304: 76 (1981).
18. P. Alessandrini, P. Avogaro, G. Bittolo Bon, P. Patrignani and C. Patrono, Physiologic variables affecting thromboxane B$_2$ production in human whole blood, Thromb. Res, in press.
19. A.K. Pedersen, M.L. Watson and G.A. FitzGerald, Inhibition of thromboxane biosynthesis in serum: limitations of the

measurement of immunoreactive 6-keto-PGF$_{1\alpha}$, Thromb.Res. 33: 99 (1984).

20. G.J. Roth, N.S. Stanford and P.W. Majerus, Acetylation of prostaglandin synthetase by aspirin, Proc. Natl. Acad. Sci. USA 72: 3073 (1975).

21. F.J. Van der Ouderaa, M. Buytenhek, D.H. Nugteren and D.A. Van Dorp, Acetylation of Prostaglandin endoperoxide synthetase with acetylsalicylic acid, Eur. J. Biochem. 109:1 (1980).

22. J.W. Burch, N. Stanford and P.W. Majerus, Inhibition of platelet prostaglandin synthetase by oral aspirin, J. Clin. Invest. 61:314 (1978).

23. C.Patrono, G. Ciabattoni, P. Patrignani, F. Pugliese, P. Filabozzi, F. Catella, G. Davi and L. Forni, Clinical Pharmacology of platelet cyclooxygenase inhibition, Circulation in press.

24. A.K. Pedersen and G.A. FitzGerald, Dose related kinetics of aspirin: presystemic acetylation of platelet cyclooxygenase in man, N. Engl. J. Med., in press.

25. G. Di Minno, M.J. Silver, and S. Murphy, Monitoring the entry of new platelets into the circulation after ingestion of aspirin, Blood 61:1081 (1983).

26. H.R. Harter, J.W. Burch, P.W. Majerus, N. Stanford, J.A. Delmez, C.B. Anderson and C.A Weerts, Prevention of thrombosis in patients on hemodialysis by low-dose aspirin, N. Engl. J. Med. 301:577 (1979).

27. H.D Lewis, J.W. Davis, D.G. Archibald, W.E. Steinke, T.C. Smitherman, J.E. Doherty, H.W. Schnaper, M.M. LeWinter, E. Linares, J.M. Pouget, S.C. Sabharwal, E. Chesler and H. DeMots, Protective effects of aspirin against acute myocardial infarction and death in men with unstable angina. Results of a Veterans Administration Cooperative Study, N. Engl. J. Med. 309:396 (1983).

28. R.L. Lorenz, M. Weber, J. Kotzur, K. Theisen, C.V. Schacky, W. Meister, B. Reichardt and P.C. Weber, Improved aortocoronary bypass patency by low-dose aspirin (100 mg daily). Effects on platelet aggregation and thromboxane formation, Lancet I:1261 (1984).

29. H.D. Lewis Jr. and J.W. Davis, Aspirin and the risk of myocardial infarction, N. Engl. J. Med. 310:122 (1984).

30. P.M. Steele, J.H. Chesebro and V. Fuster, The natural history of arterial balloon angioplasty in pigs and intervention with platelet-inhibitor therapy: implications for clinical trials, Clin. Res. 32:209A (abstract) (1984).

31. G.A. FitzGerald, B. Smith, A.K. Pedersen and A.R. Brash, Increased prostacyclin biosynthesis in patients with severe atherosclerosis and platelet activation, N. Engl. J. Med. 310: 1065 (1984).

32. R. De Caterina, D. Giannessi, W. Bernini, P. Gazzetti, C. Michelassi, A. L'Abbate, L. Donato, P. Patrignani, P. Filabozzi and C. Patrono, Low-dose aspirin in patients recovering from myocardial infarction. Evidence for a selective inhibition

of thromboxane-related platelet function, Am. J. Cardiol.
in press.

33. B.B. Weksler, K. Tack-Goldman, V. Subramanian and W.A. Gay jr.,
Cumulative inhibitory effect of low-dose aspirin on vascular
prostacyclin and platelet thromboxane production in patients
with atherosclerosis, Circulation, in press.

34. G. Boysen, A. Hasager Boss, N. Odum and J.S. Olsen, Prolongation
of bleeding time and inhibition of platelet aggregation by
low-dose acetylsalicylic acid in patients with cerebrovascular disease, Stroke 15:241 (1984).

35. B.B. Weksler, J.L. Kent, D. Rudolph, P. Scherer and D.E. Levy,
Effects of low dose aspirin on platelet function in patients
with recent cerebral ischemia. Stroke, in press.

36. L. Roy, H.R. Knapp, R.M. Robertson and G.A. FitzGerald, Endogenous biosynthesis of prostacyclin during cardiac catheteriza-
tion and angiography in man, Circulation, in press.

37. G.A. FitzGerald, A.R. Brash, P. Falardeau and J.A. Oates, Estimated rate of prostacyclin secretion into the circulation of
normal man, J. Clin. Invest. 68:1272 (1981).

38. S. Chierchia, C. Patrono, F. Crea, G. Ciabattoni, R. De Caterina,
G.A. Cinotti, A. Distante and A. Maseri, Effects of intravenous prostacyclin in variant angina, Circulation 65:470
(1982).

39. V. Bertelè, A. Falanga, M. Tomasiak, E. Dejana, C. Cerletti and
G. de Gaetano, Platelet thromboxane synthetase inhibitors
with low doses of aspirin: possible resolution of the "aspirin
dilemma", Science 220:517 (1983).

40. M.A. Orchard, I.A. Blair, C.T. Dollery and P.J. Lewis, Blood
can synthesize prostacyclin, Lancet II:565 (1983).

MANIPULATION OF PRO- AND ANTIAGGREGATING PROSTAGLANDINS:

NEW ANTITHROMBOTIC STRATEGIES

H. Deckmyn, P. Gresele, J. Arnout and J. Vermylen

Centre for Thrombosis and Vascular Research
Department of Medical Research
K.U.Leuven, Leuven, Belgium

A number of cyclooxygenase products have potent actions on platelets : thromboxane A_2 (TXA_2), the cyclic endoperoxides prostaglandins G_2 and H_2 (PGG_2, H_2) and to some extent PGE_2 are pro-aggregatory, whereas prostacyclin (PGI_2) and PGD_2 inhibit platelet activation. Attempts to change the balance in favour of the antiaggregatory PG's therefore could be of benefit in thrombotic situations, and can be done at different levels : selective inhibition of platelet cyclooxygenase, stimulation of the PGI_2 synthesis, inhibition of TXA_2 synthesis or blockage of the TXA_2 receptor.

SELECTIVE INHIBITION OF PLATELET CYCLOOXYGENASE

Inhibition of cyclooxygenase blocks not only the formation of PGG_2, PGH_2, TXA_2 and other PG's formed by the platelets but also PGI_2 production by the endothelial cells. Aspirin irreversibly acetylates the enzyme and therefore has different effects on platelets and endothelium : TXA_2 formation by platelets is blocked for the life of a human platelet, endothelial cyclooxygenase however can be resynthesized, and thus will recover much more quickly. This has led to low-dose and to prolonged low-dose aspirin regimens, the latter causing a cumulative inhibition of platelet cyclooxygenase, apparently maintaining endothelial cyclooxygenase intact.[1] This method however might be cumbersome because the optimal dose may well differ between subjects.

STIMULATION OF PROSTACYCLIN FORMATION

A number of compounds, such as the "prostacyclin stimulating plasma factor"[2] and nafazatrom (Bay g 6575),[3] have been said to

141

stimulate prostacyclin formation, which effect however mainly was seen with so-called "exhausted cells", cells which by themselves no longer produce prostacyclin, f.i. after prolonged incubation in buffer. This exhaustion is due to the inactivation of the cyclooxygenase : prostacyclin formation is restored when cyclic endoperoxides but not arachidonic acid are added to these cells.[4]

Accumulating peroxides most probably are responsible for the progressive inactivation of cyclooxygenase : reduced glutathione is able to delay the exhaustion, while hydrogen peroxide, 1,3-bis-(2-chloro-ethyl)-1-nitrosoureum,[5] an inhibitor of glutathione reductase or N-ethylmaleimide, which reacts with reduced gluta-thione, accelerate it.[4]

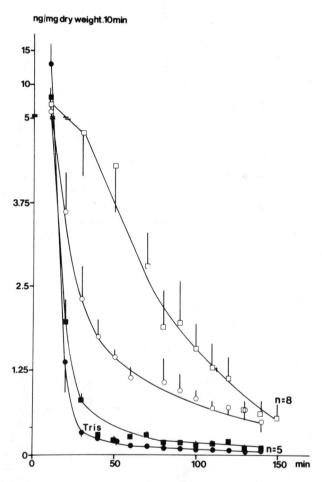

ng/mg dry weight.10min

Fig. 1. 6-keto $PGF_{1\alpha}$-formation ($\pm$ SEM) during consecutive 10 min incubation periods by aortic rings from control rats (closed symbols) or from rats pretreated with 10 mg/kg nafazatrom 1 h before (open symbols) in Tris.HCl buffer (o) or human plasma (□).

142

We found that low molecular weight component(s)[6] of normal human plasma, nafazatrom (Fig. 1) and also dipyridamole[6] delay the self-inactivation of cyclooxygenase. All these compounds furthermore produce dose-dependent inhibition of the hydrogen peroxide-initiated guaiacol co-oxidation by horse radish peroxidase or cyclooxygenase peroxidase from ram seminal vesicle microsomes. We therefore concluded that these products protect the prostacyclin-forming system from vessel wall by acting as reducing cofactors for the cyclooxygenase peroxidase, thus keeping the peroxides below their inhibitory concentration (Fig. 2).

An in vivo equivalent for these phenomena exists. When a thread is inserted into a rabbit vein, the irritation causes local prostacyclin formation, that ceases after some hours. This "exhaustion" can be overcome by enhancing the local production of cyclic endoperoxides of platelet origin (with a thromboxane synthase inhibitor[7]) and can partially be prevented by administering nafazatrom.

THROMBOXANE SYNTHASE INHIBITION

Selective thromboxane synthase inhibitors (TSI) not only block the production of TXA_2, but simultaneously will cause accumulation[8] and reorientation of the metabolism of cyclic endoperoxides.

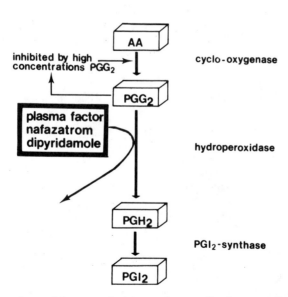

Fig. 2. The prostacyclin regulating plasma factor, nafazatrom, and dipyridamole protect the PGI_2-forming system by acting as reducing cofactors for the cyclooxygenase hydroperoxidase.

Dazoxiben, a TSI, however, inhibits arachidonic acid induced aggregation in platelet-rich plasma from some donors only ("responders").[9] When serum albumin, which increases the production of antiaggregatory PGD_2 from cyclic endoperoxides,[10,11] was added, "non-responder" platelets responded[12] (Fig. 3). On the other hand, when low levels of serum albumin are present, as in the plasma from nephrotic patients, platelets nearly invariably failed to respond to dazoxiben (in preparation). The ratio between PGD_2 and TXB_2 + PGE_2 formed was crucial in determining the response of human platelets to dazoxiben : whenever this ratio was high, platelet aggregation was inhibited. SQ 22536, an adenylate cyclase inhibitor and N 0164, a PGD_2 antagonist, reversed the inhibition by dazoxiben in human platelet-rich plasma, stressing the importance of a PGD_2 mediated rise of cyclic AMP for the effectiveness of a thromboxane synthase inhibitor.

However, the beneficial reorientation by a TSI is not limited to PGD_2, also prostacyclin formation can be increased. When dazoxiben-treated platelets are stimulated in the presence of

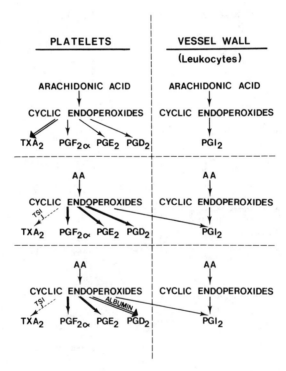

Fig. 3. Inhibition of TXA_2 synthase will cause reorientation towards the classical PG's and PGI_2. The reorientation towards the antiaggregatory PGD_2 can be enhanced by serum albumin.

144

leukocytes as in whole blood,[13] or in the presence of aspirinated endothelial cells[8] a marked increase of prostacyclin formation can be observed.

We furthermore could demonstrate that this reorientation actually also can occur in vivo,[7] using again the rabbit model with the thread in the vein : in control conditions local prostacyclin formation is increased, but declines with time, thromboxane levels are elevated and remain high. When dazoxiben is infused, local TXA_2 production drops, and PGI_2 formation no longer decreases, but tends to increase. This beneficial effect is observed where it is most needed, namely where platelets are activated and endothelial cells risk becoming exhausted.

THROMBOXANE RECEPTOR ANTAGONISM

The antithrombotic drug BM 13.177 inhibits in a competitive way the in vitro aggregation induced by endoperoxide analogues and by TX_2 produced by dog platelets stimulated with arachidonic acid.[14] This compound also specifically inhibits the contraction of isolated rabbit femoral arteries induced by endoperoxide analogues. Differently from all previously described TX-receptor antagonists, this substance is non-toxic and can safely be administered to man. One single 800 mg oral dose of BM 13.177 is effective in inhibiting ex vivo platelet aggregation induced via the thromboxane receptor (low-dose collagen, arachidonic acid, U44069, U46619, second wave ADP). A slight but statistically significant prolongation of the bleeding time was observed 4 hours after the intake of the drug. No significant modifications in plasma or serum PG's were detected.

COMBINATION OF THROMBOXANE SYNTHASE INHIBITION AND TX-RECEPTOR ANTAGONISM

Although a TSI reorients endoperoxide metabolism towards antiaggregatory PGD_2 and eventually towards PGI_2, its effect on platelet aggregation is variable. Part of the explanation could be that cyclic endoperoxides, which accumulate after TX-synthase inhibition, can occupy and activate the TX-receptor. Furthermore, they "turn off" platelet adenylate cyclase, thereby neutralizing the antiaggregatory effect of PGD_2 and prostacyclin, that exert this activity precisely by "turning on" this enzyme and increasing intracellular cyclic AMP. A competitive receptor blocker, such as BM 13.177, prevents both TXA_2 and cyclic endoperoxide-binding, but does not increase the formation of antiaggregatory PG's. Combining the two should solve the problems of each drug, without affecting their advantages. In a number of in vitro studies, we were able to demonstrate the synergism between dazoxiben and BM 13.177 on platelet aggregation, whereas the PG reorientation induced by dazoxiben was unchanged.[15]

145

The formation of TXA_2 is only one of the pathways involved in platelet activation. However, PGI_2 and PGD_2, by rising cyclic AMP-levels, will impede all known pathways of platelet activation. Increasing these PG's by protecting endothelial cyclooxygenase or by reorienting endoperoxide metabolism using a TSI, eventually together with a TX-receptor blocker, could therefore have major antithrombotic potential.

REFERENCES

1. P. Patrignani, P. Filabozzi, and C. Patrono, Low-dose aspirin is a selective inhibitor of platelet cyclo-oxygenase activity in healthy subjects, in: "Advances in Prostaglandin, Thromboxane, and Leukotriene Research, Vol. 11", B. Samuelsson, R. Paoletti, and P. Ramwell, eds., Raven Press, New York, p. 259 (1983).

2. G. Remuzzi, M. Livio, A.E. Cavenaghi, D. Marchesi, G. Mecca, M.B. Donati, and G. de Gaetano, Unbalanced prostaglandin synthesis and plasma factors in uraemic bleeding. A hypothesis, Thromb. Res. 13: 531 (1978).

3. J. Vermylen, D.A.F. Chamone, and M. Verstraete, Stimulation of prostacyclin release from vessel wall by Bay g 6575, an antithrombotic compound, Lancet i: 518 (1979).

4. H. Deckmyn, C. Zoja, J. Arnout, A. Todisco, F. Vanden Bulcke, L. D'Hondt, N. Hendrickx, P. Gresele, and J. Vermylen, Partial isolation and function of the prostacyclin regulating plasma factor. (submitted).

5. J.R. Babson and D.J. Reed, Inactivation of glutathione reductase by 2-chloroethyl nitrosourea-derived isocyanates, Biochem. Biophys. Res. 83: 754 (1978).

6. H. Deckmyn, P. Gresele, J. Arnout, A. Todisco, and J. Vermylen, Prolonging prostacyclin production by nafazatrom and dipyridamole, Lancet ii: 410 (1984).

7. H. Deckmyn, E. Van Houtte, M. Verstraete, and J. Vermylen, Manipulation of the local thromboxane and prostacyclin balance in vivo by the antithrombotic compounds dazoxiben, acetylsalicylic acid and nafazatrom, Biochem. Pharmacol. 32: 2757 (1983).

8. J. Vermylen, G. Defreyn, L.O. Carreras, S.J. Machin, J. Van Schaeren, and M. Verstraete, Thromboxane synthetase inhibition as antithrombotic strategy, Lancet i: 1073 (1981).

9. S. Heptinstall, J. Bevan, S.R. Cockbill, S.P. Hanley, and M.J. Parry, Effects of a selective inhibitor of thromboxane synthetase on human blood platelet behaviour, Thromb. Res. 20: 219 (1980).

10. T. Watanabe, S. Narumiya, T. Shimizu, and O. Hayaishi, Characterization of the biosynthetic pathway of prostaglandin D_2 in human platelet-rich plasma, J. Biol. Chem. 257: 14843 (1982).

11. M. Hamberg and B.B. Fredholm, Isomerization of prostaglandin H_2 into prostaglandin D_2, <u>Biochim. Biophys. Acta</u> 431: 189 (1976).

12. P. Gresele, H. Deckmyn, E. Huybrechts, and J. Vermylen, Serum albumin enhances the impairment of platelet aggregation with thromboxane synthase inhibition by increasing the formation of prostaglandin D_2, <u>Biochem. Pharmacol.</u> 33: 2083 (1984).

13. G. Defreyn, H. Deckmyn, and J. Vermylen, A thromboxane synthetase inhibitor reorients endoperoxide metabolism in whole blood towards prostacyclin and prostaglandin E_2, <u>Thromb. Res.</u> 26: 389 (1982).

14. P. Gresele, H. Deckmyn, J. Arnout, J. Lemmens, W. Janssens, and J. Vermylen, BM 13.177, a selective blocker of platelet and vessel wall thromboxane receptors is effective in man, <u>Lancet</u> i: 991 (1984).

15. P. Gresele, E. Van Houtte, J. Arnout, H. Deckmyn, and J. Vermylen, Thromboxane synthase inhibition combined with thromboxane receptor blockade: a step forward in antithrombotic strategy?, <u>Thromb. Haemost.</u> (in press).

FLAVONOIDS - LIPOXYGENASES - PLATELET AGGREGATION

R.J.Gryglewski, J.Robak, and J.Święs

Department of Pharmacology
N.Copernicus Academy of Medicine in Cracow
31-531 Cracow, Poland

INTRODUCTION

Flavonoids including flavonols (e.g.quercetin and rutin)are widespread in the plant kingdom and they are concentrated by bees in honey and propolis. Flavonoids interact with many macromolecules in animal cells, change the activity of mammalian enzymes and influence permeability of cell membranes. Controlled trials on the therapeutical efficacy of flavonoids were relatively few, although flavonoids were consistently claimed to show anti-bleeding, anti-thrombotic, anti-inflammatory, anti-allergic, analgesic, cytoprotective, oestrogenic, virusostatic and many other pharmacological actions (Havsteen,1983). In clinical practice, in addition to bioflavonoids, a number of semisynthetic flavonoids has been used.

Flavonoids structurally resemble nucleosides, isoalloxazine, pteroiloglutaminic acid, nordehydroguaiateric acid and disodium cromoglycate. One of these similarities is usually proposed as a basis for hypothetical mechanism of inhibitory action of flavonoids on enzymes (Havsteen, 1983). However, there is a class of enzymes that includes arachidonic acid oxygenases, the activity of which seems to be influenced by electrochemical potential of polyphenolic flavonols, that leads to scavanging of free radicals which play a double role of activators and inhibitors of arachidonic acid oxygenases (Kulmacz and Lands, 1983).

Flavonoids have been claimed to inhibit various enzymes which are involved in running of arachidonic acid cascade, such as phospholipase A_2 (Lee et al.,1982) and prostaglandin 9-hydroxydehydrogenase (Griffiths et al.,1983; Moore et al.,1983). The main two branching enzymes in the arachidonic acid metabolism, i.e.cyclo-oxygenase and lipoxygenase were investigated most thoroughly. There are pronounced differences among various flavonoids in their action on both enzymes. E.g.flavone and chrysin inhibit cyclo-oxygenase and stimulate lipoxygenase whereas quercetin and myricetin inhibit preferentially lipoxygenase in thrombin stimulated platelets (Landolfi et al.,1984; Mower et al.,1984). The effect of flavonoids on cyclo-oxygenase activity was reported to be either stimulatory (Sekiya and Okuda,1982; Sekiya et al.,1982; Święs et al.,1984) or inhibitory (Bauman and Bruchhausen,1979; Baumann et al.,1979; Baumann et al.,1980 a,b). Lipoxygenase activity was consistently reported to be inhibited by flavonols (Baumann et al., 1980 a; Fiebrich and Koch, 1979; Sekiya and Okuda,1982; Sekiya et al.,1982; Hope et al.,1983; Landolfi et al., 1984; Święs et al.1984).

Metabolism of arachidonic acid in blood platelets involves its cyclo-oxygenation to endoperoxides (PGG_2 and PGH_2) and its lipoxygenation to 12-hydroperoxyeicosatetraénoic acid (HPETE). Whereas the biological role of cyclo-oxygenase products in platelets is more or less clarified (Hammarström,1980), the role of lipoxygenase pathway remains obscure (Dutilh et al.,1980; Sun et al., 1980; Sams et al.,1982; Maclouf,1983). Flavonoids were reported to inhibit platelet aggregation (Pollock and Heath,1975; Beretz et al.,1982 a,b; Mower et al.,1984; Święs et al.1984) and one of feasible mechanisms of this action is a modification of arachidonic acid oxidative metabolism in platelets (Landolfi et al.,1984). On the other hand flavonols are known to modify functioning of polymorphonuclear leukocytes (Lee et al., 1982) and once again an interference with phospholipid (Lee et al.,1982) or oxidative metabolism (Hope et al., 1983; Tauber et al.,1984) has been postulated. A possibility of biochemical interaction between 12-lipoxygenase and 5-lipoxygenase pathways in platelets and leukocytes has been recently shown (Marcus et al.,1982; Maclouf et al.,1983). It may well be that a product(s) of the above interaction influences platelet function. PAF-acether constitutes another biochemical link between leukocytes and platelets (Vargaftig et al.,1982). Therefore, we have decided to scrutinize inhibitory action of several flavonoids on enzymatic oxidation of arachidonic acid in vitro and, then, to investigate their anti-aggregatory activity in vivo, where interaction between platelets and leukocytes occurs in the most natural environment.

METHODS

Lipoxygenases

15-Lipoxygenase from soybean (Sigma) and 12-lipo-
xygenase from human or horse platelets were used as
a source of the enzyme.
Soybean Lipoxygenase. The activity of the enzyme was
measured polarographically as previously described
(Robak,Duniec,1980). In principle a mixture of 2.9 ml
of the enzyme solution (5 μg/ml) and 0.1 ml of a flavonoid solution or solvent were stimulated with 100 μM of
sodium arachidonate. The activity was expressed in terms
of oxygen consumption by a sample during 3 min. Inhibition of the enzyme by a flavonoid was calculated from
a regression line. In addition, the enzyme activity was
measured by generation of 15-HETE using HPLC. The same
samples after 3 min of incubation were acidified to pH 3
and extracted with 6 ml of ethyl acetate. Organic phase
was evaporated to dryness, dissolved in 0.1 ml of methanol and 10 μl of that solution was used for HPLC analysis. A Beckman instrument model 110A with an ultrasphere ODS reversed phase column (4.6 x 250 mm) was used.
Flow rate was 1 ml/min, pressure 1000 psi, solvent system methanol:water:acetic acid (80:20:0.1). Absorption
was registered at 234 nm. 15-HETE standards were run in
parallel. Area under peaks was used for calculation.
Blood Platelet Lipoxygenase. High-speed horse platelet
microsome supernatant (Robak,Duniec,1980) was used as
a source of 12-lipoxygenase for polarographic measurement of the enzyme activity in a way described above
and reported previously (Robak,Duniec,1980). Another
source of 12-lipoxygenase constituted washed human
platelets (Vargas et al.,1982). Platelet suspension
was incubated in the presence of 33 μM of sodium arachidonate at 37°C during 3 min. After acidification to
pH 4 the remaining procedure was the same as that described for HPLC measurements of the soybean lipoxygenase activity. 12-HETE standard was used.

Cyclo-oxygenase

Freeze-dried ram seminal vesicle microsomes(RSVM)
were used as a source of the enzyme. Polarographic
measurement of the enzyme activity was described previously (Robak et al.,1981). Activity of the enzyme
was assessed in terms of oxygen consumption during 3
minutes after instillation of sodium arachidonate at

Table 1.   Structures and producers of the studied flavonoids

Flavonols

	R_1	R_2	R_3	R_4	R_5	Producer
Kaempferol	H	OH	OH	OH	OH	Fluka
Quercetin	OH	OH	OH	OH	OH	Lachema
Quercitrin	OH	OH	O-rhamnose	OH	OH	Fluka
Rutin	OH	OH	O-rutinose	OH	OH	Koch-Light
Troxerutin (Venoruton)	OH	O-CH$_2$CH$_2$OH	O-rutinose	O-CH$_2$CH$_2$OH	O-CH$_2$CH$_2$OH	Zyma
Diosmin (Daflon)	OH	OMe	OH	H	O-rhamnose	Servier
Benzquercine (Parietrope)	Bz-O	Bz-O	Bz-O	Bz-O	Bz-O	Biosedra

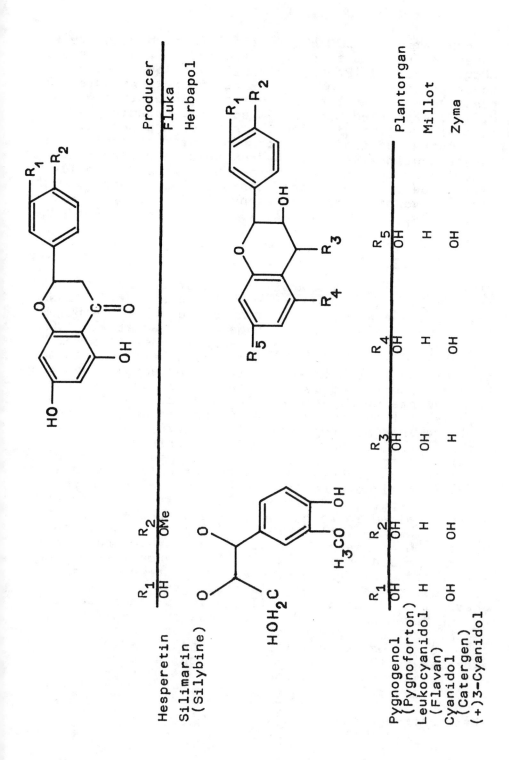

	R_1	R_2	Producer
Hesperetin	OH	OMe	Fluka
Silimarin (Silybine)			Herbapol

	R_1	R_2	R_3	R_4	R_5	Producer
Pygnogenol (Pygnoforton)	OH	OH	OH	OH	OH	Plantorgan
Leukocyanidol (Flavan)	H	H	OH	H	H	Millot
Cyanidol (Catergen)	OH	OH	H	OH	OH	Zyma
(+)3-Cyanidol						

concentration of 100 μM. Initial reaction velocity was assessed from the tangent of tracing curves. In radio-chemical method (Robak,Duniec,1982) a low substrate concentration (1.6 μM of ^{14}C-arachidonate was used. The reaction mixture after 5 minutes of incubation was aci-dified, extracted with ethyl acetate, organic phase eva-porated, residue dissolved in ethanol and separated on TLC plates. Radioactivity corresponding to individual prostaglandin standards, hydroxyacids and unreacted arachidonic acid was determined by a liquid scintil-lation spectrometer Intertechnique SL-30. Samples with added flavonoids were run in parallel to samples with added solvent (Świȩs et al.,1984).

Platelet aggregation

Platelet aggregation in vitro. The effect of flavonoids on platelet aggregation in rabbit platelet rich plasma (PRP) aggregated with sodium arachidonate (50 - 80 μM) was assayed in a Born aggregometer (Robak et al.,1981). Platelet aggregation in vivo. Thirty three cats (either sex, body weight 2 - 3 kg) were anaesthetized with so-dium pentobarbital (30 mg/kg i.p.). Arterial blood pres-sure was registered by a Stadham transducer from right carotid artery. Heparin at a dose of 2500 units/kg was injected intravenously. An Achilles tendon of a rabbit (collagen strip)(Gryglewski et al.,1978) was superfused with arterial blood withdrawn by a peristaltic pump (3 ml/min) from thoracic aorta. After superfusion blood was returned to the venous system of animal. When super-fused with blood a collagen strip was covered with pla-telet aggregates and embedded leukocytes and, therefore, a strip gained in weight as it was described original-ly (Gryglewski et al.,1978). Changes in weight (from 250 to 300 mg) were recorded through a Harvard trans-ducer type 384 on a Watanabe multirecorder. After the weight of a collagen strip reached plateau (20 min) superfusion was stopped, platelet aggregates were wa-shed with 3 ml of saline, flavonoids or their solvent or a reference compound - acetylsalicylic acid were in-jected i.v. and 10 min.later blood superfusion of a col-lagen strip was reconstituted for next 20 min. In some experiments this procedure was repeated several times. A difference in deposition of platelet clumps over a collagen strip before and after treatment with fla-vonoids was calculated and considered as an index of their anti-aggregatory activity in vivo.

Drugs

Apart from quercetin and rutin which were available in crystalline form, other flavonoids (Table 1) were available as pharmaceutical preparations (tablets or dragées). Those flavonoids were extracted with hot ethanol and recrystallized. In biological experiments all of flavonoids were dissolved in ethanol. A corresponding volume of ethanol was used in control experiments.

RESULTS

Inhibition of 15-lipoxygenase from soybean and 12-lipoxygenase from horse platelets by 6 active flavonoids is shown in Table 2. Their inhibitory effect was measured by the polarographic techniques. The following flavonoids had no influence on the enzyme activity at the highest concentrations studied: troxerutin (4000 μM), diosmine and leukocyanidol (1000 μM) and benzquercine (100 μM). Cyanidol and pygnenol inhibited the enzymes in less than 50% when used at concentrations of 1000 μM. Higher concentrations of those flavonoids were not used because of limitation in solubility.

Table 2. Inhibition of soybean and horse platelet lipoxygenase activities by flavonoids

Flavonoid	Soybean lipoxygenase				Horse platelet lipoxygenase			
	IC_{50}	b	r	n	IC_{50}	b	r	n
Quercetin	13 μM	59	0.93	18	1.3 μM	35	0.94	8
Kaempferol	220 μM	37	0.81	12	118 μM	67	0.90	6
Silimarin	405 μM	70	0.96	8	382 μM	42	0.93	7
Quercitrin	1126 μM	68	0.99	5	136 μM	62	0.99	5
Rutin	1596 μM	36	0.86	20	113 μM	45	0.89	6
Hesperetin	1669 μM	53	0.87	8	288 μM	56	0.91	5

IC_{50} was calculated from a regression equation
b - slope of regression line; r - regression coefficient
n - number of experiments

The most active flavonoid - quercetin was tried as an inhibitor of 15-lipoxygenase from soybean and 12-lipoxygenase from washed human platelets using the techniques in which end products of the reaction 15-HETE or 12-HETE were measured by HPLC. IC_{50} values were: 14$\pm$ 0.6 μM (n=11) and 4.4$\pm$ 0.9 μM (n = 6)(mean $\pm$ S.E.), respectively.

Out of seven flavonoids which were studied on their effect on cyclo-oxygenase activity in the presence of a high concentration of the substrate (100 μM) five flavonoids stimulated oxygen consumption by the enzyme and other two were inactive (Silimarin and Troxerutin)(Table 3). The stimulation of the oxygen outburst by flavonoids reached its maximum within a few seconds after the substrate was added. Thereby stimulation of the enzyme when calculated from the initial reaction reaction velocity was higher than that calculated from oxygen consumption during 3 min (Table 3). Again quercetin was among the most active stimulators of cyclo-oxygenase activity. The effect of quercetin and rutin on cyclo-oxygenase activity was also assayed radiochemically in the presence of a low concentration of the substrate (1.6 μM). Rutin at a concentration of 100 μM hardly influenced conversion of arachidonic acid to prostaglandins or to hydroxyacids whereas quercetin at a concentration of 10 μM was a potent inhibitor of transformation of arachidonic acid to both prostaglandins and to hydroxyacids (Table 4).

Table 3. The influence of flavonoids on the oxygen consumption by ram seminal vesicle microsomes in the presence of 100 μM of AA

Flavonoid	Concentration μM	Percent of control (100%)[x] calculated from:	
		Initial reaction velocity	O_2 consumption during 3 min
Quercetin	10	562+39 (n=5)	198+ 9 (n=5)
	100	860+51 (n=4)	256+12 (n=4)
Rutin	100	826+125(n=5)	250+18 (n=5)
Quercitrin	100	1014+47 (n=4)	287+13 (n=5)
Silimarin	100	110+ 8 (n=4)	101+ 5 (n=4)
Kaempferol	300	330 (n=2)	225 (n=2)
Hesperetin	300	465 (n=2)	150 (n=2)
Troxerutin	1000	110+16 (n=4)	105+12 (n=4)

[x]Mean $\pm$ S.E.

Table 4. The influence of rutin and quercetin on on cyclo-oxygenase activity from ram seminal vesicle microsomes in the presence of 1.6 μM of ^{14}C AA

	Start	Percent radioactivity recovered in zones:					
		6-oxo PGF$_{1\alpha}$	PGF$_{2\alpha}$	PGE$_2$	PGD$_2$	hydro xy- acids	AA
Control	4.7	3.3	18.4	22.4	13.5	30.3	7.4
Rutin 100 μM	4.3	4.1	20.4	28.0	9.8	25.1	8.2
Quercetin 10 μM	2.8	2.8	8.4	7.8	3.0	13.1	61.3

In rabbit PRP the anti-aggregatory action of seven studied flavonoids was weak. In some samples of PRP it was not reproducible and, therefore, we felt unable to present the statistical analysis of those data in vitro. On average, IC_{50} (μM) for studied flavonoids was as follows: quercetin (40); kaempferol (50); hesperetin (110); rutin (200); silimarin (340); quercitrin (450) and troxerutin ($>$ 500) for at least 5 experiments for each flavonoid.

Three flavonoids: quercetin, rutin and troxerurin were studied in vivo for their anti-aggregatory activity. Quercetin and rutin showed a powerful inhibition of platelet aggregation in vivo ten minutes after their intravenous injection. This inhibition was strictly dose-dependent (Fig.1). IC_{50} calculated from the regression equation was for quercetin 1.6 ± 0.03 μg/kg (mean $\pm$ S.E.; n = 15; r = 0.94) and for rutin 20.4 ± 0.05 μg/kg (mean $\pm$ S.E.; n = 12; r = 0.95). In the same experimental model the reference compound acetylsalicylic acid had IC_{50} = 6840 ± 470 μg/kg (mean $\pm$ S.E.; n = 9; r = 0.78). Troxerutin inhibited platelet aggregation at a range of doses of 0.1 - 1.0 mg/kg i.v. while at higher doses (3 - 100 mg/kg i.v.) this effect was waning (Fig.1) and, therefore, calculation of IC_{50} was impossible. Fig.2 shows the reversibility of anti-aggregatory action of quercetin and rutin.

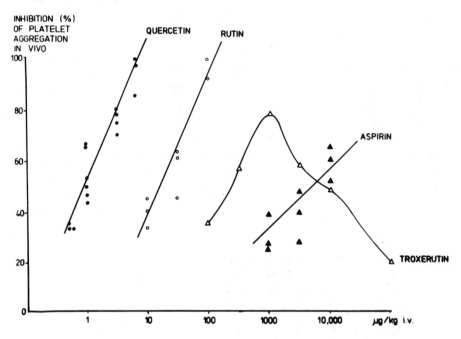

Fig. 1.   In vivo anti-aggregatory action of flavonols (quercetin, rutin and troxerutin)
and acetylsalicylic acid (aspirin).
Ordinate - percent of inhibition of platelet aggregation over blood-superfused collagen strips in anaesthetized cats.
Abcissa - doses (μg/kg in logarithmic
scale) of drugs that were injected intravenously 10 minutes before aggregation
started.
Each point represents a separate experiment.

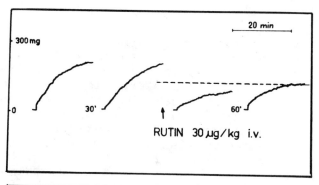

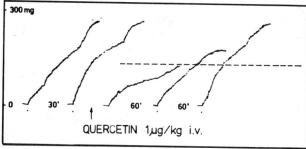

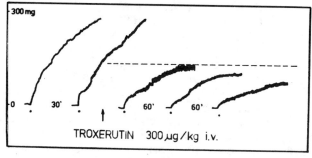

Fig. 2.   Comparison of longevity of the _in vivo_
anti-aggregatory action of flavonols in
anaesthetized cats. Original tracings of
platelet aggregation (0 - 300 mg) over
blood superfused collagen strips. Two control aggregations were separated by a 30
min period, in between of which solvent was
injected i.v., then rutin (30 μg/kg i.v.)
or quercetin (1 μg/kg i.v.) or troxerutin
(300 μg/kg i.v.) were administered 10 min
before the next aggregation. Following aggregations were separated by 60 min periods.
Note a slow recovery of platelet aggregabi-
lity in case of rutin and quercetin and po-
tentialization of anti-aggregatory action of
troxerutin with the relapse of time.

DISCUSSION

Among twelve flavonoids studied the most active in all of our experimental systems was 5,7,3,4'-tetra-hydroxyflavonol - quercetin followed by its 3-rutino-side - rutin. Hydroxylated flavonols such as quercetin and rutin that possess a catechol ring or a pyrogallol ring (e.g.myricetin) have structural features required for free radical scavengers. Indeed, those flavonols share their free radical scavenging properties (Cavallini et al.,1978; Baumann et al.,1980 b) with various phenols, catechols, dihydroxynaphtalens, butylated hydroanisole and MK 447 (Kuehl et al.,1977; Baumann et al.,1980 a; Egan et al.,1980).

Inhibition of 12-lipoxygenase and 15-lipoxygenase by quercetin and other flavonols seems to depend on the prevention of the free radical initiation of oxidation of arachidonic acid (Dirks et al.,1982) rather than on chelating of heavy metal ions by flavonols (Sekiya and Okuda,1982). We have presently shown that quercetin inhibits lipoxygenases at a following order of potency: 12-lipoxygenase from high-speed horse platelet microsome supernatant (IC_{50} = 1.3 μM), 12-lipoxygenase from washed human platelets (IC_{50} = 4.4 μM) and soybean 15-lipoxygenase (IC_{50} = 13 μM). Hope et al.(1983) have recently reported the same IC_{50} value for quercetin inhibition of 12-lipoxygenase from human platelets. Most interestingly these authors have shown a strong inhibition of 5-lipoxygenase from rat basophilic leukemia cells by quercetin (IC_{50} = 0.2 μM). Even more recently Landolfi et al.(1984) have shown that out of 18 various bioflavonoids only two flavonols: quercetin (with a catechol ring) and myricetin (with a pyrogallol ring) at a concentration of 10 μM inhibit platelet lipoxygenase by 88% and by 68%, respectively. Kaempferol and morin (flavonols with phenol and resorcinol rings) are by far less potent inhibitors of lipoxygenase whereas flavones and flavonones are inactive and, if anything, they stimulate lipoxygenase most probably owing to an inhibition of cyclo-oxygenase pathway in platelets.

Would it be as simple as that - flavonoids with with phenol, catechol or pyrogallol rings owing to the free radical scavenging properties of those moieties are lipoxygenase inhibitors ? It does not seem so. Analysis of the data of Landolfi et al.(1984) and of our data shows that the lipoxygenase inhibitory properties of "phenolic" and "catecholic" flavonoids are drastically reduced or abolished if 3-hydroxyl group in the benzopyrone ring of quercetin is blocked with

a sugar (rutin,quercitrin) or if this 3-hydroxyl group
is removed (apigenin) or if flavone is changed for fla-
vonone skeleton (hesperetin) or if 4-keto group is replaced by another substituent (pygnogenol, cyanidanol).
Out of all investigated flavonoids only two flavonols,
quercetin and myricetin, are potent lipoxygenase inhibitors in vitro. Inhibitory potency of quercetin against
lipoxygenases varies between 0.2 to 13 μM (IC_{50}) and
this may indicate a certain degree of specificity of
binding of quercetin with an enzymic protein. Quercetin,
however, has been reported to perform its "free radical
scavenging" or "anti-oxidant" properties in several
other systems, e.g. inhibition of oxidizing processes
in microsomes and mitochondria (Cavallini et al.,1978),
inhibition of ascorbate-stimulated generation of lipid
peroxides in boiled rat liver microsomes (IC_{50}=9.5 μM,
our unpublished data) or inhibition of leukocyte NADPH-
oxidase activity (IC_{50} = 39 μM)(Tauber et al.,1984).
Therefore, it is difficult to judge of specific affinity of quercetin to platelet or leukocyte lipoxygenases.
Certainly more kinetic data are required in order to
decide on this point.

Even more complex is an explanation of a dual effect of quercetin on cyclo-oxygenase activity. We have
shown that quercetin stimulates cyclo-oxygenase when
a high concentration (100 μM) of the substrate is used.
At low concentration of arachidonic acid (1.6 μM) quercetin inhibits the enzyme. A possible explanation of
this fact stems from the experiments of the Lands group
(Kulmacz and Lands,1983). According to Lands, cyclo-
oxygenase activity is tuned by the presence of lipid
peroxides (PGG_2, HPETE) in a reaction mixture. Lipid
peroxides at a range of concentrations of 10^{-9}- 10^{-7}M
will initiate oxygenation of arachidonic acid, however,
when lipid peroxides are accumulating at concentrations
higher than 10^{-6}M, inhibition of cyclo-oxygenase (Kulmacz and Lands,1983) and prostacyclin synthetase (Gryglewski et al.,1976) occurs. In that way lipid peroxides
(and thus free radicals) can activate or inhibit cyclo-
oxygenase, depending on the amount of the substrate
available for their generation. The effect of free radical scavengers on cyclo-oxygenase activity (Egan et
al.,1980) will depend on the concentration of arachidonic acid available for reaction. Indeed, in our experiments quercetin behaved like a typical free radical scavenger. At a high concentration of the substrate quercetin stimulated RSVM cyclo-oxygenase as a result of removal of a surplus of inhibitory free radicals, whereas at a low concentration of the substrate
quercetin by scavenging of minute amounts of activating

free radicals showed up its inhibitory face on the enzyme activity. A similar dual mode of action on cyclo-
oxygenase activity was reported for other free radical
scavengers such as BW 755 C (Robak and Duniec,1982),
esculetin (Sekiya and Okuda,1982), chloropromazine, caffeic acid and paracetamol (Robak and Duniec,1980; Duniec et al.,1983). Another possibility is that flavone
moiety has an inherent property of inhibiting of cyclo-
oxygenase activity (Mower et al.,1984, Landolfi et al.,
1984).

In vitro quercetin has a weak and not always reproducible (compare Beretz et al., 1982 a; Landolfi et
al.,1984 and our data) anti-aggregatory action on blood
platelets.
The reported IC_{50} values were: in rabbit PRP stimulated
with arachidonate - 40 μM (this paper; in cat PRP stimulated with arachidonate - >200 uM (our unpublished
data); in human washed platelets aggregated with collagen, ADP or thrombin 55 - 330 μM (Beretz et al.,1982 a)
in human PRP aggregated by arachidonate or collagen -
18 uM and 290 uM, respectively (Landolfi et al.,1984).
This feeble anti-aggregatory action of quercetin and
other flavonoids has been attributed to inhibition of
phosphodiesterase or to a direct effect of flavonoids on
calcium ion movements across platelet membrane (Beretz
et al.,1982 a; Beretz et al.,1982 b) as well as to inhibition of cyclo-oxygenase (e.g.flavone, phloretin)
(Mower et al.,1984; Landolfi et al.,1984). Theoretically, inhibition of phospholipase A_2 (Lee et al.,1982)
might be also considered. In contrast to leukocytes inhibition of platelet lipoxygenase by quercetin does not
seem to have any functional consequences in platelets
(Landolfi et al.,1984).

In light of the above findings one is bewildered
with the powerful anti-aggregatory action of quercetin
and rutin in vivo. We have shown that in extracorporeal
circulation of anaesthetized cats those two flavonols
inhibit platelet deposition on a collagen strip. The
anti-aggregatory action of quercetin and rutin occurs
at ID_{50} of 1.6 and 20.4 μg/kg,i.v., respectively, whereas acetylsalicylic acid requires the dose of 6840 μg/kg
i.v. to achieve the same degree of anti-aggregatory
action. The in vivo anti-aggregatory action of both flavonols is fully developed ten minutes after their intravenous injection and, then, it wanes within the next
2 - 3 hours. Troxerutin, a semisynthetic derivative of
rutin (Table 1) is by far less potent, however, its anti-aggregatory action seems to increase with time. An
explanation might be that troxerutin is slowly biotrans-
formed to an active flavonol (quercetin).

A rough calculation shows that following an intravenous injection of an active anti-aggregatory dose of
quercetin its peak plasma level will vary from 0.05 to
0.1 μM. At those concentrations quercetin is unlikely
to influence the activity of any of enzymes in platelets investigated so far. The closest in vitro effective concentration of quercetin is that for inhibition of
5-lipoxygenase in basophil leukemia cells (IC_{50}= 0.2 μM)
(Hope et al.,1983). There is no experimentally founded
explanation for a discrepancy between potent anti-aggregatory action of quercetin in vivo and its weak anti-
aggregatory action in vitro. One may speculate that in vivo
quercetin interrupts a biochemical link between leukocytes
and platelets on their lipoxygenase pathways (Marcus et
al., 1982; Maclouf,1983) or that quercetin prevents the
release or action of PAF-acether (Vargaftig et al.,1982).
Our working hypothesis is that in vivo anti-aggregatory
effect of flavonols is associated with an inhibition of
biochemical interaction of platelets with other cells
within circulatory system. Leukocytes deserve a special
attention.

REFERENCES

Baumann, J., and Bruchhausen, F., 1979, (+)-cyanidol-
    3 as inhibitor of prostaglandin synthetase.Stu-
    dies on renal medulla and liver of the rat in
    vitro and in vivo. Naunyn-Schmiedeberg's Arch.
    Pharmacol., 306:85.
Baumann, J., Bruchhausen, F., and Wurm, G., 1979, A stru-
    cture-activity study on the influence of phenolic
    compounds and bio-flavonoids on rat renal prosta-
    glandin synthetase, Naunyn-Schmiedeberg's Arch.
    Pharmacol., 307:73.
Baumann, J., Bruchhausen, F., and Wurm, G., 1980 a, Fla-
    vonoids and related compounds as inhibitors of
    arachidonic acid peroxidation, Prostaglandins,
    20:627.
Baumann, J., Wurm, G., and Bruchhausen, F., 1980 b, Hem-
    murg der Prostaglandin-Synthetase durch Flavono-
    ide und Phenolderiviate im Vergleich mit deren O_2-
    Radikalfängereigenschaften, Arch.Pharmazie, 313:
    330.
Beretz, A., Cazenave, J. P., and Anton, R., 1982 a, In-
    hibition of aggregation and secretion of human
    platelets by quercetin and other flavonoids:
    structure - activity relationship, Agents and
    Actions, 12:382.

Beretz, A., Stierle, A., Anton, R., and Cazenave, J. P., 1982 b, Role of cyclic AMP in the inhibition of human platelet aggregation by quercetin, a flavonoid that potentiates the effect of prostacyclin, Biochem. Pharmacol., 31:3597.

Cavallini, L., Bindoli, A., and Siliprandi, N., 1978, Comparative evaluation of antiperoxidative action of silymarin and other flavonoids, Pharmacol. Res. Commun., 10:133.

Dirks, R. C., Faiman, M. D., and Huyser, E. S., 1982, The role of lipid, free radical initiator and oxygen on the kinetics of lipid peroxidation, Toxicol. appl. Pharmacol., 63:21.

Duniec, Z., Robak, J., and Gryglewski, R. J., 1983, Antioxidant properties of some chemicals vs their influence on cyclooxygenase and lipoxidase activities, Biochem. Pharmacol., 32:2283.

Dutilh, C. E., Haddeman, E., and ten Hoor, F., 1980, Role of the arachidonate lipoxygenase pathway in blood platelets aggregation, in: Advances in Prostaglandin and Thromboxane Research, B. Samuelsson, P. W. Ramwell, and R. Paoletti, eds., Raven Press, New York, p 101.

Egan, R. W., Gale, P. H., Beveridge, G. C., Harnett, J., and Kuehl, F. A., 1980, Direct and indirect involvement of radical scavengers during prostaglandin biosynthesis, in: Advances in Prostaglandin and Thromboxane Research, B.Samuelsson, P. W. Ramwell, and R. Paoletti, eds., Raven Press, New York, p 153.

Fiebrich, F., Koch, H., 1979, Silymarin an inhibitor of lipoxygenase, Experientia, 35:1548.

Griffiths, R. J., Lofts, F. J., and Moore, P. K., 1983, The effects of drugs on the synthesis of 6-oxo-prostaglandin E_1, Brit. J. Pharmac., 78:51P.

Gryglewski, R. J., Bunting, S., Moncada, S., Flower, R. J., and Vane, J. R., Arterial walls are protected against deposition of platelet thrombi by a substance (Prostaglandin X) which they make from prostaglandin endoperoxides, Prostaglandins, 12:685, 1976.

Gryglewski, J. R., Korbut, R., Ocetkiewicz, A., and Stachura J.1978, In vivo method for quantitation of anti-platelet potency of drugs, Naunyn-Schmiedeberg's Arch.Pharmacol, 302:25.

Hammarström, S., and Diczfalusy, U., 1980, Biosynthesis of thromboxanes, in: Advances in Prostaglandins and Thromboxane Research, B.Samuelsson, P. W. Ramwell, and R. Paoletti, eds., Raven Press, New York, p267.

Havsteen, B., 1983, Flavonoids, a class of natural products of high pharmacological potency, <u>Biochem. Pharmacol.</u>, 32:1141.

Hope, W. C., Welton, A. F., Fiedler-Nagy, C., Batula-Bernardo, C., and Coffey, J.W., 1983, In vitro inhibition of the biosynthesis of slow reacting substance of anaphylaxis (SRS-A) and lipoxygenase activity by quercetin, <u>Biochem. Pharmacol.</u>, 32:367.

Kuehl, F. A., Humes, J. L., Egan, R. W., Ham, E. A., Beveridge, G. C., Van Arman, C. G., 1977, Role of prostaglandin endoperoxide PGG_2 in inflammatory process, <u>Nature</u>, 265:170.

Kulmacz, R. J., and Lands, E. M., Characteristics of prostaglandin H synthese, <u>in</u>: Advances in Prostaglandin, Thromboxane and Leukotriene Research, B. Samuelsson, R. Paoletti, and P. W. Ramwell, Raven Press, New York, 1983, p 93.

Landolfi, R., Mower, R. L., and Steiner, M., 1984, <u>Biochem. Pharmacol.</u>, 33:1525.

Lee, T. P., Mateliano, M. L., and Middleton, E., Effect of quercetin on human polymorphonuclear leukocyte lysosomal enzyme release and phospholipid metabolism, 1982, <u>Life Sci</u>, 31:2765.

Maclouf, J., Fruteau de Laclos, B., and Borgeat, P., 1983, Effects of 12-hydroxy and 12-hydroperoxy 5,8,10,14-eicosatetraenoic acids on the synthesis of 5-hydroxy-6,8,11,14-eicosatetraenoic acid and leukotriene B_4 in human blood leukocytes, <u>in</u>: Advances in Prostaglandin, Thromboxane and Leukotriene Research, B. Samuelsson, R. Paoletti, and P. W. Ramwell, eds., Raven Press, New York, p 159.

Marcus, A. J., Brockman, J., Safier, L. B., Ullman, H. L., and Islam, N., 1982, Formation of leukotrienes and other hydroxy acids during platelet-neutrophil interactions in vitro, <u>Biochem. Biophys. Res. Commun.</u>, 109:130.

Moore, P. K., Griffiths, R. J., and Lofts, F. J., 1983, The effects of some flavone drugs on the conversion of prostacyclin to 6-oxo-prostaglandin E_1, <u>Biochem. Pharmacol.</u>, 32:2813.

Mower, R. L., Landolfi, R., and Steiner, M., 1984, Inhibition in vitro of platelet aggregation and arachidonic acid metabolism by flavone, <u>Biochem. Pharmacol.</u>, 33:257.

Pollock, J., and Heath, H., 1975, Studies on the effects of $\beta\beta$-iminadiproprionitrile and b-(β-hydroxyethyl)-rutoside on ADP-activated aggregation of rat platelets in relation to the development of diabetic microangiopathy, <u>Biochem.Pharmacol.</u>, 24:397.

Robak, J., and Duniec, Z., 1980, The influence of chlor-
promazine on lipoxidases, Biophys. Biochim. Acta,
620:59.
Robak, J., and Duniec, Z., 1982, The influence of some
3-amino-2-pyrazoline derivatives on cyclooxygenase and lipoxidase activities, Biochem. Pharmacol., 31:1955.
Robak, J., Duniec, Z., Grodzińska, L., and Zachwieja,
Z., 1981, The influence of some cinnamic acid
derivatives on cyclooxygenase and lipoxidase activities, Pol. J. Pharmacol. Pharm., 33:521.
Sams, A. R., Sprecher, H., Sankarppa, S. K., and Needleman, P., 1982, Selective inhibitors of platelet
arachidonic acid metabolism: aggregation independent of lipoxygenase, in: Leukotrienes and
other Lipoxygenase Products, B. Samuelsson, and
R. Paoletti, eds., Raven Press, New York, p 19.
Sekiya, K., and Okuda, H., 1982, Selective inhibition
of platelet lipoxygenase by baicalein, Biochem.
Biophys. Res. Commun., 105:1090.
Sekiya, K., Okuda, H., and Arichi, S., 1982, Selective
inhibition of platelet lipoxygenase by exculetin,
Biophys. Biochim. Acta, 713:68.
Sun, F. F., McGuire, J. C., Wallach, D. P., and Brown,
V. R., 1980, Study on the property and inhibi-
tion of human platelet arachidonic acid 12-lipo-
xygenase, in: Advances in Prostaglandin and
Thromboxane Research, B. Samuelsson, P. W. Ram-
well, and R. Paoletti, eds., Raven Press, New
York, p 111.
Święs, J., Dąbrowski, L., Duniec, Z., Michalska, Z.,
Robak, J., and Gryglewski, R. J., 1984, Anti-
aggregatory effects of flavonoids in vivo and
their influence on lipoxygenase and cyclooxyge-
nase in vitro, Pol. J. Pharmacol. Pharm.,in press.
Tauber, A. J., Fay, J. R., and Marletta, M. A., 1984,
Flavonoid inhibition of the human neutrophil
NADPH-oxidase, Biochem. Pharmacol., 33:1367.
Vargaftig, B. B., Chignard, H., Lefort, J., Wal, F.,
le Couedic, J. P., and Benveniste, J., 1982,
Platelet aggregation independent of prostaglandin formation: Pharmacological properties and
the hypothetical role of platelet activating
factor, in: Cardiovascular Pharmacology of the
Prostaglandins, A. G. Herman, P. M. Vanhoutte,
H. Denolin, and A. Goossens, eds., Raven Press,
New York, p 161.
Vargas, J. R., Radomski, M., and Moncada, S., 1982, The
use of prostacyclin in the separation from plasma
and washing of human platelets, Prostaglandins,
23:929.

TRANSFORMATION OF 15-HYDROPEROXYEICOSAPENTAENOIC ACID INTO MONO-

AND DIHYDROXYEICOSAPENTAENOIC ACIDS BY HUMAN PLATELETS

Bing Lam, Ewa Marcinkiewicz** and Patrick Y-K Wong*+

Department of Pharmacology
New York Medical College
Valhalla, New York   10595

SUMMARY

[1-^{14}C]-15-hydroperoxyeicosapentaenoic acid was incubated with suspensions of washed human platelets. Two dihydroxy and one mono-hydroxy metabolites were isolated and purified by RP-HPLC and SP-HPLC. GC/MS analysis revealed that the three metabolites were: 8,15-dihydroxyeicosapentaenoic acid, 14,15-dihydroxyeicosapenta-enoic acid and 15-hydroxyeicosapentaenoic acid. In addition, the non-enzymatic generation of an allylic hydroxy-epoxide metabolite (13-hydroxy-14,15-epoxyeicosapentaenoic acid) was identified. Furthermore, 15-HEPE was demonstrated to be a potent inhibitor of f-MLP-induced neutrophil aggregation. Thus, transformation of the 15-lipoxygenase product of eicosapentaenoic acid by platelets may generate biologically active compounds that modulate neutrophil function.

Abbreviations Used: EPA, 5,8,11,14,17-eicosapentaenoic acid; 15-HPEPE, 15-hydroperoxyeicosapentaenoic acid; 15-HPETE, 15-hydroper-oxyeicosatetraenoic acid; 15-HEPE, 15-hydroxyeicosapentaenoic acid; 15-HETE, 15-hydroxyeicosatetraenoic acid; LTC, 5(S)-hydroxy-6(R)-S-glutathionyl-7,9-trans-11,14-cis-eicosapentaenoic acid; HPLC, high performance liquid chromatography; RP, reverse-phase; SP, straight-phase; PMNL, polymorphonuclear leukocytes; f-MLP, N-formyl-L-methionyl-L-leucyl-L-phenylalanine.

*Recipient of NIH Research Career Development Award (HL-00811)
+To whom all correspondence should be addressed
**Polish-U.S. Scientific Exchange Fellow

INTRODUCTION

Eicosapentaenoic acid (EPA) has been shown to be a substrate for cyclo-oxygenase on the synthesis of the trienoic series of prostaglandins, thromboxane and prostacyclin (1,2). Recently, Ochi et al. demonstrated that EPA was also a better substrate for the 5-lipoxygenase in guinea-pig peritoneal polymorphonuclear leukocytes (PMNL) for the synthesis of 5-hydroperoxy-6,8,11,14,17-eicosapentaenoic acid (5-HPEPE), a precursor for leukotrienes A_5 and B_5 (3,4).

It has been reported that EPA can be incorporated into cell membrane phospholipids similarly to arachidonic acid and other polyunsaturated fatty acids (5) which, upon stimulation, can be released and utilized by 5-lipoxygenase to yield pentaene 5-lipoxygenase products (6). In the presence of exogenous EPA, mouse mastocytoma cells challenged with ionophore A-23187 generated LTC_5 and LTB_5 in addition to LTC_4 and LTB_4 (6,7). LTC_5 was found to be equipotent to LTC_4 in contracting guinea-pig pulmonary parenchymal strips and ileal tissues (8). However, LTB_5 was 30- to 60-fold less potent than LTB_4 in eliciting neutrophil chemotaxis. Recently, it has been shown that EPA and its oxygenated products inhibit LTB_4 formation, the site of its inhibitory action being perhaps at the level of LTA_4-hydrolase (9). Although there are intensive studies of metabolism of EPA via the cyclo-oxygenase and the 5-lipoxygenase pathways in neutrophils and other cellular systems, the biotransformation of EPA via 15-lipoxygenase pathways is still unknown. In this communication we describe the biotransformation of 15-hydroperoxyeicosapentaenoic acid (15-HPEPE) by human platelets.

MATERIALS AND METHODS

Materials

[1-^{14}C]-EPA (specific activity, 55 mCi/nmole) was purchased from New England Nuclear, Boston, MA.,5,8,11,14,17-eicosapentaenoic acid and soybean lipoxygenase I (EC 1,13,11,12) were purchased from Sigma Co. Eicosapentaenoate ethyl ester was a generous gift from Dr. Y. Tamura, Chiba University, Chiba, Japan. Platelet concentrates were obtained from Hudson Valley Blood Services, Valhalla, N.Y.

Preparation of 15-HPEPE

15-HEPE was generated by incubation of [1-^{14}C]-EPA (20 µCi/10 µM) with soybean lipoxygenase I similarly to the preparation of 15-HPETE as described by Hamberg and Samuelsson (10). After diethyl ether extraction, the 15-HPEPE was purified by silicic acid column chromatography (CC-7, Mallinkrodt, St. Louis, MO) as described (10). The sample was applied to the column in 2 ml of diethyl ether/hexane (5/95, v/v) and the hydroperoixde of EPA was wluted

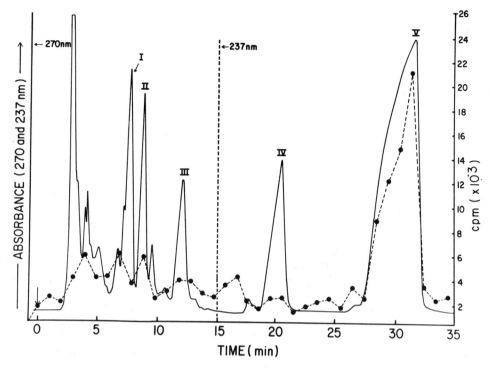

Fig.1. RP-HPLC chromatogram of [1-14C]-HPEPE metabolites isolated after incubation of human platelets and [1-14C]-HPEPE. Solid line (———————) shows U.V. absorption at 270 nm and 237 nm. Broken line (------) shows radioactivity in each fraction estimated by liquid scintillation counting.

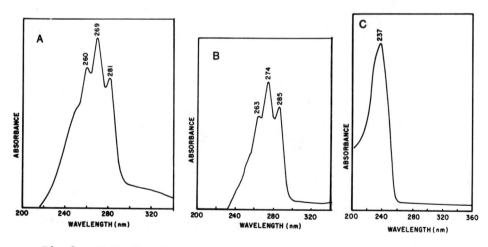

Fig.2. U.V. Spectra of compound I (A), III (B) and V (C).

with diethyl ether/hexane (15/85, v/v). The chromatographically pure material was stored in absolute ethanol at -70°C. The identity and purity of the product was determined by co-chromatography with 15-HPETE on TLC using a solvent system:diethyl ether:petroleum ether:acetic acid (50/50/0.05, v/v) (11) and by RP-HPLC after reduction to 15-HPETE with sodium borohydride (12).

Preparation of Washed Platelets and Incubation

Newly expired human platelets (5 to 10 units) were centrifuged at 600 x g for 20 min. The platelet pellets were resuspended in 25 ml of saline Tris buffer (0.15 M NaCl at pH 7.4; 25 mM Tris-HCl; 0.2 mM EDTA). These platelet suspensions were centrifuged for 20 min at 650 x g.

The final pellet of washed platelets was resuspended in Dulbecco's phosphate buffered saline, pH 7.4, to a final platelet count of 1.5×10^6 platelets/μl. Indomethacin (10 μM) was added to the platelets before incubation with 15-HPEPE. After pre-warming the platelet suspension to 37°C, 15-HPEPE was added to a final concentration of 150 μM and incubated for 30 min at 37°C with constant shaking. The amount of ethanol needed to dissolve 15-HPEPE never exceeded 0.1% of the incubation volume. The incubation was terminated by the addition of two volumes of ethanol.

Extraction and Purification

The incubation precipitate was filtered, and the ethanolic filtrate was evaportaed to dryness. The residue was dissolved in 5 ml of distilled water and acidified to pH 3.5 with 1 N HCl. The solution was then extracted with 10 volumes of ethyl acetate. The ethyl acetate fraction was rotor evaporated to dryness under vacuum. The residue was dissolved in 200 μl of solvent A and separated by HPLC on a Waters' Associates Dual Pump System equipped with a RP ultrasphere ODS column (C_{18}-ODS, 5μ, 4.6 mm x 25 cm, Beckman, Palo Alto, CA), a U-6K injector and a 481 variable wavelength detector. The products were eluted with a linear gradient of methanol/water/acetic acid (50:50:0.05, v/v) (solvent A) to methanol (solvent B) for 45 min at a flow rate of 1 ml/min (13). Column effluents were monitored with a Waters' Associates 481 λmax variable wavelength detector set at 270 (0 to 14 min) and 237 nm (14 to 45 min). Fractions of 1 ml were simultaneously collected with an on-line fraction collector and a portion of each fraction was removed for estimation of recovered radioactivity.

PGB_2 and 15-HETE were used as standards for di-HETEs and mono-HETEs. The day-to-day variations in retention times were determined to be less than 5%.

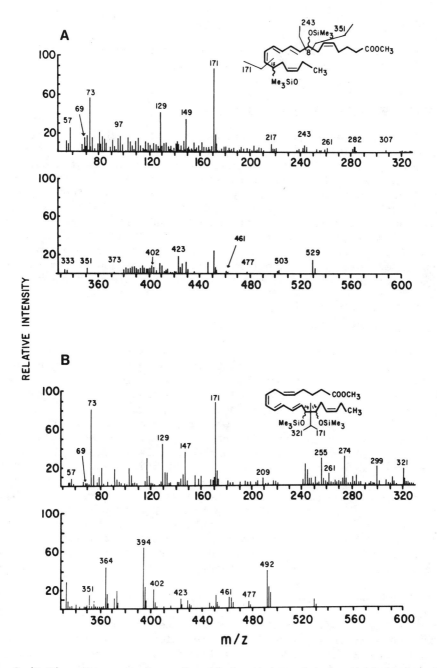

Fig.3 (A,B). Mass spectra of methyl ester and trimethylsilylated products of compound I (8,15-DHEPE); compound III (14,15-DHEPE); isolated from RP-HPLC and purified by SP-HPLC.

U.V. Spectroscopy

Samples eluted from the HPLC were rotor evaporated to dryness, dissolved in absolute ethanol and examined with a Hewlett-Packard 8450-A UV/Vis spectrophotometer.

Gas-Chromatography-Mass-Spectrometry

The methyl ester of compounds I to V (Fig. 1) (10 µg each) were converted to trimethylsilyl ethers by addition of 25 µl of pyridine followed by 50 µl of trimethylchlorosilane and 50 µl of hexamethyl-disilazane (Supelco). The mixtures were kept at room temperature for 20 min and evaporated to dryness with N_2. Next, the samples were dissolved in hexane (25 µl) and injected into the gas-chromato-graph-mass-spectrometer (Hewlett-Packard 5895-B) equipped with a glass column (1.5 cm x 4 mm) packed with 1% SE-30 on chromosorb W (HP), 80/100 mesh. The helium flow was set at 40 ml/min, with the oven temperature, injection temperature and ion source temperature set at 200, 260 and 200°C, respectively. The electron energy was set at 70 eV.

Neutrophil Aggregation

Neutrophils were obtained from Wistar rats 24 hours after an intra-peritoneal injection of an 8% casein solution. Contaminating red blood cells were removed by hypotonic lysis. The cells were washed in 0.9% saline before being resuspended at 15 x 10^6 cells/ml in Hank's Balanced Salt Solution containing Ca^{2+} (1.5 mM) and Mg^{2+} (0.7 mM). Neutrophils (0.5 ml) were pipetted into siliconized glass cuvettes containing stirring bars. Aggregation studies were performed in a Payton Dual Aggregation Module (Buffalo, N.Y.). Dose-response curves to the agonist f-MLP (dissolved in Tris buffer) were performed before each experiment and the lowest concentration of f-MLP producing maximal aggregation was used to test the inhibi-tory effects of the metabolites of 15-HPETE and 15-HPEPE (dissolved in minimal amounts of ethanol and diluted in Tris buffer). Total additions of f-MLP and inhibitors never exceeded a volume of 5 µl. The final ethanol concentration was always less than 0.1% and had no effect on neutrophil aggregation.

RESULTS AND DISCUSSION

RP-HPLC analysis of the ethyl acetate extract of human plate-lets incubated with [^{14}C]-15-HPEPE revealed five major products (Fig. 1, solid line). The radioactivity of each fraction indicated that these metabolites were derived from [1-^{14}C]-15-HPEPE. All five components (compounds I to V) were subsequently isolated and dried under N_2. The residue of each fraction was methylated with excess diazomethane for 20 min at room temperature. The methyl esters of compounds I to V were further purified by SP-HPLC using

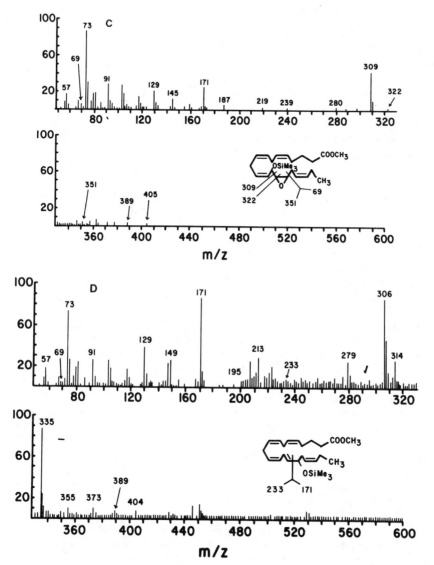

Fig.3 (C,D). Mass spectra of methyl ester and trimethylsilylated products of compound IV (13-Oh,14,15,epoxide-EPA) and compound V (15-HEPE) isolated from RP-HPLC and purified by SP-HPLC.

a step gradient of solvent I (hexane:isopropanol:acetic acid, 990: 10:0.1, v/v) and II (hexane:isopropanol:acetic acid, 940:60:0.2; v/v) as described (14). Compounds I and II were combined, methylated and separated by SP-HPLC into 2 major and 5 minor components. Two major compounds, Ia and Ib, had retention times of 38.6 and 40.6 min, respectively. The five minor compounds demonstrated by SP-HPLC had retention times of 29.5, 31.0 and 32.8, 34.2 and 37.2 min. Compounds Ia Me and Ib Me displayed a conjugated triene U.V. spectrum with λ_{MAX}^{EtOH}=269.5nm with shoulders at 260 and 281nm (Fig.2A). All five minor components displayed similar U.V. spectra indicating that they are probably stereoisomers of compounds Ia and Ib. The methyl ester trimethylsilyl derivatives of compounds Ia and Ib were analyzed by gas-chromatography and mass-spectrometry. Compounds Ia and Ib showed equivalent chain lengths (C-value) of 23.1 and 23.6, respectively. Their mass-spectra were identical and were characterized by the major ion at M/Z:492 [M^+], 477 [M-15], 461 [M-31], 423 [M-69, loss of CH_2 $(CH_2)_2$ CH_3], 402 [M-90, loss of Me_3SIO], 351 [$M-CH_2$ $(CH)_2$ $(CH_2)_3$ $COOCH_3$], 243 [loss of $CH_3SiO-CH_2$ $(CH)_2$ $(CH_2)_3$ $COOCH_3$], 171 [base peak, loss of $Me_3SiO-CH_2$ $(CH)_2$ $(CH_2)_2$ CH_3] and 69 [loss of CH_2 $(CH)_2$ $(CH_2)_2$ CH_3] (Fig.3A).

The major hydroxyl groups were identified at C-8 and C-15 based on the following ions of 171, 321 and 423 (M-69], suggesting the fragmentation of C_{17} to C_{20} with a C_{17-18} double bond of EPA. Thus, based on the GC/MS and U.V. data, compounds Ia and Ib were identified as 8,15-dihydroxyeicosapentaenoic acid (8,15-DHEPE).

The methyl ester of compound III was analyzed similarly by SP-HPLC. Two major components, compounds IIIa and IIIb, with retention times of 33.0 and 39.2 min, respectively, were isolated and purified. Their U.V. absorption spectra were identical with λ_{MAX}^{EtOH}=273.5nm with shoulders at 263 and 285nm (Fig.2B). Using gas chromatography the methyl ester trimethylsilyl ether of compounds IIIa and IIIb showed a C-value of 24.1 and 24.6, respectively. Their mass-spectra were identical with major ions at M/Z:492 [M^+], 477 [M-15], 461 [M-31], 423 [M-69], 421 [M-71], 402 [M-90], 351 [M-141, loss of CH_2 $(CH)_2$ $(CH_2)_3$ $COOCH_3$], 261 [M-(141+90)], 394 [rearrangement ion of C-1 to C-14, $Me_3SiO-CH$ $(CH)_6$ CH_2 $(CH)_2$ $(CH_2)_3$ $C-OMeO$ $SiMe_3$)] (17), 321 [M-171] and 171 [base peak, loss of $Me_3SiO-CH_2$ $(CH)_2$ CH_2CH_3]. The position of the hydroxy groups at C-14 and 15 were determined by ions appearing at M/Z, 171 and 321 as well as the rearrangement ion of 394, a characteristic ion of 14,15-dihydroxy compounds (17,18). Based on the U.V. absorption spectra and the GC/MS data, it is concluded that compounds IIa and IIb were 14,15-dihydroxyeicosapentaenoic acid (14,15-DHEPE) (Fig.3B).

Compound IV, which displayed a U.V. spectrum of λ^{EtOH}_{MAX}=237nm, was derivatized to trimethylsilyl methyl ester as described above. GC revealed that the trimethylsilyl methyl ester derivative had a C-value of 22.8.

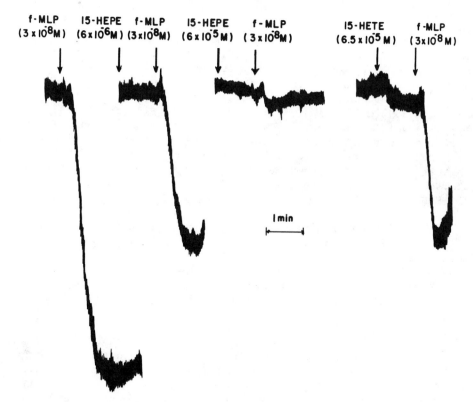

Fig.4. Bioassay of compound V (15-HEPE) on neutrophil aggregation induced by f-MLP as compared to 15-HETE.

The mass spectrum showed prominent ions at M/Z: 405 [M-15], 389 [M-31], 351 [M-69], 322 [M-C(CH-OSiMe3) - (CH)$_2$ CH$_2$ (CH)$_2$ CH$_2$ (CH)$_2$ - (CH$_2$)$_3$ - COOCH$_3$], 309 [Major ion, M - CH - OSiMe3 (CH)$_2$ CH$_2$ (CH)$_2$ CH$_2$ (CH)$_2$ (CH$_2$)$_3$ - COOCH$_3$], 219, 142, 73 and 69.

Although the molecular ion was not observed in the mass spectrum, the molecular weight was deduced to be 420 by the presence of ions at 405 [M-15] and 389 [M-317]. Ions at 351 and 69 indicated the cleavage at C_{15-16} with the loss of the fragment of C_{16-20} containing an W-3 double bond (17). According to the RP-HPLC and SP-HPLC retention times, C-value and mass spectrum compound IV was identified as 13-hydroxy-14,15-epoxy-5,8,11,17-eicosapentaenoic acid which is analogous to the 13-hydroxy-14,15-epoxy-5,8,11-eicosatetraenoic acid derived from 15-HPETE as reported by Bryant et al. and Narumiya et al. (17,18) (Fig. 3C).

The methyl ester of compound V, after purification by SP-HPLC (retention time 12.5 min), was further derivatized to trimethyl-silyl methyl ester and analyzed by GC/MS. With gas-chromatography, compound IV displayed a C-value of 21.6 suggesting that it was a mono-hydroxy fatty acid. The U.V. spectrum showed a $\lambda_{MAX}^{EtOH} = 237$ nm suggesting a pair of conjugated double bonds (14). The mass-spectrum of compound IV was characterized by major ions at M/Z: 404 [M+], 389 [M-15], 373 [M-31], 335 [M-69], 314 [M-90], 233 [M-171] and 171 [base peak]. The mass spectrum of compound IV was similar to that of 15-HETE except that there were two mass-units less due to the presence of a W-3 double bond in 15-HPEPE. Taking together its U.V. spectrum, MS spectrum and RP-HPLC and SP-HPLC data, compound V was identified as 15-hydroxyeicosapentaenoic acid (15-HEPE) (Fig. 3D).

The biological activity of 15-HEPE was examined with neutrophil aggregation. 15-HEPE displayed potent inhibition on f-MLP induced neutrophil aggregation at low micromolar concentrations (Fig. 4) (0.5 to 5 μM, IC_{50} = 4.7 μM) (19). Furthermore, our studies demonstrated that 15-HEPE is at least tenfold more potent than 15-HETE on the inhibition of neutrophil aggregation (Figs. 4A,B,C,D) (19).

This report describes the formation of a new group of mono- and di-hydroxy compounds derived from 15-HPEPE in human platelets. Their structural elucidations were based on their chromatographic behavior on RP-HPLC, SP-HPLC, U.V. spectrum, C-values and finally by GC/MS. Although there are four isomers of 14,15-DHEPE and at least 7 isomers of 8,15-DHEPE, only two major isomers of the 8,15-

DHEPE were identified by GC/MS at this time; all the other isomers were only detected by SP-HPLC and U.V. spectroscopy. Due to their thermal instability, GC/MS analysis must wait for the availability

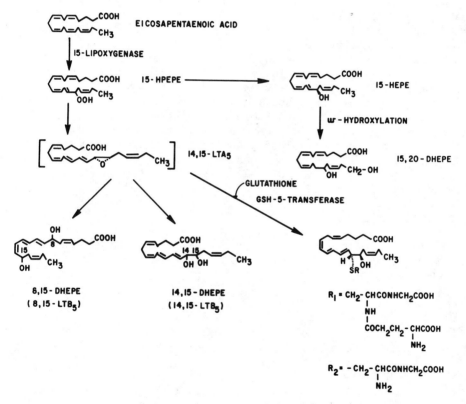

Fig.5. Proposed metabolic pathway of EPA by 15-lipoxygenase.

of larger quantities of each isomer. The stereo-chemistry of the conjugated double bonds and hydroxy-groups of 8,15-DHEPE and 14,15-DHEPE, as well as their biological activities, are now being examined in this laboratory.

It is interesting to note that 15-HEPE is a potent inhibitor of neutrophil aggregation induced by f-MLP. 15-HETE has been shown to be an inhibitor of other lipoxygenases including the 12-lipoxygenase in platelets and 5-lipoxygenase in PMNL (20). In a certain experimental model, 15-HETE has been shown to inhibit the inflammatory response by blocking the synthesis of the chemotactic agent LTB$_4$ by PMNL (21). Furthermore, the general anti-lipoxygenase action of 15-HETE was proposed to be functionally important in the control of the level of inflammatory mediators (22) (Fig.5).

In this study, we demonstrated that 15-HEPE was the major metabolite of 15-HPEPE in human platelets and exhibited a more potent biological activity than 15-HETE on neutrophil aggregation as provoked by the chemotactic peptide f-MLP. In addition to PMNL, it has been demonstrated that 15-lipoxygenase activity also exists in human platelets (23). Thus, it is possible that during nutritional manipulation, diets enriched in EPA may result in the change of the biological spectra of eicosanoids derived from platelets and other cell types. Therefore, diets enriched in 20:5W-3 polyunsaturated fatty acids may result in the generation of substances which can lower blood pressure (24), reduce the incidence of myocardial infarctions and render platelets less sensitive to aggregatory stimuli (24), as well as to delay the onset of certain auto-immune diseases (25).

ACKNOWLEDGMENTS

We wish to thank Dr. Y. Tamura of Chiba University, Japan, for ethyl ester of eicosapentaenoic acid. This work was supported by NIH grant HL-25316-05.

REFERENCES

1. P. Needleman, A. Raz, M. S. Minkes, J. A. Ferrendelli, H. Sprecher, Triene prostaglandins: prostacyclin and thromboxane biosynthesis and unique biological properties, Proc. Natl. Acad. Sci. 76:944 (1979).
2. M. O. Whitaker, A. Wyche, F. Fitzpatrick, H. Sprecher and P. Needleman, Triene prostaglandins: prostaglandin D3 and eicosapentaenoic acid as potential antithrombotic substances, Proc. Natl. Acad. Sci. 76:5919 (1979).
3. K. Ochi, T. Yoshimoto, S. Yamamoto, K. Taniguchi and T. Miyamoto, Arachidonate 5-lipoxygenase of guinea-pig peritoneal polymorphonuclear leukocytes. Activation by adenosine, J. Biol. Chem. 258:5754 (1983).

4. R. C. Murphy, W. C. Pickett, B. R. Culp and W. E. M. Lands, Tetraene and pentaene leukotrienes: selective production from murine mastocytoma cells after dietary manipulation, Prostaglandins 22:613 (1981).

5. T. W. Weiner and H. Sprecher, Arachidonic acid 5,8,11-eicosatetrienoic acid and 5,8,11,14,17-eicosapentaenoic acid. Dietary manipulation of the levels of these acids in rat liver and platelet phospholipids and their incorporation into human platelet lipids, Biochim. Biophys. Acta 792: 293 (1984).

6. S. Hammarstrom, Biochim. Biophys. Acta 663:575 (1981).

7. L. Orning, R. Bernstrom and S. Hammarstrom, Formation of leukotrienes E_3, E_4 and E_5 in rat basophilic leukemia cells, Eur. J. Biochem. 120:41 (1981).

8. A. G. Leitch, T. H. Lee, E. W. Ringel, J. D. Prickett, D. R. Robinson, E. J. Corey, J. M. Drazen, K. F. Austen and R. A. Lewis, Immunologically induced generation of tetraene and pentaene leukotrienes in peritoneal cavities of menhaden-fed rats, J. Immunol. 132:2559 (1984).

9. S. M. Prescott, The effect of eicosapentaenoic acid on leukotriene B production by human neutrophils, J. Biol. Chem., 242:5329 (1967).

10. M. Hamberg and B. Samuelsson, On the specificity of the oxygenation of unsaturated fatty acids catalyzed by soybean lipoxidase, J. Biol. Chem. 242:5329 (1967).

11. G. Graff, Preparation of 15-L-hydroperoxy-5,8,11,13-eicosatetraenoic acid (15-HPETE), in: "Methods in Enzymology," W. E. M. Lands and W. L. Smith, eds., Academic Press, New York (1982).

12. M. Hamberg and B. Samuelsson, Prostaglandin endoperoxides. Novel transformations of arachidonic acid in human platelets, Proc. Natl. Acad. Sci. 71:3400 (1974).

13. F. F. Sun and J. C. McGuire, Characterization of the enzymatic reactions that lead to the synthesis of leukotriene B_4, Biochim. Biophys. Acta 794:56 (1984).

14. P. Y-K Wong, P. Westlund, M. Hamberg, E. Granstrom, P. H-W Chao and B. Samuelsson, ω-Hydroxylation of 12-L-hydroxy-5,8,10,14-eicosatetraenoic acid in human polymorphonuclear leukocytes, J. Biol. Chem. 259:2683 (1984).

15. R. W. Bryant and J. M. Bailey, Rearrangement of 15-hydroperoxy-eicosatetraenoic acid (15-HPETE) during incubations with hemoglobin: a model for platelet lipoxygenase metabolism, Proc. Lipid Res. 20:279 (1981).

16. S. Marumiya, J. S. Salmon, F. H. Cottee, B. C. Weatherley and R. J. Flower, Arachidonic acid 15-lipoxygenase from rabbit peritoneal polymorphonuclear leukocytes. Partial purification and properties, J. Biol. Chem. 256:9583 (1981).

17. G. Eglington, D. H. Hunneman and A. McCormick, in: "Organic Mass Spectrometry," Academic Press, New York (1968).

18. W. Jubiz, O. Radmark, J. K. Lindgren, C. Malmsten and B. Samuelsson, Novel leukotrienes: products formed by initial oxygenation of arachidonic acid at C-15, Biochem. Biophys. Res. Commun. 99:976 (1981).

19. P. Y-K Wong, R. A. Hughes and B. Lam, Lipoxene: A new group of trihydroxy pentaene of eicosapentaenoic acid derived from porcine leukocytes, Biochem. Biophys. Res. Commun., submitted (1984).

20. J. Y. Vanderhoek, R. W. Bryant and J. M. Bailey, Inhibition of leukotriene biosynthesis by the leukocyte product 15-hydroxy-5,8,11,13-eicosatetraenoic acid, J. Biol. Chem. 255:10064 (1980).

21. J. Y. Vanderhoek, R. W. Bryant and J. M. Bailey, 15-hydroxy-5,8,11,13-eicosatetraenoic acid: a potent and selective inhibitor of platelet lipoxygenase, J. Biol. Chem. 255: 5996 (1980).

22. J. M. Bailey, R. W. Bryant, C. E. Low, M. B. Pupillo and J. Y. Vanderhoek, Regulation of T-lymphocyte mitogenesis by the leukocyte product 15-hydroxy-eicosatetraenoic acid (15-HETE), J. Cell. Immunol. 67:112 (1982).

23. P. Y-K Wong, P. Westlund, E. Granstrom, M. Hamberg, P. H-W Chao and B. Samuelsson, Effects of bradykinin (BK) on the metabolism of arachidonic acid (AA) in human platelets and polymorphonuclear leukocytes: Formation of 15-lipoxygenase products, Thromb. Haemostas. 50:389 (1983).

24. J. Dyerberg, H. O. Bang, E. Stofferson, S. Moncada and J. R. Vane, Eicosapentaenoic acid and prevention of thrombosis and atherosclerosis, Lancet 2:117 (1978).

25. J. D. Prickett, D. R. Robinson and A. D. Steinberg, Dietary enrichment with the polyunsaturated fatty acid eicosapentaenoic acid prevents proteinuria and prolongs survival in NZBXNZW F1 mice, J. Clin. Invest. 68:556 (1981).

METABOLISM OF ARACHIDONIC ACID BY 12- AND 15-LIPOXYGENASES IN

HUMAN PLATELETS AND POLYMORPHONUCLEAR LEUKOCYTES

Patrick Y-K Wong+*, Par Westlund, Mats Hamberg,
Elisabeth Granstrom, Patricia H-W Chao
and Bengt Samuelsson

+*Department of Pharmacology
New York Medical College
Valhalla, NY 10595
Department of Physiological Chemistry
Karolinska Institutet
S-104 01 Stockholm, Sweden

SUMMARY

The metabolism of arachidonic acid by human polymorphonuclear leukocytes and indomethacin-treated washed human platelets was investigated. $[1-^{14}C]$-arachidonic acid (AA) was extensively converted to mono-HETEs and DHETEs in these cell types. These mono-HETEs and DHETEs were identified as oxidative products of AA via the 12- and 15-lipoxygenase pathways and DHETEs were exclusively generated from 15-lipoxygenase pathway. Incubation of AA or $12-L_s$-hydroxy-5, 8, 10, 14-eicosatetraenoic acid (12-HETE) with suspensions of human polymorphonuclear leukocytes led to the formation of $12-L_s$, 20-dihydroxy-5, 8, 10, 14-eicosatetraenoic acid (12, 20-DHETE). The structure of this new metabolite was assigned by physical methods and by chemical degradation. Thus, during platelet and leukocyte interaction, "transcellular metabolism" of various lipoxygenase products of AA may generate new compounds of biological importance.

INTRODUCTION

In 1974, Hamberg and Samuelsson discovered that human platelet lipoxygenase catalyzes the conversion of arachidonic acid into $12-L_s$-hydroperoxy-5, 8, 10, 14-eicosatetraenoic acid (12-HPETE) which is rapidly reduced to 12-HETE (1). However, the metabolic fate of this compound has not been further clarified. Human poly-morphonuclear leukocytes (HPMNL) possess an enzyme system that
+All corespondence should be sent to this address

catalyzes the ω-hydroxylation of leukotrienes and leukotriene-related compounds (2). Thus, "transcellular metabolism" of platelet lipoxygenase products by the leukocyte ω-hydroxylase may generate new compounds during platelet-leukocyte interactions.

Recently, various triene metabolites of arachidonic acid or 15-hydroperoxyeicosatetraenoic acid (15-HPETE) were discovered after incubation with human platelets and leukocytes (3, 4). Four DHETEs were isolated and assigned the structures 14, 15-dihydroxy-5, 8, 10, 12-eicosatetraenoic acid (14, 15-DHETE, two isomers) and 8, 15-dihydroxy-5, 9, 11, 13-eicosatetraenoic acid (8, 15-DHETE, two isomers). These trienes were proposed to be derived from 14, 15-LTA$_4$ which in turn is formed from 15-HPETE (5). Furthermore, these conjugated trienes have been tentatively identified after incubation with dihomo-γ-linolenic acid (6). These reports suggest the possible occurrence of a 15-lipoxygenase in human platelets. However, the conversion of exogenous arachidonic acid into 14, 15- and 8, 15-DHETE via the 15-lipoxygenase pathway in human platelets has not been conclusively demonstrated. The present paper is concerned with the following observations: (1) the isolation and identification of a novel metabolite of arachidonic acid formed by sequential action of platelet lipoxygenase and the ω-hydroxylation system of polymorphonuclear leukocytes during platelet and leukocyte interaction; (2) the isolation and identification of seven 15-lipoxygenase metabolites in human platelets, i.e.: 15-HETE, 14, 15-DHETE (three isomers) and 8, 15-DHETE (three isomers). Thus, the presence of a 15-lipoxygenase activity in human platelets can be conclusively established.

MATERIALS AND METHODS

Cell Preparation and Incubations

Human leukocytes obtained from peripheral blood were prepared as previously described by Borgeat et al. (8). The cell preparations were contaminated with platelets (7) and with mononuclear leukocytes. The leukocytes were suspended in Dulbecco's phosphate buffered saline (PBS), pH 7.4, and adjusted to 100 x 10^6 cells/ml. The viability of the cells as measured by the trypan blue exclusion test was found to be greater than 90%. [1-^{14}C]-Arachidonic acid(AA) was from Amersham, and [1-^{14}C]-12-HETE was prepared as described by Hamberg and Samuelsson (1). The cell suspension in 5 ml volume was incubated for 10 min at 37°C with [1-^{14}C]-arachidonic acid (final conc., 13 μM; specific activity, 57.6 μCi/μmole) or [1-^{14}C]-12-HETE (final conc., 62.5 μM; specific activity, 1.25 μCi/μmole) both dissolved in 100 and 50 μl ethanol, respectively, under a normal atmosphere, and the reactions were terminated by additions of 3 volumes of ethanol. For larger preparations, 50 ml of leukocyte suspensions were used under identical conditions.

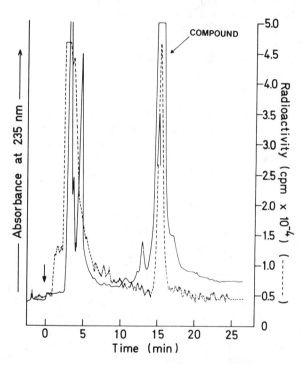

Fig. 1A. Straight-phase HPLC separation of the lipid extract of the incubation of HPMNL (5 ml) with exogenous (1-14C)-AA (13 μM) for 10 min at 37°C. Elution was isocratic with solvent system I (hex-ane: isopropanol:acetic acid (94/6/0.01)). The solid line shows UV absorption at 235 nm and the broken line (----) shows the radio-activity of the effluent.

Preparation of Washed Human Platelets and Incubation with Arachidonic Acid

Blood (500 ml) of healthy donors who had not taken any drugs for one week was collected with 7.5% (v/v) of 77 mM sodium EDTA and centrifuged at 200 x g for 15 min. The platelet rich plasma was further centrifuged at 650 x g for an additional 20 min. The platelet pellet obtained from 40-50 ml of platelet rich plasma was suspended in 25 ml of 0.15 M NaCl:25 mM Tris-HCl buffer, pH 7.4, containing 0.2 mM EDTA, and centrifuged for 20 min at 650 x g. This washing was repeated twice. The final pellet of washed platelets was suspended in PBS to a final platelet count of 1.2×10^6 platelets/μl. To this suspension was added either indomethacin (final conc., 10 μM) or aspirin (final conc., 0.3 mM).

The suspension of washed platelets was preincubated at 37°C for 10 min followed by the addition of $[1-^{14}C]$-arachidonic acid (final conc., 13 μM, or unlabeled, final conc., 13-300 μM). Incubation was done with shaking for 10 min at 37°C, and the reaction was terminated by the addition of 3 vols of ethanol.

Extraction and Purification

The incubation precipitate after addition of 3 vol. of ethanol was filtered, and the ethanolic filtrate was evaporated to dryness. The residue was dissolved in 5 ml of distilled water and acidified to pH 3.5 with 0.1 N HCl. The solution was then extracted with 10 volumes of ethyl acetate. The ethyl acetate fraction was evaporated to dryness, dissolved in methanol, treated with diazomethane and separated by a SP-HPLC column, (25 cm x 5 mm), packed with Nucleosil 50-5μ, SiO$_2$, (Macherey-Nagel, Duren, West Germany). AA metabolites were eluted isocratically with solvent system I, hexane/isopropyl alcohol/acetic acid, (94:6:0.01, v/v). Alternatively, HETE and DHETE were separated using solvent system II, hexane/isopropyl alcohol/acetic acid, (99:1:0.02, v/v) for 20 min followed by solvent system I for an additional 40 min. Solvent was delivered by an LDC-HPLC pump equipped with a Rheodyne injector. Fractions of 1 ml were collected every minute with an on-line fraction collector, and UV absorption at 235 nm was simultaneously monitored using an LDC-III variable wavelength detector. Radioactivity was monitored by a radioactivity detector (Berthold LB 5026). Material present in peaks of radioactivity was collected, dried and stored at -20°C under N$_2$.

Incubation of 12-HETE with Human Polymorphonuclear Leukocytes (HPMNL)

$[1-^{14}C]$-12-HETE (final conc., 62.5 μM) was added to 50 ml of an HPMNL cell suspension, and incubated at 37°C for 10 min. The re-

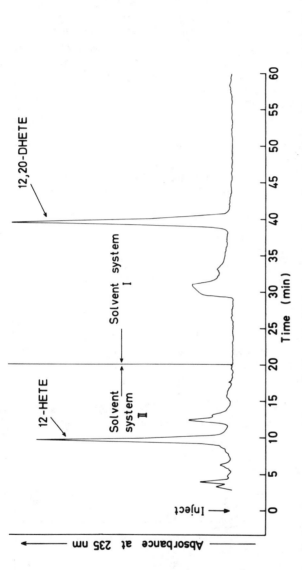

Fig. 1B. Straight-phase separation of the lipid extract of an incubation of HPMNL (5 ml) with (1-14C)-12-HETE (62.5 μM) for 10 min at 37°C. Elution was isocratic with solvent system II (hexane:isopropanol:acetic acid (99/1/0.01)) for 20 min followed by solvent system I for 40 additional minutes. UV absorption was monitored at 235 nm.

action was terminated and $[1-^{14}C]$-12-HETE and its metabolite were extracted, separated and purified as described above.

Chemical Degradation of AA Metabolites

AA metabolites and a 12-HETE metabolite (Compound A), isolated from platelets of PMNL, were hydrogenated as described by Falardeau et al. (6). The hydrogenated derivative of Compound A was then further oxidized by CrO_3 oxidation as described by Wong et al. (7). The resulting compounds were treated with diazomethane and further examined by GC/MS. Oxidative ozonolysis of AA metabolites was also performed as described (7).

RESULTS

Straight-phase HPLC analysis of the ethyl acetate extract obtained from human polymorphonuclear leukocytes with UV detection at 235 nm gave an HPLC profile as shown in Fig. 1A (solid line). In addition to arachidonic acid and monohydroxy fatty acids (5-HETE, 12-HETE and 15-HETE), which eluted with the solvent front, a major labeled compound appeared in the dihydroxy acid region with a retention time of 16.0 ± 1.5 min (Compound A). The radioactivity tracing showed two major peaks of radioactivity which co-chromatographed with the mono-hydroxy acid fraction and the unknown Compound A, respectively (Fig. 1A, broken line).

After incubation with $[1-^{14}C]$-12-HETE with HPMNL, a step gradient solvent system was used to separate 12-HETE and its metabolite. In this system, 12-HETE had a retention time of 9.5 ± 0.5 min and Compound A a retention time of 40 ± 1 min (Fig. 1B). Under these experimental conditions, the transformation of 12-HETE to Compound A was $45 \pm 5\%$ (3 experiments). Using either chromatographic system, Compound A appeared after the same retention times, regardless of whether it was derived from arachidonic acid or 12-HETE.

GC/MS Analysis of Compound A

The ultraviolet spectrum of Compound A showed $\lambda_{max}^{EtOH} = 237$ nm which suggested the presence of a pair of conjugated double bonds. The mass spectrum was similar to the corresponding derivative of 12-HETE (1), but the C-value suggested that it was a hydroxylated derivative of 12-HETE. After catalytic hydrogenation, Compound A-Me-Me$_3$Si showed one major gas chromatographic peak (about 80%) with an equivalent chain length of 25.6, suggesting that the additional hydroxyl group was located near the methyl end ($\omega 1$ or $\omega 2$). In order to locate the exact position of the extra hydroxyl group of Compound A, CrO_3 oxidation of the saturated derivative was performed (Fig. 2A). After hydrogenation followed by oxidation, and methyl esterification, Compound A was identified as dimethyl 12-keto-

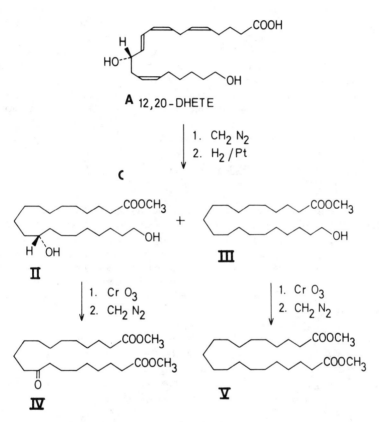

Fig. 2A. Catalytic hydrogenation and oxidation of Compound A for structural analysis.

eicosane-1, 20-dioate (Fig. 2A, IV), as shown by mass spectrometry (Fig. 2B). Ions of high intensity were observed at m/z: 384 (M); 369 (M-15, loss of CH_3); 353 (M-31, loss of OCH_3); 321 (M-(31+32)); 311 (M-73, loss of CH_2COOCH_3); 242 (M-142, loss of CH_2=CH-$(CH_2)_4COOCH_3$, β-cleavage); 227 (M-157, loss of $(CH_2)_7COOCH_3$, α-cleavage); 200 (M-184, loss of CH_2=CH-$(CH_2)_7COOCH_3$, β-cleavage); and 185 (M-199, loss of $(CH_2)_{10}COOCH_3$, α-cleavage) (7). The four ions at 242, 227, 200 and 185 were the characteristic α- and β-cleavages, at a 12-keto group; in the case of the β-cleavages with the McLafferty rearrangement, Compound A isolated from the incubations of either [1-^{14}C]-AA or [1-^{14}C]-12-HETE gave identical mass spectra. This was found with derivatives prepared both before and after hydrogenation and CrO_3 oxidation. The ozonolysis products obtained from Compound A contained the (-)menthoxycarbonyl derivative of dimethyl L-malate, demonstrating that the hydroxyl group at C-12 had the "L_s" configuration (i.e., the same as 12-HETE) (1). From the results of the oxidative ozonolysis, mass spectrometric and ultraviolet spectrometric data localized three of the four double bonds of Compound A at Δ^8, Δ^{10} and Δ^{14}. Thus, the structure of Compound A is: 12-L_s, 20 dihydroxy- 5, 8, 10, 14-eicosatetraenoic acid (12, 20-DHETE).

HPLC Analysis of the Dihydroxy Acid Fractions from Incubation of AA with Human Platelets

After washed human platelets had been incubated with arachidonic acid, the diazomethane-treated ethyl acetate extract was chromatographed on HPLC. The chromatogram from an experiment with 40 µM arachidonic acid is shown in Fig. 3. Analysis of the radioactivity showed that over 70% was found in the region corresponding to 12-HETE. In the more polar dihydroxy acid region of the chromatogram, four major peaks of UV absorbing material were seen: they were designated I through IV (absorbance at 270 nm recorded). Material from peaks I through IV was collected and rechromatographed separately using solvent system of methanol:water:acetic acid; (70:30:0.1, v/v, pH 4.2). In this RP-HPLC system, peaks II and III clearly separated into two components (designated IIa and b, and IIIa and b, respectively). UV spectra were recorded for the material in each peak. All were found to display the triplets characteristic of conjugated triene structures (4). Compound I had three absorption bands at 262.5, 272.5 and 283.5 nm, Compound IIa at 261, 270 and 281 nm, and Compound IIb at 263, 272 and 283 nm. All the remaining metabolites, IIIa, IIIb and IV, displayed very similar UV spectra with λ_{max}^{MeOH} at 268-269 nm, shoulders at 259-260 and 279-280 nm (Table I).

GC-MS analysis was performed on the Me-Me$_3$Si derivatives of all these metabolites as well as their hydrogenated counterparts. Compounds I- and IIb-Me-Me$_3$Si both appeared as two gas chromatographic peaks, whereas the remaining compounds were homogenous. The HPLC, UV and GC/MS data are compiled in Table I. The mass spectra of

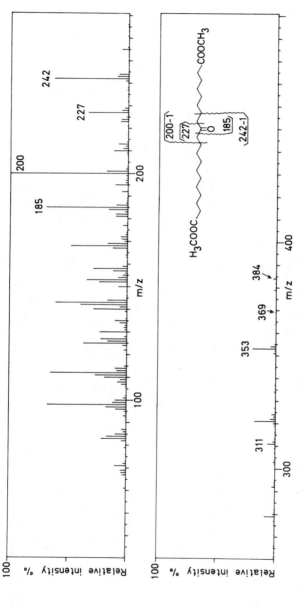

Fig. 2B. Mass spectrum of dimethyl 12-keto-eicosane-1,20-dioate, the major product formed by catalytic hydrogenation and CrO_3 oxidation of Compound 1-Me.

Compounds I-, IIa- and IIb-Me-Me₃Si were essentially identical and similar to data previously published on isomers of 14, 15-dihydroxy-eicosatetraenoic acid (4, 5, 9, 10, 11). The difference in retention

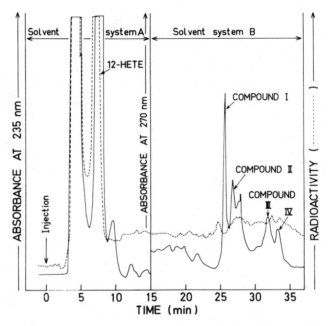

Fig. 3. Straight-phase HPLC separation of the diazomethane treated lipid extract of human platelets incubated with exogenous $(1-^{14}C)$-arachidonic acid (40 μM, final con.) for 10 min at 37°C. Elution was isocratic in two steps, with solvent system A and B (hexane: isopropanol:acetic acid, 99/1/0.02 and 97/3/0.02, by vol.). Solid line: UV absorption at 235 nm (systemA) and at 270 nm (system B). Broken line: radioactivity.

volumes indicated that Compound I was likely to be erythro-14 (R), 15 (S)-dihydroxy-5, 8, (Z), 10, 12 (E)-eicosatetraenoic acid and Compound IIb, analogously, was three-14 (R), 15 (S)-dihydroxy-5, 8 (Z), 10, 12 (E)-eicosatetraenoic acid (Table I) (4). The UV spectrum of Compound IIa suggested that it was an 8 (Z) isomer of 14, 15-dihydroxy-eicosatetraenoic acid (11).

The remaining metabolites, IIIa, IIIb and IV, displayed great similarities in their GC/MS data (Table I). Comparison with previously reported data indicated that all these compounds were likely to be isomers of 8, 15-dihydroxy-eicosatetraenoic acid. Differences in C-values and UV spectra were almost negligible and, therefore, no conclusions could be drawn concerning double-bond geometry or stereochemistry of hydroxyl groups from these data alone. However, comparison of chromatographic behaviour and UV data with previously published data (4, 9, 10, 11) suggested that these were all trans isomers with respect to double-bond geometry of the triene structure. Certain differences in retention volumes in RP-HPLC further indicated that Compound IIIa might be 8 (R), 15 (S)-dihydroxy-5, (Z), 9, 11, (E)-eicosatetraenoic acid and Compound IV, by the same criteria, the corresponding 8 (S) isomer. The structural identification of all these 14, 15- and 8, 15-dihydroxy metabolites was further supported by analysis of their hydrogenated derivatives (Table I). Analysis of the monohydroxy fatty acid fraction revealed the major component of this fraction to be 12-HETE and its isomers (12), and the minor component (less than 1% of the 12-HETE) was identified as 15-HETE by HPLC and GC/MS.

DISCUSSION

A novel metabolite of 12-HETE, i.e., 12, 20-DHETE (Compound A), was isolated and identified from incubations of human leukocytes with [1-^{14}C]-AA or [1-^{14}C]-12-HETE. It has been reported that preparations of leukocytes from peripheral blood contain a mixture of platelets and leukocytes (13, 14). Thus the formation of 12, 20-DHETE may be the result of an interaction between platelets and leukocytes as suggested (7). The platelets probably served as the source of 12-HETE, and the leukocytes provided the enzyme for ω-hydroxylation. When 12-HETE was incubated with washed platelets alone (leukocyte contamination, less than 0.3%), there was no conversion into 12, 20-DHETE. However, the addition of [1-^{14}C]-12-HETE to human leukocytes led to the formation of 12, 20-DHETE. It is likely that 12-HETE formed in platelets was further metabolized by ω-hydroxylation in the leukocytes.

Table I. Chromatographic, UV and GC/MS data of Compounds I-IV

Compound	HPLC retention times in min (Me-esters, system D)	max (Me-esters in HPLC grade methanol)	GC/MS-data (1% SE-30)			
			Me-Me$_3$Si derivatives		Hydrogenated Me-Me$_3$Si derivatives	
			C-value	Characteristic ions	C-value	Characteristic ions
I	36.5	262.5, 272.5, 283.5	23.9 24.9	494(M), 479(M-15), 463(M-31), 394(M-100; rearrangement ion)(18); 321(M-173; loss of Me$_3$SiO-CH-(CH$_2$)$_4$CH$_3$), 173	23.7	487(M-15), 471(M-31), 402(M-100), 329(M-173), 173(base peak)
IIa	37.5	261.0, 270.0, 281.0	24.9		23.9	
IIb	47.0	263.0, 272.0, 283.0	23.9 24.9		23.9	
IIIa	22.5	258.5, 268.5, 279.5	24.9	494(M), 479(M-15), 463(M-31), 423(M-71), 404(M-90; loss of Me$_3$SiOH, 353(M-141; loss of CH-CH=CH-(CH$_2$)$_3$COOMe) 263 (353-90), 243(MeSiO$^+$=CHCH$_2$CH=CH(CH$_2$)$_3$COOMe, 173, 125(base peak)	24.3	487(M-15), 431(M-71), 341(M-(71+90)), 269(M-(143+90)), 245(Me$_3$SiO=CH(CH$_2$)$_6$-COOMe), 173 (base peak)
IIIb*	28.0	258.5, 268.5, 279.5	24.9		N.A.	
IV	27.5	259.0, 268.5, 279.5	24.9		24.3	

* Tentatively identified
N.A.: not analyzed

12-HETE has been found to be chemotactic and chemokinetic for human neutrophils and eosinophils (15, 16), and to stimulate the influx of leukocytes to the peritoneal cavity of guinea pigs (17). Furthermore, 12-HETE enhanced the expression of C_3b receptors on both neutrophils and eosinophils (17) and lysosomal enzyme release (18). It was recently reported that 20-hydroxy-LTB_4 retained most, if not all, of the smooth muscle stimulating activity of LTB_4 but lost most of its chemotactic activity (19). Therefore, it will be of interest to investigate the biological activity of 12, 20-DHETE.

Human platelets contain two enzymes for the oxidative metabolism of arachidonic acid: the cyclooxygenase which converts arachidonic acid to PGG_2, and the 12-lipoxygenase which converts it into 12-HPETE (1). In the present study we demonstrate that arachidonic acid can also be converted into several other lipoxygenase products in human platelets, viz., three 14,15-DHETEs, three 8,15-DHETEs and one 15-HETE. The structures of these compounds were confirmed by UV and GC/MS data. Our study clearly demonstrated that the second lipoxygenase activity can convert arachidonic acid into 15-lipoxygenase products, although the 12-lipoxygenase product, 12-HETE, is the dominating one. It has been reported that 15-lipoxygenase products are biologically active; i.e., 15-HPETE inhibits PGI_2 formation, 15-HETE inhibits the 5-lipoxygenase in leukocytes (20), 8, 15-DHETE has potent chemotactic activity (21), and 8, 15-dihydroperoxy-eicosatetraenoic acids have been shown to inhibit platelet aggregation (22). Thus, the presence of 15-lipoxygenase in human platelets may generate biologically active products from AA. Furthermore, 15-lipoxygenase in platelets may play an important role in the conversion of arachidonic acid into lipoxins A and B, recently discovered (23).

ACKNOWLEDGMENTS

This work was supported by grants from the Swedish Medical Research Council (proj. no 03X-05915, 03P-5804, 03X-5170 and 03X-00217), by the swedish National Association against Rheumatism, and by NIH (HL-25316 and 00811).

REFERENCES

1. M. Hamberg and B. Samuelsson. Prostaglandin Endoperoxides: Novel Transformations of Arachidonic Acid in Human Platelets. Proc. Natl. Acad. Sci. USA, 71:3400-3404, 1974.
2. B. Samuelsson. Leukotrienes: A New Class of Mediators of Intermediate Hypersensitivity Reactions and Inflammation. In: "Adv. Prostaglandin Thromboxane Leukotriene Res." B. Samuelsson, R. Paoletti and P. Ramwell, eds. Raven Press, N.Y. vol 11:1-13 (1983).
3. W. Jubiz, O. Radmark, C. Malmsten, G. Hansson, J.A. Lindgren, J. Palmblad, A.M. Uden and B. Samuelsson. A Novel Leukotriene Produced by Stimulation of Leukocytes with formyl-methionyl-leucyl-

phenylalanine (fMLP). J. Biol. Chem. 257:6106-6110, 1982.

4. R.L. Maas, A.R. Brash. Evidence for a Lipoxygenase Mechanism in the Biosynthesis of Epoxide and Dihydroxy Leukotrienes from 15 (S)-Hydroperoxyeicosatetraenoic Acid by Human Platelets and Porcine Leukocytes. Proc. Natl. Acad. Sci. USA 80:2884-2888, 1983.

5. D.-E. Sok, C.-O. Han, W.-R. Shien, B.-N. Zhou and C.J. Sih. Enzymatic Formation of 14, 15-leukotriene A and C (14)-sulfur-linked peptides. Biochem. Biophys. Res. Commun. 104:1363-1370, 1982.

6. P. Falardeau, M. Hamberg and B. Samuelsson. Metabolism of 8, 11, 14-eicosatrienoic acid in Human Platelets. Biochim. Biophys. Acta 441:193-200, 1976.

7. P.Y-K. Wong, P. Westlund, E. Granstrom, M. Hamberg, P.H-W Chao, and B. Samuelsson. ω-Hydroxylation of 12-L-Hydroxy-5, 8, 10, 14-eicosatetraenoic acid in Human Polymorphonuclear Leukocytes. J. Biol. Chem. 259:2683-2686, 1984.

8. P. Borgeat and B. Samuelsson. Transformations of Arachidonic Acid by Rabbit Polymorphonuclear Leukocytes. Formation of Novel Dihydroxyeicosatetraenoic Acid. J. Biol. Chem. 254:2643-2646, 1979.

9. W. Jubiz, O. Ridmark, J.A. Lindgren, C. Malmsten and B. Samuelsson. Novel Leukotrienes: Products Formed by Initial Oxygenation of Arachidonic Acid at C-15. Biochem. Biophys. Res. Commun. 99:976-986, 1981.

10. U. Lundberg, O. Radmark, C. Malmsten and B. Samuelsson. Transformation of 15-hydroperoxy-5, 9, 11, 13-eicosatetraenoic acid into Novel Leukotrienes. FEBS Lett. 126:127-132, 1981.

11. R.L. Maas, A.R. Brash and J.A. Oates. A Second Pathway of Leukotriene Biosynthesis in Porcine Leukocytes. Proc. Natl. Acad. Sci. USA 78:5523-5527, 1981.

12. P.Y-K. Wong, P. Westlund, M. Hamberg, E. Granstrom, P.H-W Chao and B. Samuelsson. 15-lipoxygenase in Human Platelets. J. Biol. Chem. (submitted for publication, 1984).

13. P. Borgeat, S. Picard, J. Drapeau and P. Vallerand. Metabolism of Arachidonic Acid in Leukocytes: Isolation of a 5, 15-dihydroxy-eicosatetraenoic acid. Lipids 17:676-681, 1982.

14. J. Maclouf, F.D. Laclos and P. Borgeat. Stimulation of Leukotriene Biosynthesis in Human Blood Leukocytes by Platelet-derived 12-hydroperoxy-eicosatetraenoic acid. Proc. Natl. Acad. Sci. USA 79:6042-6046, 1982.

15. S.R. Turner, J.A. Tainer and W.S. Lynn. Biogenesis of Chemotactic Molecules by the Arachidonate Lipoxygenase System of Platelets. Nature 257:680-681, 1975.

16. E.J. Goetzl, H.R. Hill and R.R. Gorman. Unique Aspects of the Modulation of Human Neutrophil Function by 12-L-hydroperoxy-5, 8, 10, 14-eicosatetraenoic acid. Prostaglandins 19:71-85, 1980.

17. E.J. Goetzl, J.M. Woods and R.R. Gorman. Stimulation of Human Eosinophil and Neutrophil Polymorphonuclear Leukocyte Chemotaxis and Random Migration by 12-L-hydroxy-5, 8, 10, 14-eicosatetraenoic acid. J. Clin. Invest. 59:179-182, 1977.

18. W.F. Stenson and C.W. Parker. Monohydroxyeicosatetraenoic Acids (HETEs) Induce Degranulation of Human Neutrophils. J. Immunol 124: 2100-2104, 1980.

19. A.W. Ford-Hutchinson, A. Rackham, R. Zamboni, J. Rokach and
S. Roy.   Comparative Biological Activities of Synthetic Leukotriene
B_4 and its Omega-oxidation Products.   Prostaglandins 25:29-37, 1983.
20. J.Y. Vanderhoek, R.W. Bryant and J.M. Bailey.   15-hydroxy-5, 8,
11, 13-eicosatetraenoic acid: A Potent and Selective Inhibitor of
Platelet Lipoxygenase.   J. Biol. Chem. 255:5996-5998, 1980.
21. S. Shak, D.H. Perez and I.M. Goldstein.   A Novel Dioxygenation
Product of Arachidonic Acid Possesses Potent Chemotactic Activity
for Human Polymorphonuclear Leukocytes.   J. Biol. Chem. 250:14948-
14953, 1983.
22. G.S. Bild, S.G. Bhat and B. Axelrod.   Inhibition of Aggregation
of Human Platelets by 8, 15-dihydroperoxides of 5, 9, 11, 13-eico-
satetraenoic and 9, 11, 13-eicosatrienoic acids.   Prostaglandins
16:795-800, 1978.
23. C.W. Serhan, M. Hamberg and B. Samuelsson.   Lipoxins: Novel
Series of Biologically Active Compounds Formed from Arachidonic
Acid in Human Leukocytes.   Proc. Natl. Acad. Sci. 81:5335-5339, 1984.

EPOXIDATION OF ARACHIDONIC ACID AND PROSTACYCLIN IN THE KIDNEY

Patrick Y-K. Wong[+], John C. McGiff,
Michal Schwartzman and F.F. Sun[*]

New York Medical College, Valhalla, N.Y. 10595
*The Upjohn Company, Kalamazoo, MI, 49001

SUMMARY

The renal epoxygenase has been demonstrated to be an active pathway for the conversion of arachidonic acid (AA) to 11,12-epoxide, 19-hydroxy and 20-hydroxy-eicosatetraenoic acids. The epoxygenase activity was found to be located predominantly in the renal cortex. This renal epoxygenase pathway also transformed PGI_2 to a new, previously unreported, metabolite. This metabolite was isolated and identified by radio gas chromatography and gas chromatography-mass spectrometry as 5-hydroxy-6-keto-$PGF_{1\alpha}$. Its structure was further confirmed by comparison of the mass-spectra to that of the synthetic standard. The formation of 5-hydroxy-6-keto-$PGF_{1\alpha}$ in the kidney suggested epoxidation of prostacyclin via the renal epoxygenase as an alternative pathway of PGI_2 metabolism.

Abbreviations: PGI_2, prostacyclin;
6-keto-$PGF_{1\alpha}$, 6-keto-prostaglandin $F_{1\alpha}$;
HPLC, High Performance Liquid Chromatography;
GC-MS, Gas chromatography-mass spectrometry;
mHETE, mono-hydroxyeicosatetraenoic acid
OTMS, methylester-trimethyl-silyl ether;
$NOCH_3$, O-methyl-oxime;
3-MC, 3-methylcholanthrene;
β-NF, β-naphthoflavone

[+] To whom all correspondence should be addressed

INTRODUCTION

The generation of prostaglandins and other oxygenated metabolites of arachidonic acid (AA) is a complex process initiated by
the release of esterified AA from cellular lipids. Once liberated
from the membrane lipids by diverse stimuli - peptide hormones,
neurotransmitters and mechanical disruption - the free AA is rapidly
metabolized. Metabolism of AA involves three enzymatic systems:
cyclo-oxygenase, lipoxygenases and cytochrome P450 mixed-function
oxidases. The pathway by which AA will be transformed will depend
on the tissue, the kind of stimulus, cofactor availability, inhibitors, etc. Cyclo-oxygenase and lipoxygenase pathways, both in
the presence of oxygen, will facilitate the sequence of hydrogen
removal, double-bond rearrangement and inclusion of an oxygen
moiety to yield one of several unstable hydroperoxy fatty acids
(HPETEs). Most HPETEs (i.e., 5, 8, 11 and 15) formed by the action
of lipoxygenase may then form their corresponding hydroxy fatty
acids (HETEs). Alternatively, the 5-HPETE forms a labile 5,6 epoxide (LTA$_4$) which is the precursor of the leukotrienes. The third
pathway by which AA may be oxygenated in vivo is the cytochrome
P450-dependent mono-oxygenases, a mixed-function oxidase system
strictly dependent on molecular oxygen and NADPH. This system can
metabolize AA by three types of reactions:

1) allylic oxidation leading to the formation of all mono-
hydroxyeicosatetraenoic acids (mHETEs);

2) olefin epoxidation leading to the formation of four different epoxyeicosatrienoic acids (EETs) which can undergo hydrolysis by epoxide hydrolase to form the corresponding diol metabolites - the dihydroxyeicosatrienoic acids (DETs); and

3) oxidation at ω and ω-1 positions to form the 20- and 19-
HETEs, respectively. Since cytochrome P450 exists in multiple
forms, the predominance of one of these reactions over others may
be controlled by the isoenzyme composition of each tissue or cell
type.

The cytochrome P450 mixed-function oxidase system is comprised
of three components: cytochrome P450 as the hemoprotein, a flavo-
protein reductase identified as the NADPH-dependent cytochrome C
reductase and phosphatidylcholine which serves to facilitate electron transfer in microsomal systems. Cytochrome P450, as the terminal oxidase of the drug metabolizing enzyme system, exists in
multiple forms which differ in substrate specificity, positional
specificity and stereospecificity (1). Although the hepatic cytochrome P450 system is well characterized, less is known concerning
the renal cytochrome P450. The distribution of the components and
activities of the mixed-function oxidase system have been studied
in the rabbit kidney (2). The highest level of cytochrome P450 was

198

present in kidney cortex. Furthermore, Oliw et al. (3) and
Capdevila et al.(4,5)have demonstrated the conversion of AA to
several oxygenated metabolites by hepatic and renal cortical

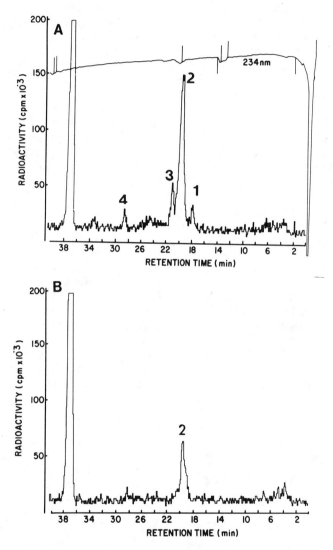

Figure 1: HPLC tracing of incubation of renal cortex
microsomes with [14C]-arachidonic acid in the
presence of NADPH (A, upper panel) in the
absence and (B, lower panel) in the presence
of SKF-525A (100μM).

microsomes and by a reconstituted, purified, cytochrome P450 system in the presence of NADPH. While the role of prostaglandins in the regulation of renal function has been well studied, the renal functional effects of AA metabolites arising from either lipoxygenase or cytochrome P450-dependent mono-oxygenases are virtually unknown. Initial studies suggest that products of AA arising from cytochrome P450-dependent enzymes exert actions on the vasculature (6) and participate in the regulation of hormonal secretion (7). Jacobson et al. (8) have recently demonstrated that 5, 6 EET, when injected into perfused rabbit cortical collecting tubules, was able to inhibit sodium transport.

In this communication we summarize our recent results on the metabolism of AA by the cytochrome P450 enzyme system in the rabbit renal cortex, as well as the discovery of a new, previously unreported metabolite of PGI_2 via the cytochrome P450 enzyme system in the isolated perfused rabbit kidney.

MATERIALS AND METHODS

Radiolabeled [9-^{3}H] PGI_2 methyl ester with specific activity of 15 µCi/umole and [1-^{14}C]-AA (50 µCi/umole) were purchased from New England Nuclear, Boston, Massachusetts. The purity of the PGI_2 methyl ester was established by thin-layer chromatography (TLC plate, 0.25 mm thick, 5 x 20 cm silica gel precoated plastic sheets, Brinkman) with hexane:acetone (1:1, v/v) as solvent. Radiochromatogram scans showed a single peak of PGI_2 methyl ester on TLC plates with an Rf value of 0.68. The methyl ester of [9-^{3}H] PGI_2 was converted to the PGI_2 sodium salt the day before use by mild alkaline hydrolysis and diluted with authentic PGI_2 sodium salt (Upjohn) to a specific activity of 12.76 µCi/µmole as described (9).

Biosynthesis of Cytochrome P450 Products of AA by Kidney Cortex Microsome

The rabbit renal cortex was homogenized using a Potter-type teflon glass homogenizer in ice-cold, phosphate buffered saline (PBS), pH 7.4 (3 ml/g wet weight of tissue). The cortical homogenates were centrifuged twice at 9,000 x g for 20 min and the pellet was discarded. The supernate was centrifuged at 105,000 x g for 90 min. The microsomal pellet was resuspended in PBS, centrifuged at the same force for 60 min and resuspended again in PBS. The microsomal suspension was used as the enzyme source for cytochrome P450. Protein was determined by the method of Lowry (10). Microsomal fractions (300 µg protein concentration) were incubated with [1-^{14}C]-AA (10 µM) and NADPH (1 mM) in the presence of SKF-525A (100 µM).

The incubations were stopped at 10 min by acidification with 1N HCl to pH 4.5, and extracted twice with 3 ml of ethyl acetate.

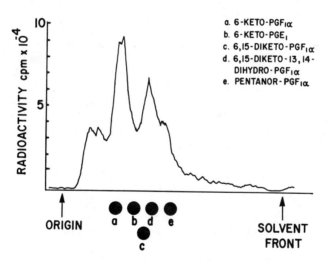

Figure 2:   Radiochromatograph scan of radioactive products extracted from the venous effluent of the rabbit kidney after infusion of $[9-^3H]-PGI_2$ Radioactive metabolites were extracted, separated and identified as described under "Methods".

201

The extracts were dried under N_2 and subjected to separation by RP-HPLC with a C_{18}-Bondapak column using a gradient from $CH_3CN:H_2O:HAc$ (50:50:0.1, v/v) to $CH_3CN:HAc$ (100:0.1, v/v) at a rate of 1.25%/min and flow rate of 1 ml/min.

Kidney Perfusion

Male New Zealand rabbits were anesthetized with sodium pento-barbitol (30 mg/kg). After midline laparotomy, the kidneys were exposed. The renal artery and ureter were cannulated and the kidney was flushed with Tyrode's solution, removed from the animal, and placed in a thermostatically-controlled chamber. The kidney was perfused through the renal artery with oxygenated Tyrode's solution (37°C) at a rate of 10 ml/min. 10.0 μCi of $[9-^3H]$ PGI_2 Na salt (12.76 μCi/mole) was infused into the kidney through the arterial cannula over a period of 5 min. The venous and ureteral effluents were acidified with 1N HCl to pH 3.0 and extracted three times with equal volumes of ethyl acetate. The acetate extract was evaporated to dryness _in vacuo_.

Chromatographic Method

Thin-layer chromatography was performed with Brinkman precoated silica gel G-25 plates and solvent system A9 (organic phase of ethyl acetate:acetate acid:iso-octane:H_2O (55:10:25:50, v/v). The radio-active products were detected with a Packard model 7320 radiochro-matogram scanner. High-performance liquid chromatography (HPLC) was carried out with a 6000A pump (Waters Associates, Milford, MA) system and an ultrasphere - ODS reverse-phase column maintained at a flow rate of 0.5 ml/min and monitored by a model GM770 variable wave length detector set at 192 nm. The compounds were eluted iso-cratically with acetonitrile:water (30:70, v/v, pH 2.95). The column effluent was collected in 0.5 ml fractions and an aliquot of 50 μl each was assessed for radioactivity.

Radiometric Gas Chromatography and Mass Spectrometry (GC-MS)

The radioactive products were converted to methyl ester, 0-methyl-oxime trimethylsilyl ether (11) before analyses by radio-metric GC coupled with MS. The final derivative was dissolved in a small aliquot of acetone before injection. GC was carried out on a Varian 2700 GC coupled with a Packard 894 radioactivity detector for simultaneous recording of mass and radioactivity. GC-MS analysis was carried out by LKB-9000 mass spectrometer. The 6-foot column

[1% SE30 on Chromosorb-H (HP)] was kept at 210°C, the flash heater at 240°C, and the separator at 250°C. Electron energy was set at 22.5 eV (11).

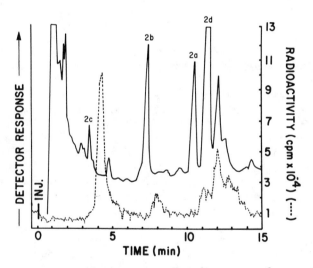

Figure 3: Radio-gas chromatograph of $[9-^3H]-PGI_2$ metabolites recovered from zones 2 and 3; GC detector as broken line (----). Note that the radioactive detector responses were one minute later than those of the GC detector.

RESULTS

AA Metabolism in Rabbit Kidney Cortex

Fig. 1a (upper panel) shows a radioactive RP-HPLC chromatogram of the lipid material recovered from the incubation of $[1-^{14}C]$-AA with rabbit cortical microsomal fractions. Compounds I and IV had no absorbance at 234 nm nor at 280 nm and were identified as 11, 12-diol and 11, 12-epoxide-AA by GC-MS (12), compound II was identified as 19-OH-AA (12) and compound III as 20-OH-AA. Fig. 1b (lower panel) shows the radioactive HPLC-chromatography of the lipid material recovered from the control experiments where SKF-525A, a cytochrome P450-dependent enzyme(s) inhibitor, was included in the incubation mixture. The addition of SKF-525A (100 μM) resulted in 90-95% inhibition of the formation of 11, 12-diol, 11, 12-epoxide and 20-OH-AA (the formation of 19-OH-AA was inhibited by SKF-525A by 70%). The formation of compounds I, II, III and IV were dependent on the presence of NADPH as cofactor.

PGI$_2$ Metabolites in Rabbit Kidney Perfusate

Figure 2 represents a typical radiochromatogram scan of a thin-layer chromatogram of the extract from rabbit kidney perfusate. Two major and one minor radioactive zones were observed. Of the total radioactive $[9-^3H]$ injected, 95% was recovered in the renal effluent (average of three experiments); 34% migrated in zone 1, which corresponds to the mobility of 6-keto PGF$_{1\alpha}$, and 44% migrated to zones 2 and 3 which correspond to the mobility of pentanor PGF$_{1\alpha}$ and 6, 15-diketo-13, 14-dihydro PGF$_{1\alpha}$. However, when zones 2 and 3 were eluted from the TLC plate and subjected to radiometric GC analysis, five radioactive peaks were observed (Fig. 3). Compounds 2a and 2b were identified as 6-keto PGF$_{1\alpha}$ and 2, 3-dinor PGF$_{1\alpha}$, respectively. Compounds 2c and 2d are novel metabolites and their structural characteristics were carried out by RP-HPLC analysis and GC-MS.

Gas chromatographic analysis of the trimethylsilyl derivative of compound 2c showed the radioactive peak with equivalent chain length of C-20.3. The spectrum resembled that reported for the TMS derivative of 9, 11, 15-trihydroxy-pentanor prosta-13-enoic acid γ-lactone or pentanor PGF$_{1\alpha}$ γ-lactone (13). Subsequently, structural comparison with the authentic standard confirmed the structrual assignment as that previously reported (13). Approximately 25% of the radioactivity in both zones 2 and 3 (Fig.3, lower tracing) was accounted for by compound 2d and was detected by radioactive GC because of imcomplete separation by TLC. Compound 2d was slightly more polar than 6-keto PGF$_{1\alpha}$ as it eluted off the reverse-phase column before 6-keto PGF$_{1\alpha}$. The retention time of the methyl ester, 0-methoxime-TMS derivative of 2d, had a C-value of 25.3. In the mass spectrum (Fig. 4), the molecular ion was

204

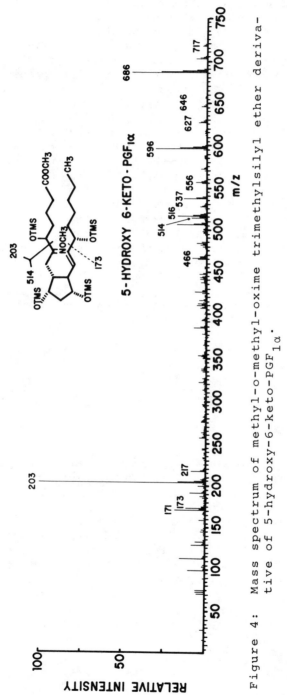

Figure 4: Mass spectrum of methyl-o-methyl-oxime trimethylsilyl ether derivative of 5-hydroxy-6-keto-PGF$_{1\alpha}$.

found at m/e 717. Fragment ions were found at 702[M-15], 686[M-31], 646[M-71], 627[M-90], 596[M-90+31], 556[M-90+71], 537[M-2x90], 516[M-201], 514[M-203], 466[M-2x90+71], 203 (base peak) and 171. The molecular ion and most of the prominent fragments at the high mass end are in accord with the formation of a 6-keto-PGF$_{1\alpha}$ derivative with an additional hydroxyl group. A series of [M-71] fragments indicate that the compound is not a 19 or 20-hydroxyl compound and the spectrum differs from the corresponding spectrum from similar derivatives of 19 or 20-hydroxy-6-keto-PGF$_{1\alpha}$. The base peak at m/e 203 and the M-203 fragment at m/e 514 suggested that the most probable position of the extra hydroxyl group is at C-5 because of the favorable cleavage between the adjacent -OTMS and -NOCH$_3$ groups. Based on this information, we concluded that compound 2d was a new metabolite of PGI$_2$:5-hydroxy-6-keto-PGF$_{1\alpha}$. Further, structural conformation was provided by oxidative cleavage by periodic acid. About 50 µg of compound 2d was treated with 0.5 ml of 2 mg/ml aqueous periodic acid for 16 hours. The product was converted to methyl ester TMS derivative and analyzed by GC-MS. The compound was qualitatively converted to the 15 carbon pentanor PGF$_{2\alpha}$ γ-lactone, therefore confirming the adjacent keto/alcohol functions at C-5 and C-6. 5-hydroxy-6-keto-PGF$_{1\alpha}$ was subsequently prepared by direct epoxidation of PGI$_2$ with m-chloroperoxybenzoic acid to form the 5, 6-epoxide, followed by ring opening with diluted aqueous acid (14). The product has identical chromatographic and mass spectral characteristics as the biological material.

Similar to our previous report (11), the urinary effluent obtained from the isolated perfused kidney, during infusion of [9-^{3}H]-PGI$_2$ and thereafter (three experiments), did not show appreciable (less than 0.1%) radioactivity nor contain any tritiated water.

DISCUSSION

We have previously reported that renal metabolism of PGI$_2$ is extensive; the major metabolites in venous effluent have been isolated and identified as 7, 9-dihydroxy, 4, 13-diketo-dinor-PGF$_{1\alpha}$, dinor-6-keto-PGF$_{1\alpha}$, suggesting that a substantial portion of the infused [9-^{3}H]-PGI$_2$ was metabolized via the 15-hydroxyprostaglandin dehydrogenase followed by Δ 13, 14 reductase, as well as by β-oxidation (11, 13). Radioactive metabolites were not detected in the urine, suggesting that exogenous PGI$_2$ was not secreted by the proximal tubular secretory system. PGI$_2$, unlike PGE$_2$, is a poor substrate for the organic acid secretory system (15).

In this report, we have demonstrated the identification of the new metabolite, 5-hydroxy-6-keto-PGF$_{1\alpha}$, probably generated from an unstable intermediate, "epoxide-ether": "5, (6)-oxido-PGI$_1$" by the renal epoxygenases. The "epoxide-ether", "5, (6)-oxido-PGI$_1$", is subsequently hydrolyzed to 5-hydroxy-6-keto-PGF$_{1\alpha}$ by the addition of H$_2$O. (Fig. 5)

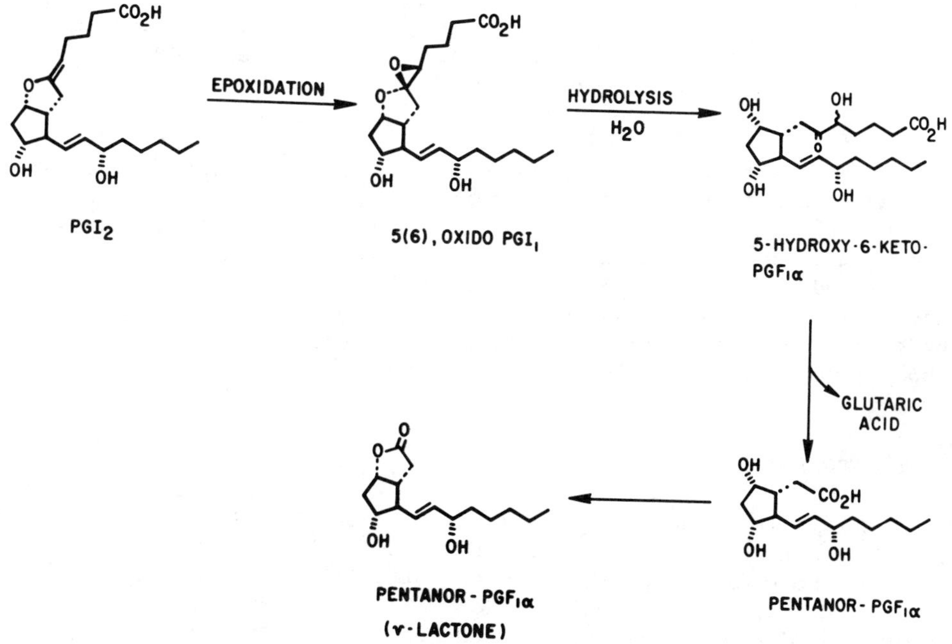

Figure 5: Proposed metabolic pathways of epoxygenation of prostacyclin in the rabbit kidney.

The occurrence of a cytochrome P450-dependent mono-oxygenase/epoxygenase system in renal microsomes has been demonstrated by Oliw et al. (12) and by Manna et al. (16). Recently, this enzyme system was demonstrated in the cells isolated from the thick ascending limb of Henle's loop (17). In this report we also showed the formation of 11, 12-epoxide and its corresponding diol metabolites by cortical microsomes previously shown to be formed by cytochrome P450-dependent mono-oxygenase. In addition, cortical microsomes contain ω and ω-1 hydroxylation, an NADPH-dependent cytochrome P450 activity, as demonstrated by the formation of 19 and 20-OH-AA. The formation of these metabolites was inhibited by SKF-525A, indicating the involvement of cytochrome P450. Further, we were able to demonstrate the correlation between cytochrome P450 system and AA metabolism in renal tissue (18). Drugs which caused the depletion of cytochrome P450, like $CoCl_2$, reduced the formation of the above metabolites. Induction of cytochrome P450 system by 3-MC and β-NF caused an increase of cytochrome P450-dependent metabolites. Since the discovery of this new epoxygenase pathway, a new group of epoxygenase products of AA have been isolated and identified. The biological properties of these products of AA have been studied by Capdevila and coworkers (7,19). All of these epoxides of AA were found to be potent stimulators of polypeptide hormone release at low concentrations. Furthermore, the 5, 6-epoxide of AA was found to be a potent inhibitor of ion transport (8) as well as of Na^+/K-ATPase activity (20). In view of the potent biological effect of various unstable AA metabolites, e.g., PGI_2, PGH_2 and 5, 6 LTA_4, the postulated intermediate, "5, (6) oxido-PGI_1", may also be biologically active.

More recently, Oliw (21) reported that 5, (6) oxido-C-20:3 can be used as substrate for the ram seminal vesicle cyclo-oxygenase to generate two new products, namely 5-hydroxy-$PGI_{1\alpha}$ and 5-hydroxy-$PGI_{1\beta}$ (two isomers). In this study we demonstrated that PGI_2 can be metabolized by the renal epoxygenase enzyme system and transformed into a series of new products, including 5-hydroxy-6-keto-$PGF_{1\alpha}$. The biological significance of the products of this pathway in the kidney remains to be defined.

ACKNOWLEDGMENTS

We wish to thank Dr. J.E. Pike for the generous gift of prostaglandins, and 5-hydroxy-6-keto $PGF_{1\alpha}$ and for his valuable suggestions and comments on the development of this project, and Dr. D.R. Morton for the synthesis of various intermediates. The assistance of Mrs. Sallie McGiff and Mrs. Doreen Carrigan-Friary in the preparation of this manuscript is gratefully acknowledged. This work was supported by grants from NIH, HL-25316 (Dr. P. Y-K Wong), HL-25394 (Dr. J.C. McGiff). Dr. Wong is a recipient of an NIH Research Career Development Award (HL-00811).

REFERENCES

1. A.Y.H. Lu and S.B. West. Multiplicity of mammalian microsomal cytochromes P-450. Pharmacol. Rev. 31:277-295, 1980.

2. T.V. Zenser, M.B. Mattamal and B.B. Davis. Differential distribution of the mixed function oxidase activities in rabbit kidney. J. Pharmacol. Exp. Ther. 207:719-725, 1978.

3. E.H. Oliw, F.P. Guengerich and J.A. Oates. Oxygenation of arachidonic acid by hepatic monooxygenases: Isolation and metabolism of four epoxide intermediates. J. Biol. Chem. 257:3771-3781, 1982.

4. J. Capdevila, L. Parkhill, N. Chacos, R. Okita, B.S.S. Masters and R.W. Estabrook. The oxidative metabolism of arachidonic acid by purified cytochrome P-450. Biochem. Biophys. Res. Commun. 101:1357-1363, 1981.

5. J. Capdevila, N. Chacos, J. Werringloer, R.A. Prough and R.W. Estabrook. Liver microsomal cytochrome P-450 and oxidative metabolism of arachidonic acid. Proc. Natl. Acad. Sci. USA 78:5362-5366, 1981.

6. H.A. Singer, J.A. Saye and M.J. Peach. Effect of cytochrome P450 inhibitors on endothelium-dependent relaxation in rabbit aorta. Blood Vessels 21:223-230, 1984.

7. G.D. Snyder, J. Capdevila, N. Chacos, S. Manna and J.R. Falck. Action of luteinizing hormone-releasing hormones: Involvement of novel arachidonic acid metabolites. Proc. Natl. Acad. Sci. USA 80:3504-3507, 1983.

8. H.R. Jacobson, S. Corona, J. Capdevila, N. Chacos, S. Manna, A. Womack and J.R. Falck. 5,6 epoxyeicosatrienoic acid inhibits sodium absorption and potassium secretion in rabbit cortical collecting tubule. Kidney Int. 25:330, 1984 (abstract)

9. R.A. Johnson, F.H. Lincoln, E.G. Nidy, H.P. Schneider, J.L. Thompson and U. Axen. Synthesis and characterization of prostacyclin, 6-keto-prostaglandin $F_{1\alpha}$, prostaglandin I_1, and prostaglandin I_3. J. Amer. Chem. Soc. 100:7690-7693, 1980.

10. O.H. Lowry, N.J. Rosebrough, L.A. Farr and R.J. Randall. Protein measurement with the folic phenol reagent. J. Biol. Chem. 193:265-275, 1951.

11. P.Y-K Wong, J.C. McGiff, L. Cagen, K.U. Malik and F.F. Sun. Metabolism of prostacyclin in the rabbit kidney. J. Biol. Chem. 254:12-14, 1979.

12. E.H. Oliw, J.A. Lawson, H.R. Brash, J.A. Oates. Arachidonic acid metabolism in rabbit renal cortex: Formation of two novel dihydroxyeicosatrienoic acids. J. Biol. Chem. 256:9924-9931, 1981.

13. P.Y-K Wong, K.U. Malik, D.M. Desiderio, J.C. McGiff and F.F. Sun. Hepatic metabolism of prostacyclin (PGI2) in the rabbit: formation of a potent novel inhibitor of platelet aggregation. Biochem. Biophys. Res. Commun. 93:486-494, 1980.

14. J.C. Sih, R.A. Johnson, E.G. Nidy and D.R. Graber. Synthesis of the four isomers of 5-hydroxy-PGI$_1$. Prostaglandins 15:409-421, 1978.

15. M.J.S. Miller, E.G. Spokas and J.C. McGiff. Metabolism of prostaglandin E2 in the isolated perfused kidney of the rabbit. Biochem. Pharmacol. 31:2955-2960, 1982.

16. S. Manna, J.R. Falck, N. Chacos and J. Capdevila. Synthesis of arachidonic acid metabolites produced by purified kidney cortex microsomal cytochrome P-450. Tetrahedron Letters 24:33-36, 1983.

17. N.R. Ferreri, M. Schwartzman, N.G. Ibraham, P.N. Chander and J.C. McGiff. Arachidonic acid metabolism in a cell suspension isolated from rabbit renal outer medulla. J. Pharmacol. Exp. Ther. 231, in press (1984).

18. M. Schwartzman, N.R. Ferreri, M. Carroll, N. Ibraham, R.D. Levere and J.C. McGiff. Arachidonic acid metabolism in isolated cells from the thick ascending limb of Henle's loop. Clin. Res. 32:456A, 1984 (abstract).

19. J. Capdevila, N. Chacos, J.R. Falck, S. Manna, A. Negro-Vilar and S.R. Ojeda. Novel hypothalamic arachidonate products stimulate somatostatin release from the median eminence. Endocrinology 113:421-423, 1983.

20. M. Schwartzman, M.C. Carroll, N.R. Ferreri and J.C. McGiff. Renal arachidonic acid metabolism, the third pathway. Submitted, Hypertension, 1984.

21. E.H. Oliw. Metabolism of 5 (6) oxidoeicosatrienoic acid by ram seminal vesicles: Formation of two stereoisomers of 5-hydroxyprostaglandin I$_1$. J. Biol. Chem. 259:2716-2721, 1984.

THE EFFECT OF 9α-FLUOROHYDROCORTISONE ON THE URINARY EXCRETION OF 6-KETO-PGF$_{1\alpha}$ IN MAN

P. Minuz, G. Capuzzo[◊], M. Degan[◊], C. Lechi[◊◊],
G. Covi[◊], G.P. Velo and A. Lechi[◊]

Istituto di Farmacologia, Clinica Medica[◊] and
Cattedra di Chimica e Microscopia Clinica[◊◊]
Università di Verona, Italy

The exogenous administration of pharmacological doses of mineralocorticoids causes a transient sodium retention which is followed after a few days by a return to a new sodium balance. This latter phenomenon, known as escape from the sodium-retaining effects of mineralocorticoids, is characterized by an increased urinary volume and sodium excretion. At the same time increased renal blood flow, glomerular filtration rate and reduced renal vascular resistance are observed[1]. Besides the haemodynamic factors, prostaglandins (PGs) and kallikrein-kinin system have been suggested as being responsible, at least partly, for the escape phenomenon.

Renal prostaglandins and prostacyclin (PGI$_2$) in particular, which is the main product of renal vasculature, have a vasodilatory effect and show natriuretic properties in vivo[2]. Moreover, a direct inhibition of tubular sodium transport by PGI$_2$ has been observed in the rat in vitro[3]. Kinins, which are released intra-renally by kallikrein produced at tubular level, share several properties with PGI$_2$, such as natriuresis and vasodilation[4]. They also stimulate renal PGI$_2$ synthesis[5].

In this study we evaluated the effect of 9α-fluorhydrocortisone (9α-FF, Florinef[R]) on the urinary excretion of 6-keto-PGF$_{1\alpha}$ in normal subjects, as an index of renal prostacyclin production. We also measured the urinary excretion of kallikrein, aldosterone, sodium and potassium.

MATERIALS AND METHODS

Seven healthy male volunteers, aged 26 to 43 years, mean age $\pm$ SD: 28.8 $\pm$ 5.9 years, were studied before and during oral administration of 1 mg of 9α-fluoro-hydrocortisone for 10 days at a constant sodium intake (150 mg/day). Urinary excretion of sodium, potassium, aldosterone, kallikrein and 6-keto-PGF$_{1\alpha}$ was measured initially and after 3, 6 and 9 days of administration of the drug.

24-hour specimens of urine were collected and stored at -20°C until analysis. Urinary kallikrein was measured by an enzymatic method based on the cleavage of the chromophore p-nitroaniline from the chromogenic tripeptide substrate S-2266[6]. Urinary aldosterone was determined by radioimmunoassay (RIA), (Aldo RIA Kit, Sorin Biomedica, Saluggia, Italy). 6-keto-PGF$_{1\alpha}$ was measured by RIA after high pressure liquid chromatography (HPLC); the following procedure was used: 20 ml of each urinary sample was centrifuged at 1000 g for 10 minutes and then acidified to pH 3.2 by the addition of diluted formic acid. About 1500 CPM of ^{3}H-6-keto-PGF$_{1\alpha}$ (specific activity 120-180 Ci/mM, New England Nuclear, Boston, USA) was added to each sample, and an initial chromatography was carried out by passing the urine through a pre-packed reverse-phase chromatography column (Sep Pak C18 Cartridge, Waters Associetes, Milford, Mass., USA) which had been pretreated with ethanol, 20 ml (the solvents used were RPE ACS or HPLC grade, Carlo Erba, Milano, Italy), followed by water, 20 ml. Each cartridge was rinsed successively with water (20 ml), ethanol:water (15:85, 20 ml), petrol-ether (20 ml) and methyl formate (10 ml) (method developed by Powell)[7]; this last solvent containing the 6-keto-PGF$_{1\alpha}$ was collected and dried under nitrogen. The residue was dissolved in benzene: ethyl acetate:methanol (60:40:2, 1 ml), and then passed through a Sep Pak Silica cartridge (Waters Associated,

Milford, USA) which had been prepared with benzene:ethyl acetate (60:40, 5 ml), benzene:ethyl acetate:methanol (60:40:20, 5 ml) and 1 ml of 60:40 benzene:ethyl acetate again. The cartridge was washed with benzene:ethyl acetate (60:40, 20 ml) and, finally, 6-keto-PGF$_{1\alpha}$ was eluted with benzene:ethyl acetate:methanol (60:40:20, 5 ml) and dried under nitrogen. The dried extract was dissolved in 200 µl of water:acetonitrile (70:30); 100 µl were then subjected to HPLC using the Beckman 112 solvent delivery module and HPLC octodecyl (ODS) reverse-phase column (Altex Ultrasphere ODS, 5µ, 4.6 mm x 15 cm). The fractions were collected utilizing a LKB 7000 Ultra-rac collector. 6-keto-PGF$_{1\alpha}$ was eluted isocratically from ODS reverse-phase column with water:acetonitrile (70:30) + 0.02 M phosphoric acid. Flow rate was 1 ml/min. 1 ml fractions were collected and 6-keto-PGF$_{1\alpha}$ was identified by detection of the tritiated 6-keto-PGF$_{1\alpha}$ previously added to each sample. The samples containing 6-keto-PGF$_{1\alpha}$, collected after HPLC, were extracted with ethyl acetate (2 ml), dried under nitrogen and resuspended in 1 ml of phosphate buffer (pH 7.4, 0.02 M). The recovery of the ^{3}H-6-keto-PGF$_{1\alpha}$, expresed as mean $\pm$ SD, was 40.4 $\pm$ 12.9% at the end of the purification process.

The radioimmunoassay was performed by incubating in a polistyrene tube: 100 µl of phosphate buffer (pH 7.4, 0.02 M) with about 2500 CPM of ^{3}H-6-keto-PGF$_{1\alpha}$, 500 µl of phosphate buffer containing bovine albumine (1.5 g/l) and specific antiserum (0.5 µl, diluted 1:10) and 100 µl of phosphate buffer with 6-keto-PGF$_{1\alpha}$ standard (Upjohn Company, Kalamazoo, Michigan, USA) or 50-100 µl of the sample. Phosphate buffer (0.02 M, pH 7.4) was added to achieve a final volume of 1 ml. Two different volumes (50 and 100 µl) of each sample were assayed in duplicate. Specific antiserum to 6-keto-PGF$_{1\alpha}$ was obtained in our laboratory by immunizing rabbits with 6-keto-PGF$_{1\alpha}$-human albumin conjugate[8]. One of the antisera obtained was used for the RIA procedure. This antiserum showed a K$_A$ of 0.53 x 10^{-11} M/l. Cross-reactivity was 0.3% with PGE$_2$, 1.5% with PGF$_{2\alpha}$ and 0.015% with Thromboxane B$_2$. The final dilution of antiserum in the assay was 1:20,000 (B$_0$= 43%) and the sensitivity (IC$_{50}$) was 52 pg. The radioimmunoassay was validated performing dilution and recovery tests (Fig. 1) and comparing the results with those obtained using a different antiserum, kindly provided us by Prof. G. Folco (Istituto di Farmacologia e Farmacognosia, Università di Milano, Italy).

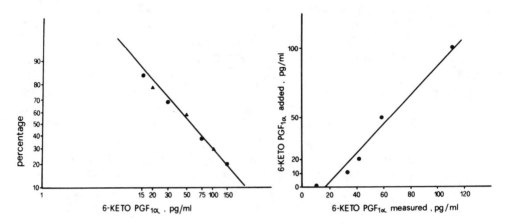

Fig. 1. Dilution of two samples of urine (●, ▲); straight line represents standard curve (left). Recovery by RIA of 6-keto-PGF$_{1\alpha}$ added to a sample of urine (right).

RESULTS

Urinary electrolyte excretion and 24-hour urinary volume variations are shown in Fig. 2. Urinary volume was slightly reduced at day 3 of drug administration and increased at days 6 and 9; however, these variations were not statistically significant. Mean urinary sodium excretion increased significantly at day 6 ($P < 0.05$). The highest sodium excretion was observed at day 6 in 5 subjects and at day 9 in the remaining two subjects. Maximal sodium urinary excretion and negative sodium balance were considered the index of the "escape" phenomenon. Urinary potassium excretion increased significantly at day 3 ($P < 0.05$) and returned subsequently to basal values.

During the whole period of 9α-FF administration urinary aldosterone was reduced ($P < 0.01$), while urinary

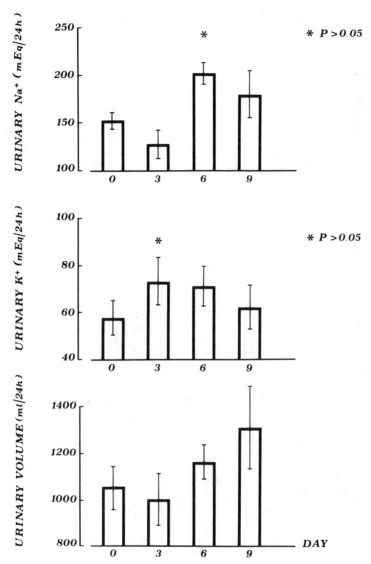

Fig. 2. Urinary excretion of sodium, potassium and
urinary volume before (0) and at day 3, 6 and
9 of 9α-fluorohydrocortisone administration.
Values are expressed as mean ± standard error.
Statistical analysis was performed using the
Student's t test for paired data.

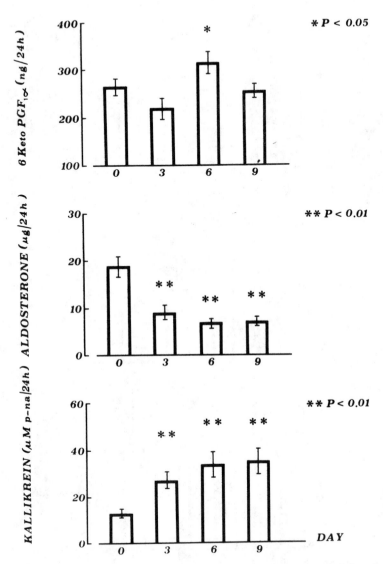

Fig. 3. Urinary excretion of 6-keto-PGF$_{1\alpha}$, aldosterone
and kallikrein before (0) and at day 3, 6 and
9 of 9α-fluorohydrocortisone administration.
Values are expressed as mean ± standard error.
Statistical analysis was performed using the
Student's t test for paired data.

kallikrein was increased (P<0.01), as shown in Fig. 3.

Urinary 6-keto-PGF$_{1\alpha}$ excretion was slightly reduced at day 3, significantly increased at day 6 (P<0.05) and back to basal values at day 9 (Fig. 3). At day 3 there was a significant correlation between urinary 6-keto-PGF$_{1\alpha}$ and urinary sodium variations (r = 0.81, P<0.05). No other correlations were found between the other parameters studied.

DISCUSSION

The increase in urinary volume and sodium excretion indicates that the escape from the sodium-retaining action of 9α-FF takes place between day 6 and day 9. However, there are great interindividual differences in this phenomenon.

As expected, we observed a decrease of aldosterone and an increase of kallikrein in the urine. These two effects are probably due to 9α-fluorohydrocortisone, which, like other mineralocorticoids, directly stimulates urinary kallikrein production[9,10].

Urinary 6-keto-PGF$_{1\alpha}$ excretion was reduced at day 3 and this correlates with the sodium excretion decrease. The reduction of renin and angiotensin release, caused by volume expansion, might be responsible for this effect. In fact, it is well known that angiotensin directly stimulates PGI$_2$ production in the kidney[2,11]. Subsequently 6-keto-PGF$_{1\alpha}$ excretion increased during the escape; nevertheless no significant correlations were observed between the increase of sodium, kallikrein and 6-keto-PGF$_{1\alpha}$. Dürr et al. observed that urinary excretion of PGF$_{2\alpha}$, PGE$_2$ and kallikrein increases during 9α-FF treatment in normal subjects and that the peak excretion of the two prostaglandins occurs concomitantly to the sodium escape[12]. However, they did not observe any significant statistical correlation between PG increase and sodium excretion. Indomethacin, a PG inhibitor, does not reduce kallikrein excretion but causes a delay in the escape phenomenon and only a transient sodium retention[12].

This might suggest that PGs could be at least partly responsible for the escape.

On the contrary, Zipser et al.[13] did not observe any variation in PGE_2 levels after desoxycorticosterone acetate (DOCA) administration and suggested that the increased release of kallikrein was principally responsible for the escape phenomenon. However, Nasjletti et al.[10] showed that the administration of DOCA to rats produces an increase in urinary volume, kallikrein and PGE_2. Aprotinin, a kallikrein inhibitor, reduces PGE_2 and sodium excretion, therefore indicating a cooperative action of kallikrein-kinin and prostaglandin systems.

In our study we did not find any significant correlation between sodium increase and $6\text{-keto-PGF}_{1\alpha}$ increase during escape. This could be explained by the presence of other factors, such as the secretion of natriuretic factors[14] and the modifications in renal haemodynamics, in particular the enhancement of renal perfusion pressure[15], which may contribute largely to sodium excretion during escape.

Equally, the administration of mineralocorticoids increases renal kallikrein production and kinin release, hence inducing PGI_2 stimulation; on the other hand volume expansion inhibits the renin-angiotensin system. These two different events (increased kinins and inhibition of angiotensin) make the evaluation of the role of PGI_2 problematic and may explain the different results reported in the literature.

Even though urinary $6\text{-keto-PGF}_{1\alpha}$ increases during escape our data do not clearly indicate that renal PGI_2 has a direct role in this phenomenon.

REFERENCES

1. F. G. Knox, J. C. Burnett Jr., D.E. Kohan, W. S. Spielman, and J. C. Strand, Escape from the sodium-retaining effects of mineralocorticoids, Kidney Int. 17:263 (1980).

2. J. G. Gerber, R. J. Anderson, R. W. Schrier, and A. S. Nies, Prostaglandins and the regulation of renal circulation and function, in: "Prostaglandins and the Cardiovascular System" Advances in Prostaglandin, Thromboxane, and Leukotriene Research vol. 10, J. A. Oates, ed., Raven Press, New York (1982).

3. Y. Iino and B. M. Brenner, Inhibition of Na transport by prostacyclin (PGI_2) in rabbit cortical collecting tubule, Prostaglandins 22:715 (1981).

4. O. A. Carretero and A. G. Scicli, The renal kallikrein-kinin system, in: "Renal endocrinology", M. J. Dunn, ed., Williams & Wilkins, Baltimore/London (1983).

5. K. M. Mullane and S. Moncada, Prostacyclin release and the modulation of some vasoactive hormones, Prostaglandins 20:25 (1980).

6. E. Amundsen, J. Pütter, P. Friberger, M. Knös, M. Larsbraten, and G. Gleason, Methods for the determination of glandular kallikreins by means of a chromogenic tripeptide substrate, Adv. Exp. Med. Biol. 120:83 (1979).

7. W. S. Powell, Rapid extraction of oxygenated metabolites of arachidonic acid from biological samples using octadecylsilyl silica, Prostaglandins 20: 947 (1980).

8. B. M. Jaffe, J. W. Smith, W. T. Newton, and C. W. Parker, Radioimmunoassay for prostaglandins, Science 171:494 (1971).

9. M. J. Dunn and V. L. Hood, Prostaglandins and the kidney, Am. J. Physiol. 233:F169 (1977).

10. A. Nasjletti, J. C. McGiff, and J. Colina-Chourio, Interrelations of the renal kallikrein-kinin system and renal prostaglandins in the conscious rat: Influence of mineralocorticoids, Circ. Res. 43:799 (1978).

11. M. J. Dunn, Renal prostaglandins, in: "Renal Endocrinology", M. J. Dunn, ed., Williams & Wilkins, Baltimore/London (1983).

12. J. Dürr, L. Favre, R. Gaillard, A. M. Riondel, and M.B. Vallotton, Mineralocorticoid escape in man: role of renal prostaglandins, Acta Endocrinol. 99:474 (1982).

13. R. D. Zipser, P. Zia, R. A. Stone, and R. Horton, The prostaglandin and kallikrein-kinin systems in mineralocorticoid escape, _J. Clin. Endocrinol. Metab._ 47:996 (1978).

14. H. E. De Wardener, Natriuretic hormone, _Clin. Sci._ 53:1 (1977).

15. J. E. Hall, J. P. Granger, M. J. Smith, and A. J. Premen, Role of renal hemodynamics and arterial pressure in aldosterone "escape", _Hypertension_ 6:I-183 (1984).

PROSTACYCLIN IN THERAPY OF VASCULAR DISEASE

R.J. Gryglewski and A. Szczeklik

Department of Pharmacology and
Department of Medicine
N. Copernicus Academy of Medicine in Cracow
31-531 Cracow, Poland

INTRODUCTION

In arteries of animals with experimental atherosclerosis (Gryglewski et al. 1978, DeGaetano et al.
1979, Larrue et al. 1980, 1982)and in arteries of
humans with atherosclerosis (D'Angelo et al. 1978,
Sinzinger et al. 1979) or with an exposure to risk
factors (Silberbauer et al. 1979, Dadak et al. 1981)
the generation of a prostacyclin-like activity is
severely suppressed. On the other hand it has been
recently reported that the urine excretion of prostacyclin metabolites is augmented in atherosclerosis.
The validity of a conception that prostacyclin deficiency is associated with development of atherosclerosis depends on further analytical studies, however, the
results of early experimental findings stimulated
clinicians to use prostacyclin for treatment of arterial disease (Szczeklik et al. 1979). Irrespectively to
a role that prostacyclin may play in pathogenesis of
atherosclerosis, the drug itself has a potent platelet-
-suppressant and vasodilatory actions (Szczeklik et al.
,1978). Fibrionolytic (Dembińska-Kieć et al. 1982)
and cytoprotective (for ref. see Vane, 1983) properties
of prostacyclin might be also of clinical importance.

MODE OF ADMINISTRATION

Prostacyclin (PGI_2, epoprostenol) is available as
a freeze-dried preparation (Flolan of Wellcome and
Cyclo-prostin of Upjohn) which when dissolved in

0.1 M glycine buffer pH 10.5 retains its full pharmacological activity for at least 12 hrs at room temperature (Fig. 1). In adult conscious patients prosta-

PGI$_2$

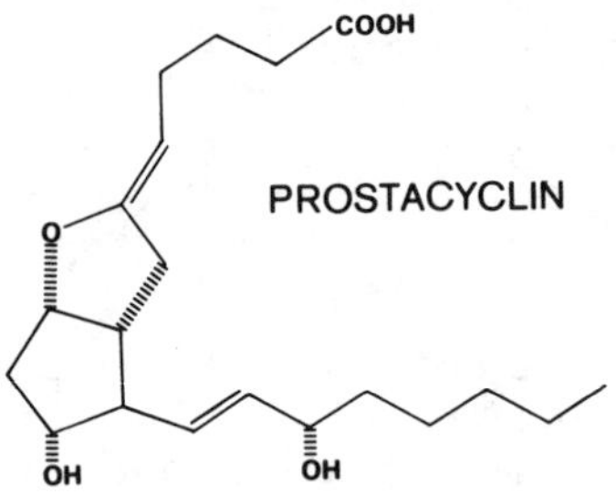

COOH

PROSTACYCLIN

EPOPROSTENOL

FLOLAN®

CYCLO-PROSTIN®

+

0.1 M GLYCINE BUFFER pH 10.5

Fig. 1   Chemical structure, generic and trade names,
and solvent for prostacyclin.

cyclin is infused i.v. or i.a. at doses ranging from
2 to 10 ng/kg/min (10 - 50 μl/min). In the first clinical trial prostacyclin was administered in a continuous
intravenous infusion for 72 hrs (Szczeklik et al. 1979).
This regimen is still being used in most trials, although
in some others the duration of infusions may vary from

222

one hour (Yui et al. 1982) up to several days (Żygulska-
-Mach et al. 1980, 1984). An intra-arterial route of
infusion was also introduced (Uchida et al. 1982,
Niżankowski et al. 1984). A long-term infusion of
prostacyclin was reported to induce a paradoxical
activation of platelets, to stimulate renin-angiotensin

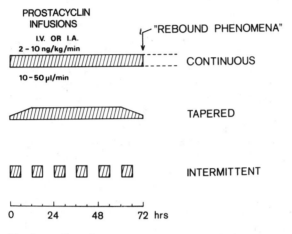

Fig. 2   Mode of administration of prostacyclin.

system and to extinguish fibrinolytic potential of
prostacyclin (Sinzinger et al. 1981, Dembińska-Kieć
et al. 1981, Silberbauer et al. 1982). In order to
avoid those "rebound" phenomena an intermittent
(Gryglewski et al. 1983) and a tapered (Henriksson
et al. 1984) regiments of prostacyclin infusions
were introduced (Fig. 2).
      Prostacyclin even at a dose as low as 2 ng/kg/min
i.v. produces facial flushing. At higher doses a moderate fall in arterial blood pressure and tachycardia
may appear. Other side effects of prostacyclin therapy
include headache, restlessness, nausea, drowsiness,
gastro-intestinal disturbances, hiperglycaemia,
articular pain and ectopic beats (Pickles and O'Grady,
1982, Niżankowski et al., 1984). Those side-effects
wane or are considerably reduced when a maximum
tolerated dose of prostacyclin is tailored individually
for each patient. Incidently, prostacyclin at doses

lower than 2 ng/kg/min i.v. may well have a therapeutic
effect equal to that of a maximum tolerated dose of the
drug. We just do not know it, since the lowest effective
dose of prostacyclin in humans has not been determined.

OPEN CLINICAL TRIALS

There are numerous open clinical trials with
prostacyclin which have not yet been followed by
controlled studies.
    Prostacyclin is a unique dienoic prostanoid that
is endowed with a vasodilatory action on pulmonary
circulation (Kadowitz et al. 1980). Vasodilatation of
pulmonary vascular bed by prostacyclin was reported
in patients with secondary pulmonary hypertension due
to mitral stenosis (Szczeklik et al. 1980 a) , in
patients with primary pulmonary hypertension (Rubin
et al. 1982), in pulmonary vascular disease (Duagni
et al. 1981), in persistent foetal circulation (Lock
et al.1979) and idiopathic pulmonary hypertension
in a child (Watkins et al. 1980).
    Dis-aggregatory and anti-aggregatory action of
prostacyclin on platelets, its protective action on
damaged capillary endothelial cells as well as its
fibrinolytic properties might be responsible for the
reported improvement of visual acuity in patients
with occlusion of retinal blood vessels (Żygulska-Mach
et al. 1980, 1984), improvement of hearing in patients
with sudden unilateral deafness of vascular origin
(Olszewski et al., 1984), decrease in platelet deposition
on prosthetic graft surface in patients with vascular
prosthetic grafting (Sinzinger et al. 1983), inhibition
of kidney transplant rejection (Leithner et al. 1981)
and improvement of patients with pre-eclampsia (Dadak
et al. 1983). Those reports have to be confirmed or
disproved in controlled studies before any conclusion
on therapeutical efficacy of prostacyclin in the above
disorders can be drawn.

CONTROLLED CLINICAL TRIALS

In three types of arterial disease prostacyclin
was tried in a controlled manner. Those are peripheral
arterial disease, coronary heart disease and ischaemic
stroke,

Peripheral arterial disease

When prostacyclin was first given to patients with
advanced peripheral arterial disease (PAD) a sustained
relief of rest pain and healing of ischaemic ulcers

were noticed (Szczeklik et al., 1979). These early observations were confirmed by several (Assal et al. 1980, Olsson, 1980, Pardy et al. 1981, Kaukinen et al. 1984) but not all (Machin et al. 1981) investigators in open clinical trials. From one controlled study (Hossman et al. 1981) a final conclusion is difficult to be drawn because of a short period of observation of patients and a cross-over design of the study.

The first random-assignment placebo-controlled study (Belch et al. 1983 a) in 28 patients with PAD has shown an immediate relief in rest pain in all of 15 prostacyclin-treated patients as compared to 3 improved patients out of placebo group. This difference is statistically significant. Although prostacyclin did not change calf blood flow still in some patients pain did not return up to 6 months of the observation period. At that time a frequency of surgical interventions was substantially higher in placebo as compared to prostacyclin group.

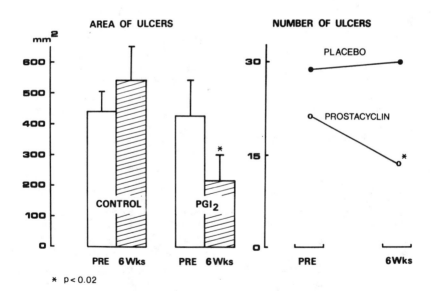

Fig. 3   The effect of prostacyclin therapy in PAD patients on area and number of ischaemic ulcers. PRE - pretreatment measurements, 6Wks- 6 weeks after treatment. Significance (p<0.02) for t unpaired test (Niżankowski et al. 1984).

225

The second random-assignment placebo-controlled
study (Niżankowski et al., 1984) was designed to study
the effect of prostacyclin on healing of ischaemic
ulcers in patients with arteriosclerosis obliterans and
thrombangiitis obliterans. Unlike in the first study
prostacyclin was administered intra-arterially, i.e.
into femoral artery. The drug (14 patients) or inert
vehicle (16 patients) were given in a continuous 72 h
infusions to patients who suffered from ischaemic
ulcers (5 sq cm) on one or both legs. Exclusions
were: patients with diabetes, gangrene and the aorto-
-iliac disease. Six weeks after prostacyclin or placebo
had been administered area and number of ulcers significantly diminished in the prostacyclin group as compared
to controls (Fig. 3).

Thus in two controlled studies it has been shown
that in PAD patients the administration of prostacyclin
relieves rest pain and promotes healing of ischaemic
ulcers.

These controlled studies as well as previous open
trials allow to draw a conclusion that PAD patients
with proximal lesions respond worse to prostacyclin
therapy than those with distal localization of the
disease affecting arteries below the knee. No response
to the therapy should be expected in patients with deep
black gangrene of the foot and in patients with grossly
infected ulcers. Concomitant diabetes seems to hinder
success of the therapy. There exists no empirical
evidence for therapeutical superiority of intra-arterial
versus intravenous route of administration of prostacyclin. In PAD patients high doses of prostaglandins
used in treatment of ischaemic ulcers might have detrimental effects. This conclusion was reached by Rhodes
and Heard, 1983 who infused prostaglandin E_1 at a dose
of 21 ng/kg/min to PAD patients. They also pointed to
the fact that the worst results with prostacyclin for
treatment of ischaemic ulcers were those of Machin et
al., 1981 who had been using the highest dosing regimen
for prostacyclin (5 - 50 ng/kg/min during 72 hrs) so
far reported.

In 14 patients with Raynaud's disease (mostly
young women with avarage 6 yrs of history of the
disease) prostacyclin or placebo were given intravenously as 5 hr infusions at weekly intervals for
3 weeks (Belch et al. 1983 b). Treatment with the drug
reduced significantly the frequency and duration of
ischaemic pain attacks and improved hand temperature
measurments. Alleviation of pain was still present 6
weeks after prostacyclin infusion. Healing was observed
in all 3 patients of the prostacyclin group who had had
digital ischaemic ulcers, whereas for the 3 patients

in the placebo group healing occured in 1 patient only.
Recently Prentice and Belch, 1984 have reported on
similar therapeutical effects of prostacyclin in next
30 patients with Raynaud´s disease.

In summary, there are available four random-assignment placebo-controlled trials on prostacyclin treatment
of patients with peripheral arterial disease. These
studies support a majority of early open clinical
trials in which it has been claimed that prostacyclin
relieves rest pain and promotes healing of ischaemic
ulcers. Further controlled, preferably multicenter
studies, are required in order to compare the therapeutical efficacy of prostacyclin with that of prostaglandin E_1 (Carlson and Eriksson, 1973) and with other
vasodilator and platelet-suppressant drugs. In any of
next controlled trials an appropriate exclusion of
poor candidates for the prostacyclin therapy should
be done on basis of hitherto existing observations.
The mechanism of beneficial long-term effect of prostacyclin in PAD patients remains unknown. One possibility is that prostacyclin "cleans" collateral circulation
from fresh platelet and fibrin deposits and thus
enables the affected endothelium to regain a capacity
to produce endogenous prostacyclin. In consequence
collateral circulation remains patent.

Coronary heart disease

Angina pectoris has not a uniform etiology. Apart
from the main division between effort angina and spontaneous angina (angina at rest) the patients can be
classified into several subgroups. At various stages
of development of the disease patients may suffer both
from effort and spontaneous angina. This complexity
in classification of patients with angina might be
partly responsible for contradictory reports on the
effectivness of prostacyclin treatment of patients
with angina.

In an attempt to summarize available data the
following can be said. In patients with effort angina
who had been submitted to atrial pacing prostacyclin
failed to protect them against chest pain and ECG
ischaemic symptoms (Szczeklik et al. 1980 b, 1981,1984),
although Bergman et al. 1981 observed some protective
action of prostacyclin in those patients. Spontaneous
angina creates even more problems. In most of patients
with variant angina (Prinzmetal angina characterized by
ST segment elevation and coronary vasospasm) prostacyclin was hardly effective (Chierchia et al. 1982,
Szczeklik et al. 1984). A similar lack of therapeutic
effect of prostacyclin was reported in patients with

spontaneous angina whose attacks were associated with
a rise in arterial blood pressure and tachycardia

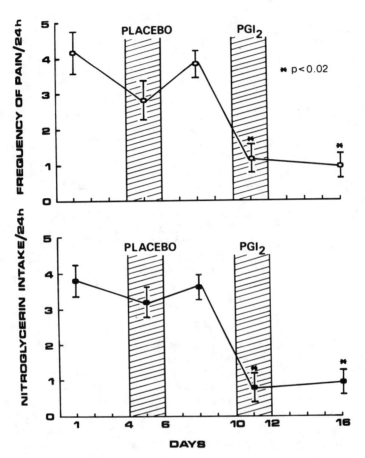

Fig. 4   A self-controlled study on the effect of
         placebo and prostacyclin infusions (48 hrs)
         on frequency of chest pain attacks and
         daily nitroglycerine intake within a group
         of 16 patients with spontaneous angina
         that was characterized by ST segment de-
         pression not accompanied by a rise in
         arterial blood pressure and tachycardia.
         Bars represent 2 S.E., asterics - signi-
         ficance at a level of p< 0.02. (Szczeklik
         et al. 1984).

(Szczeklik et al., 1984). The only subgroup of patients with spontaneous angina who benefited from prostacyclin therapy were those patients with ST segment depression whose attacks frequently occured at night and were not associated with hypertensive paroxysms and an increase in heart rate. In a self-controlled study Szczeklik et al. 1984 reported that 11 out of 16 of the above described patients had improved after administration of prostacyclin (4 ng/kg/min i.v. during 48 hrs) in contrast to treatment with placebo (Fig. 4). In "responders" this improvement lasted from 10 days to 3 months. Perhaps, activation of platelets at a site of endothelial damage in coronary arteries was responsible for symptoms of spontaneous angina in a subgroup of patients who did respond favourably to prostacyclin.

In experimental myocardial infarction prostacyclin was reported to limit infart size and to decrease mortality of infarcted animals (for ref. see Vane, 1983). Prostacyclin was well tolerated by humans when infused into coronary arteries (Hall and Dewar, 1981) and by patients with myocardial infarction when given intravenously (Edhog et al., 1983). A successful coronary recanalization was induced by intracoronary administration of prostacyclin to 9 patients with acute myocardial infarction (Uchida et al. 1982). These observations led to the first controlled clinical trial on prostacyclin in acute myocardial infarction (AMI) by Wennmalm's group (Henriksson et al. 1984).

Thirty AMI patients of less than 16 hrs duration of the infarct were randomly and in equal numbers allocated into infusions of either prostacyclin or placebo. The drug was infused intravenously in a tapered manner (Fig. 2) at maximum dose of 5 ng/kg/min during 72 hrs. None of prostacyclin patients but four patients in the placebo group developed an extention of myocardial infarction during the course of infusion. Extention of myocardial infarction was evidenced by an additional rise in plasma indicator enzymes, increase in pain and ECG changes. The difference between prostacyclin and placebo groups in limitation of myocardial infarction was statistically significant, however, a two-week follow up disclosed that 2 patients in the prostacyclin group reinfarcted compared to none in the control group. These results suggest that prostacyclin has a protective action on ischaemic myocardium as long as it is infused into patients. This assumption was also supported by the fact that in a subgroup of patients who were treated with prostacyclin within 10 hrs after the onset of symptoms there was observed a lower rise in plasma CPK-MB during the first 24 hrs infusion as compared to controls.

In summary, there are available two controlled studies on the effect of prostacyclin in patients with coronary heart disease. Most of types of angina pectoris are resistant to prostacyclin therapy. Prostacyclin alleviates chest pain and reduces frequency of attacks in a subgroup of patients with spontaneous angina, whose nocturnal attacks are not associated with hypertensive paroxysms and tachycardia and in ECG ST segment is consistently depressed. Within this group an improvement in "responders" may stay as long as few weeks. In contrast to patients with angina, AMI patients benefit from prostacyclin therapy only as long as the drug is infused, and therefore in future it will be necessery to offer to those patients a conceptually related therapy (e.g. orally active prostacyclin analogues, thromboxane synthetase inhibitors, low doses of aspirin, endogenous prostacyclin releasers etc.) after cessation of prostacyclin infusion. In both types of coronary heart disease the mode of action of prostacyclin remains unknown. Perhaps in patients with angina a dis-aggregatory effect and anti-release effect of prostacyclin on platelets is of importance, whereas in patients with acute myocardial infarction prostacyclin exerts a cytoprotective action on ischaemic myocardium.

Ischaemic stroke

Following an open clinical trial (Gryglewski et al., 1983) two random-assignment placebo-controlled studies on the effect of prostacyclin in patients with completed ischaemic stroke (CIS) have been recently presented (Martin et al.,1984, Huczyński et al.,1984). The studies included 24 and 26 patients, respectively. Patients were infused with either prostacyclin (2.5 ng/kg/min i.v.) or vehicle in an intermittent regimen (Fig. 2), i.e. 5 times for 6 hr periods with 6 hr breaks in between. Infusions started not earlier than 48 hrs and not later than 5 days after the onset of neurological symptoms. Neurological status of CIS patients was scored before infusion and then at various time intervals up to the end point which was 2 weeks after infusions. Neurological scores were ascribed to a patient by two independent observers who had not seen patients during infusions. In both trials the improvement in neurological deficit in CIS patients treated with prostacyclin was more pronounced than in controls, however in the study of Martin et al., 1984 this improvement never reached statistical significance, whereas in the study of Huczyński et al., 1984

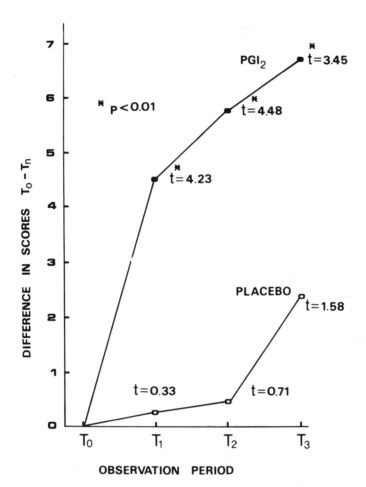

Fig. 5 Analysis of neurological status (difference in scores $T_0 - T_n$) in patients with completed ischaemic stroke (CIS), who were treated with either prostacyclin (PGI$_2$) or placebo. Time of scoring: T_0 - before infusion, T_1 - 6 hrs after infusion, T_2 - 54 hrs after infusion and T_3 - 2 weeks after infusion. t is for matched--pair Student test. Astericks are for significance at a level of $p < 0.01$. Data from Huczyński et al., 1984.

an alleviation of aphasia and hemiparesis (those two mainly contributed to neurological scores) was stati-

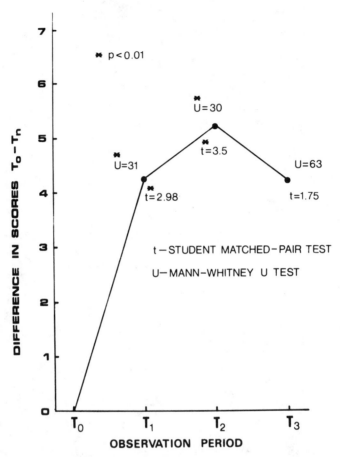

Fig. 6   Net-effect of prostacyclin treatment on neurological status (difference in scores $T_0 - T_n$) of patients with completed ischaemic stroke (CIS) in a random-assignment placebo--controlled study (Fig. 5). As indicated in this figure the final analysis was performed by both parametric and non-parametric tests. Two weeks after prostacyclin infusion (T_3) the alleviation of neurological deficit by prostacyclin was no more statistically significant.

stically significant after 6 hrs (T_1) and 54 hrs (T_2) of prostacyclin infusion as compared to controls. Two weeks later (T_3) this improvement lost its statistical significance (Fig. 5 and Fig. 6).

In summary, the results of controlled studies on the use of prostacyclin for treatment of patients with completed ischaemic stroke are not conclusive but highly encouraging to undertake further controlled trials. Like in case of AMI patients also in CIS patients the intensification and extention of beneficial effects of prostacyclin would be desirable. Options include a replacement of intermittent regimen for a continuous one (Fig. 2), a supplementation with orally active prostacyclin analogues, prostacyclin releasers, thromboxane synthetase inhibitors etc. or a use of a combined therapy with prostacyclin, heparin and indomethacin as suggested by Hallenbeck, 1984. Again, like in AMI patients or patients with retinal vein occlusion also in CIS patients it might be of crucial clinical importance to start prostacyclin infusions at the earliest possible stage of the disease. Then patients with transient ischaemic attacks will be also embraced into such trial.

CONCLUSIONS

In following vascular disoders prostacyclin was infused to patients: pulmonary hypertension, sudden blidness and sudden deafness of vascular origin, vascular prosthetic grafting, kidney transplant rejection, disseminated intravascular coagulation, congestive heart failure, peripheral vascular disease including Raynaud´s disease, coronary heart disease and ischaemic stroke. Only in the last three arterial disease the therapeutic efficacy of prostacyclin was investigated in a controlled manner. These controlled studies leave little doubt that prostacyclin exerts a long-term beneficial effect in a selected group of patients with peripheral arterial disease. Therapeutical effects of prostacyclin in patients with spontaneous angina, myocardial infarction and ischaemic stroke , although encouraging, are not yet conclusive and call for further careful controlled trials. The hitherto accumulated observations will fascilitate a design of new controlled studies. Open and controlled trials with prostacyclin in patients with vascular disease revealed its therapeutical potential which may depend on a combination of platelet-suppressant, vasodilatory, fibrinolytic and cytoprotective properties which abide in a molcule of prostacyclin.

REFERENCES

Assal, J.P., Helg, C., VonderWeld, N. et al. , 1980,
    Prostacyclin perfusions in diabetic peripheral
    arterial insufficiency, Diabetologia 19:254.
Belch, J.J.F., McArdle, B., Pollock, J.G., Forbes, C.D.,
    McKay, A., Leiberman, P., Lowe, G.D.O. and
    Prentice, C.R.M., 1983a,Epoprostenol (prostacyc-
    lin) and severe arterial disease, Lancet i:315
Belch, J.J.F., Drury, J.K., Capell, H., Forbes, C.D.,
    Newman , P., McKenzie, F., Leiberman, P.,
    Prentice, C.R.M., 1983b, Intermittent Epoprose-
    nol (prostacyclin) infusion in patients with
    Raynaud's syndrome, Lancet i:313.
Bergman,G., Daly, K., Atkinson, L., Rothman, M.,
    Richardson, P.J., Jackson, G., Jewitt, D.E.,
    1981, Prostacyclin: haemodynamic and metabolic
    effects in patients with coronary heart disease,
    Lancet i:596.
Carlson, L.A. and Eriksson, I., 1973, Femoral artery
    infusion of prostaglandin E_1 in severe periphe-
    ral vascular disease, Lancet i:155.
Chierchia, S., Patrono, C., Ciabattoni, G., De Caterina,
    R., Cinotti, G.A., Distante, A. and Maseri, A.,
    1982, Effect of intravenous prostacyclin in
    variant angina, Circulation, 65:470.
Dadak, C., Leithner, C., Silberbauer, K. and Sinzinger,
    H., Diminished prostacyclin formation in umbili-
    cal arteries of babies born to women who smoke,
    Lancet 1981, i:94
Dadak, C., and Sinzinger, H., 1983, Therapie der
    schweren EPH-Gestose mit Prostacyclin. Gyn.
    Rundschau 23:225
D'Angelo, V., Villa, S., Myśliwiec, M., Donati, M.B.
    and deGaetano, G., 1978, Defective fibrinolytic
    and prostacyclin-like activity in human athero-
    matous plaques. Thromb.Diath.Haemor. 39:535.
DeGaetano, G., Remuzzi, G., Myśliwiec, M., Donati, M.B.
    1979, Vascular prostacyclin and plasminogen
    activator sctivity in experimental and clinical
    conditions of disturbed haemostasis or thrombo-
    sis. Haemostasis 8:300.
Dembińska-Kieć, A. , Kostka-Trąbka, E. and Gryglewski,
    R.J., 1982, Effect of prostacyclin on fibrinolytic
    activity in patients with arteriosclerosis
    obliterans, Thromb.Haemostas. ,47:190.
Dembińska-Kieć, A., Żmuda, A., Grodzińska,L., Bieroń, K.,
    Basista, M., Kędzior, A., Kostka-Trąbka, E.,
    Telesz, E., Żelazny, T.,1981, Increased platelet
    activity after termination of prostacyclin
    infusion into man. Prostaglandins 21:827.

Duadagni, D.N., Ikram, H., Maslowski, R., 1981,
    Haemodynamic effects of prostacyclin (PGI$_2$) in
    pulmonary hypertension. Br. Heart J. 45:385.
Edhog, O., Henriksson.P., Wennmalm, A., 1983, Prostacyc-
    lin infusion in patients with acute myocardial
    infarction (preliminary report), New Engl.J.Med.
    308:1032.
Gryglewski, R.J., Dembińska-Kieć, A., Chytkowski, A.,
    Gryglewska, T., 1978, Prostacyclin and thrombo-
    xane biosynthetic capacities of the heart, arte-
    ries and platelets at various stages of
    experimental atherosclerosis in rabbits,
    Atherosclerosis 31:385.
Gryglewski, R.J., Nowak, S., Kostka-Trąbka, E.,
    Kuśmiderski, J., Dembińska-Kieć, A., Bieroń, K.,
    Basista, M., Błaszczyk, B., 1983, Treatment of
    ischaemic stroke with prostacyclin, Stroke
    14:197.
Hall, R.J. and Dewar, H.A., 1981, Safty of coronary
    arterial prostacyclin infusion, Lancet i:949.
Hallenbeck, J.M. , 1984, The effect of prostacyclin,
    indomethacin and heparin on postischaemic
    nerve cell function, in: Clinical Trials of
    Prostacyclin, edited by R.J. Gryglewski,
    A. Szczeklik and J.C. McGiff, Raven Press,
    New York, in press.
Henriksson, P., Edhog, O. and Wennmalm, A., 1984,
    Limitation of myocardial infarction with
    prostacyclin - a double blind study, in:
    Clinical Trials of Prostacyclin edited by
    R.J. Gryglewski, A. Szczeklik and J.C. McGiff,
    Raven Press, New York, in press.
Hossman, V., Heinen, A., Auel, H., 1981, A randomized
    placebo-controlled trial of prostacyclin (PGI$_2$)
    in peripheral arterial disease. Thromb.Res.
    22:481.
Huczyński, J., Kostka-Trąbka, E., Sokołowska, W., Bieroń,
    K., Grodzińska, L., Dembińska-Kieć, A., Pykosz-
    -Mazir, E., Peczak E. and Gryglewski, R.J.,1984
    Prostacyclin in patients with completed ischae-
    mic stroke - a controlled trial., in: Clinical
    Trials of Prostacyclin edited by R.J. Gryglew-
    ski, A. Szczeklik and I.C. McGiff, Raven Press,
    New York , in press.
Kadowitz, P.J., Spannhake, E.W., Levin , J.L., Hyman,
    A.L., 1980, Differential actions of the prosta-
    glandins on the pulmonary vascular bed, in:
    Advances in Prostaglandin and Thromboxane
    Research. vol. 7, edited by B. Samuelsson,
    P.W. Ramwell and R. Paoletti, Raven Press,
    New York, pp. 731-743.

Kaukinen, S., Pessi, T., Ylitalo, P., Krais T., and
    Vapaatalo, H., 1984, Clinical study on ZK 36374
    - a new stable prostacyclin analogue for
    treatment of peripheral vascular disease, in:
    Clinical Trials of Prostacyclin, edited by
    R.J. Gryglewski, A. Szczeklik and J.C. McGiff,
    Raven Press, New York, in press.
Larrue, J., Rigaud, M., Daret, D., Demond, J., Durand, J.
    Bricaud, H., 1980, Prostacyclin production by
    cultured smooth muscle cells from atherosclero-
    tic rabbit aorta. Nature 285:480.
Larrue, J., Leroux, C., Daret, D., Bricaud, H., 1982
    Decreased prostacyclin production in cultured
    smooth muscle cells from atherosclerotic rabbit
    aorta. Biochem.Biophys. Acta 710:257.
Leithner, C., Sinzinger, H., Schwartz, M., 1981,
    Treatment of chronic kidney transplant rejection
    with prostacyclin - reduction of platelet
    deposition in the transplant; prolongation of
    platelet survival and improvement of transplant
    function. Prostaglandins 22:783.
Lock, J.E., Olley, P.M., Coceani F., 1979, Use of
    prostacyclin in persistent fetal circulation,
    Lancet i:1343.
Machin, S.J., Defreyn, G., Chamone, D.A. , Vermylen, J.,
    1981, Clinical infusions of prostacyclin in
    advanced arterial disease, in: Clinical
    Pharmacology of Prostacyclin, edited by P.J.
    Lewis and J.M. O'Grady, Raven Press, New York,
    pp. 173 - 175.
Martin, J.F., Hamdy, N.A.T., Nicholl, J., Lewatas, N.,
    Bergvall, U., Owen, P., Whittington, D., 1984,
    Interim results from a double-blind controlled
    trial of prostacyclin in cerbral infarction,
    in: Clinical Trials of Prostacyclin, edited by
    R.J. Gryglewski, A. Szczeklik and J.C. McGiff,
    Raven Press, New York, in press.
Niżankowski, R., Szczeklik, A., Królikowski, W.,
    Bielatowicz J., Schaller, J., 1984, Prostacyclin
    for ischaemic ulcers in peripheral arterial
    disease - A random assignment, placebo-control-
    led study, in: Clinical Trials of Prostacyclin
    edited by R.J. Gryglewski, A. Szczeklik and J.C.
    McGiff, Raven Press, New York, in press.
Olsson, A.G., 1980, Intravenous prostacyclin for
    ischaemic ulcers in peripheral artery disease,
    Lancet, ii:1076.
Olszewski, E., Sekuła, J., Kstka-Trąbka, E., Grodzińska
    L., Dembińska-Kieć, A., Bieroń, K., Basista, M.
    Kędzior, A. and R.J. Gryglewski, 1984, Prosta-
    cyclin in sudden deafness of vascular origin,

in: Clinical Trials of Prostacyclin, edited by
    R.J. Gryglewski, A. Sczeklik and J.C. McGiff,
    Raven Press, New York, in press.
Pardy, B.J., Lewis, J.D, Eastcott, H.H.G., 1981,
    Preliminary experience with prostaglandins E_1
    and I_2 in peripheral vascular disease, Surgery,
    88:826.
Pickles, H. and O'Grady, J., 1982, Side effects occuring
    during administration of epoprostenol (prosta-
    cyclin, PGI_2) in man, Br.J.Clin.Pharmac., 14:
    :177.
Prentice, C.R.M. and Belch, J.J.F., 1984, Prostacyclin
    in Raynaud's syndrome, in: Clinical Trials of
    Prostacyclin, edited by R.J. Gryglewski, A.
    Szczeklik and J.C. McGiff, Raven Press, New York
    in press.
Rhodes, R.S. and Heard, S.E., 1983, Detrimental effects
    of high-dose prostaglandin E_1 in the treatment
    of ischaemic ulcers, Surgery 93:839.
Rubin, L.J., Groves, B.M., Reeves J.T., Frosolono, M;.,
    Hendel, F., Cato, A., 1982, Prostacyclin-induced
    acute pulmonary vasodilatation in primary
    pulmonary hypertension, Circulation, 66:334
Silberbauer, K., Schernthaner, G., Sinzinger, H. ,
    Piza-Katzer, H., Winter, M., 1979, Decreased
    vascular prostacyclin in juvenile-onset diabetes,
    New Eng.J.Med. 300,366.
Silberbauer, K., Sinzinger, H., Puzengruber, C., 1982,
    Long-term prostacyclin-therapy in peripheral
    vascular disease - influence on some vascular
    and platelet regulating mechanisms, in:
    Prostaglandins in Clinical Medicine - Cardio-
    vascular and Thrombotic Disorders, edited by
    K.K. Wu and P. Rossi, Yearbook Medical Publish-
    ers, Ne York, pp, 182 - 191.
Sinzinger, H., Feigl, W., Silberbauer, K., 1979,
    Prostacyclin generation in atherosclerotic
    arteries, Lancet, ii:469.
Sinzinger, H., O'Grady, J., Cromwell, M., Hofer, R.,
    1983, Epoprostenol (prostacyclin) decreases
    platelet deposition on vascular prosthetic
    grafts. Lancet, i:1275.
Sinzinger, H., Silberbauer, K., Harsch, A.K., Gall, A.,
    1981, Decreased sensitivity of human platelets
    to PGI_2 during long-term intraarterial prosta-
    cyclin infusion in patients with peripheral
    vascular disease - a rebound phenomenon,
    Prostaglandins 21:49.
Szczeklik, A., Gryglewski, R.J., Niżankowski, R.,Musiał,
    J., Piętoń, R., Mruk, J., 1978, Circulatory and
    anti-platelet effects of intravenous prostacyclin
    in healthy men. Pharmacol.Res.Commun. 10:545.

237

Szczeklik, A., Niżankowski, R., Skawiński,S., Szczeklik, J. , Głuszko, P.Gryglewski, R.J., 1979, Successful therapy of advanced arterioslerosis obliterans with prostacyclin. Lancet i:1111.

Szczeklik, A., Niżankowski, R. ,Szczeklik, J., Tabeau, J., Królikowski, W., 1984, Prostacyclin therapy in subgroups of patients with spontaneous angina, in: Clinical Trials of Prostacyclin , edited by R.J. Gryglewski, A. Szczekl k and J.C. McGiff, Raven Press, New York, in press.

Szczeklik, A., Szczeklik, J., Niżankowski, R., 1981, Prostacyclin, nitroglycerin and effort angina. Lancet i:1006.

Szczeklik, A., Szczeklik, J., Niżankowski, R., Głuszko, P., 1980 b, Prostacyclin for acute coronary insufficiency, Artery 8:7.

Szczeklik, A., Szczeklik, J., Niżankowski, R., 1980a, Prostacyclin for pulmonary hypertension, Lancet ii:1076.

Uchida, Y., Hanai, T., Hasegawa, K.,Kawamura, K., Oshima, T., 1982, Coronary recanalization induced by intracoronary administration of prostacyclin in patients with acute myocardial infarction. Circulation 66/II:Abstract No1045.

Vane, J.R., Prostaglandins and the cardiovascular system, 1983, Br.Heart J. 49:405

Watkins, W.D., Peterson, M.B., Crone, R.K., Shandon, D.C., Levine, L., 1980, Prostacyclin and prostaglandin E$_1$ for severe idiopathic pulmonary artery hypertension, Lancet i:1083.

Yui, Y., Nakajima, H., Kawai, C., Murakami, T., 1982, Prostacyclin therapy in patients with congestive heart failure, Am.J.Cardiol. 50:320.

Żygulska-Mach, H., Kostka-Trąbka, E., Mitoń, A. , Gryglewski, R.J., 1980, Prostacyclin in central retinal vein occlusion, Lancet ii:1075

Żygulska-Mach, H., Kostka-Trąbka, E., Grodzińska, L., Bieroń, K., Telesz, E., Gryglewski, R.J., 1984, Prostacyclin in therapy of central retinal vein occlusion, in: Clinical Trials of Prostacyclin, edited by R.J. Gryglewski, A. Szczeklik and J.C. McGiff, Raven Press, New York, in press.

LTC$_4$ INDUCES HYPERREACTIVITY OF THE ISOLATED VASCULAR TISSUE TO HISTAMINE, SEROTONIN AND NOREPINEPHRINE

L. Daffonchio, C. Omini, G. Brunelli and F. Berti

Institute of Pharmacology and Pharmacognosy
University of Milan, Italy

INTRODUCTION

Leukotrienes (LTs) are released from human lung "in vitro"[1,2] and they exert a potent bronchocontracturating activity in normal and asthmatic subjects[3], suggesting an important role for LTs in the allergic bronchoconstriction[4].
On the other hand anaphylactic shock is accompanied by increase in pulmonary vascular resistance[5] and both specific antigen-challenge and LTs "in vitro" induce a vasoconstriction of pulmonary vessels of different animal species[6,7]. During anaphylactic reaction the vessels of the respiratory system release a considerable amount of LTD$_4$[8,9] and its relative low pharmacological activity[10] in this vascular tissue does not rule out a possible interaction with other chemical mediators. All these observations prompted us to investigate the ability of LTs to induce vascular hyperreactivity to other vasoactive compounds. In this regard LTs have been suggested to play a role in the pathogenesis of bronchial hyperreactivity[11,12]; in addition to this, Creese and Bach[13] have shown in guinea-pig tracheal smooth muscle a clear cut potentiating action of LTD$_4$ on histamine and acetylcholine induced contractions.

MATERIALS AND METHODS

Male guinea-pigs weighing from 350 to 450 g were killed by

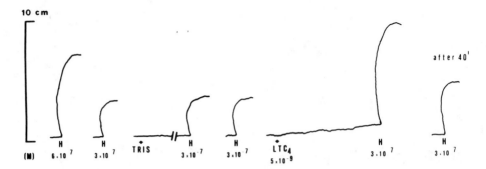

Fig. 1 - Hyperreactivity of guinea-pig pulmonary artery induced by LTC_4 on Histamine (H) activity.

LTC_4 and its solvent (TRIS) were added 15 min before H challenge.

a blow to the head and exanguinated. The main pulmonary artery (GPPA) was isolated by passing a suitable PE tube through the artery lumen from the right ventricle into the large lower lobe to the point of resistance. Descending thoracic aorta (GPTA) was dissected from aortic arch to the diaphragm; the tissues were cleaned and freed of excess fat, connective tissue and blood. Segments, cut as spirals of about 30 mm in length, were suspended in a 20 ml organ bath containing Krebs-bicarbonate buffer. Guinea-pig portal vein (GPPV) was isolated from hepatic hilum for about 1.5-2 cm of length, and suspended in 20 ml organ bath containing Ringer buffer solution. The buffer solutions bathing the tissues were mantained at 37°C and gased with 95% O_2 -5%CO_2. A load (0.8 g for GPPA; 1.5 g for GPTA; 1 g for GPPV) was applied to the tissues and usually a minimum of 60 min of equilibrium was allowed before starting the experiments.

Responses of isolated vessels were recorded via isotonic transducers (Basile 7006) on a Basile recorder (Gemini 7070). Norepinephrine (NE) 4×10^{-8} M, histamine (H) 3×10^{-7} M, and serotonin (5HT) 1.5×10^{-7} M were added to the organ bath until a constant effect was obtained. LTC_4 (5×10^{-9} M) dissolved in Tris 10mM and its solvent were added to the organ bath 15 min before

TABLE 1. - Interaction of LTC_4 ($5 \times 10^{-9}M$) with the contractile activity of histamine (H), serotonin (5HT) and norepinephrine (NE) on guinea-pig pulmonary artery (GPPA) and thoracic aorta (GPTA)

TISSUES	COMPOUNDS	contraction in mm without LTC_4 $\bar{x} \pm$ SEM	contraction in mm with LTC_4 $\bar{x} \pm$ SEM	contraction in mm at 40 min. $\bar{x} \pm$ SEM
GPPA	H, $3 \times 10^{-7}M$	28.7 ± 4.0	68.3 ± 8.0**	45.3 ± 7.1+
	5HT, $1.5 \times 10^{-7}M$	17.4 ± 2.6	48.0 ± 8.2*	17.1 ± 3.2
	NE, $4 \times 10^{-8}M$	13.7 ± 0.8	32.3 ± 1.9**	14.3 ± 1.7
	INDO + H	34.3 ± 1.1	89.3 ± 6.5**	44.5 ± 4.4
GPTA	H, $3 \times 10^{-7}M$	30.1 ± 2.7	57.8 ± 7.3**	51.3 ± 7.6

INDO = indomethacin was added to the organ bath at the concentration of $3 \times 10^{-6}M$ 1 h. before H.
Mean values ± standard error of the mean are referred to 4 replications.
** = $p < 0.01$; * = $p < 0.05$ from ANOVA two way
40 min. after LTC_4 washout, differences in contractility versus control (without LTC_4) have been statistically compared using "t" Student test for paired data. + = $p < 0.02$

241

agonist challenge. In some experiments the Krebs-solution was medicated with indomethacin (3×10^{-6} M), and the tissues were bathed for 60 min before challenge.

Data are expressed as mm of contraction induced by the agonists alone, and in presence of LTC_4. Statistical analysis was carried out according to a factorial experimental design[14]. The statistical procedure chosen, which consists in the evaluation of the effect of a single concentration of the agonist against a single concentration of LTC_4, allowed to compare the interaction among the compounds tested.

RESULTS

The contractile activity of H, 5HT and NE was evaluated on GPPA and GPTA in order to select equiactive concentrations of these compounds at submaxymal activity, and similarly a threshold concentration · of LTC_4 was chosen. LTC_4 (5×10^{-9} M) maintained in contact for 15 min to GPPA and GPTA induced a modest increase of the tonus of these preparations (Fig. 1). When H (3×10^{-7} M), 5HT (1.5×10^{-7} M) and NE (4×10^{-8} M) were tested in GPPA in presence of LTC_4 a significant potentiation of the contractile activity of the three compounds was observed (Table 1).

The positive interaction of LTC_4 with H was still significant 40 min after the washout of the peptido-leukotriene, whereas at this time, the contractile activity of both 5HT and NE returned to control values (Table 1). Similar results between LTC_4 and H have been obtained on GPTA: however in this case the time course of the phenomenon seemed to be shorter in comparison to that observed in GPPA (Table 1). Addition of FPL-55712 (10^{-5} M) to GPPA for 20 min abolished the potentiating effect of LTC_4 on H induced vasoconstriction (data not shown).

Indomethacin (3×10^{-6} M) added to the organ bath 60 min before starting the experiment, did not interfere with the LTC_4 induced hyperreactivity of GPPA to H. (Table 1). However, the phenomenon was not statistically significant 40 min away from LTC_4 washout. In contrast on GPPV the contractile activity of both NE (2×10^{-8} M) and H (10^{-5} M) was not augmented by LTC_4 (5×10^{-9} M), indicating that, at least for large peripheral veins of the guinea-pig, LTC_4 did not induce hyperreactivity to these vasoactive compounds (data not shown).

Preliminary experiments with human intralobar pulmonary artery, set up according to the laminar flow technique[15], clearly indicate that also in this human vascular tissue LTC_4

(100 pg/ml) generated hyperreactivity to H (100 ng) (Fig. 2).

DISCUSSION

The role of leukotrienes in the asthmatic syndrome and particularly their bronchocontractile activity are now well recognized[3,16]. Moreover pulmonary circulation is also affected by these lipidic compounds, and the results obtained with human pulmonary vessels indicate a preferential constrictive effect on pulmonary veins[10]. The present results, which demonstrate that LTC_4 significantly potentiates the contractile activity of H and, in a lesser extent, that of 5HT and NE on GPPA, support the hypotesis that leukotrienes may alter pulmonary vascular responsiveness in a number of pathological conditions[17,18]. Although the hyperreactivity caused by LTC_4 on GPPA seems to be a rather unspecific phenomenon, involving different types of vasoactive compounds, the H activity is certainly more sensitive to the presence of threshold concentration of LTC_4. In fact the increased responsiveness to H of this pulmonary tissue is long-lasting as compared to that observed with 5HT and NE.

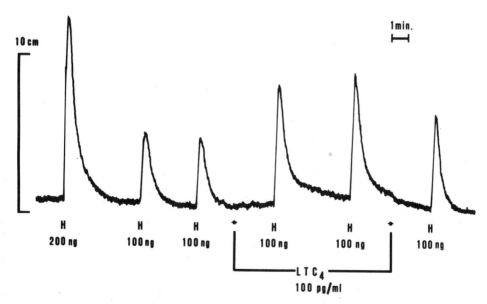

Fig. 2 - Hyperreactivity of perfused human intralobar pulmonary artery induced by LTC_4 on H activity.

The positive interaction between LTC$_4$ (and possibly other leukotrienes) and H may have some relevance in pulmonary circulation during anaphylaxis, since a dangerous viscious circle, leading to sustained pulmonary hypertension, may take place. The data obtained with GPTA preparations suggest that the vascular hyperreactivity due to LTC$_4$ is not restricted to the pulmonary circulation but seems to be a more general phenomenon which may compraise the arterial vasculature of other organs. On this line it would be of interest to examine a possible interaction between LTC$_4$ and H in coronary arteries, where leukotrienes display a pronounced constrictive effect[19] and may contribute with H, released during cardiac anaphylaxis, to the overall derangement of cardiac function[20]. The negative results obtained with GPPV preparations, where LTC$_4$ did not positively interact with both NE and H, are not surprising: the spontaneous motility and tonus of the portal-vein are not very sensitive to cysteinyl-leukotrienes[21] and therefore other venous tracts of small diameter, where the increase in permeability and tonus are coupled in the early event of the inflammatory responce, should be investigated. The increased sensitivity of GPPA for vasoactive compounds due to LTC$_4$ is antagonized by FPL-55712 but not by indomethacin. This suggests that the hyperreactivity of the vascular tissue particularly versus H is not dependent from production of prostaglandins. However, since indomethacin treatment shortenes the time course of the hyperreactivity to H, it is reasonable to speculate that the arachidonic acid metabolites of the cyclo-oxygenase pathway may contribute in some how in maintaining the status of hypersensitivity of the GPPA.

Since FPL-55712, a typical leukotriene receptor antagonist, prevents this phenomenon, which involves three different agonists, it is likely that LTC$_4$ may act through its receptors depolarizing the plasma membrane of the smooth muscle cells with reduction of the resting membrane potential as already reported for KCl[22]. In fact in tracheal smooth muscle KCl and LTC$_4$ increased the reactivity of the preparation to acetylcholine; these effects were not additive and therefore a similar mechanism of action was suggested[13]. However other mechanisms involving altered membrane binding or fluxes of Ca^{2+} may explain the hyperreactivity of GPPA and GPTA produced by leukotrienes.

The results obtained with human intralobar pulmonary artery "in vitro" are very interesting: they indicate that also in human lung vasculature LTC$_4$ induces hyperreactivity to H. We are now carefully investigating this phenomenon.

244

REFERENCES

1) S. E. Dahlén, G. Hansson, P. Hedqvist, T. Björek, E. Granstrom and B. Dahlén. Allergen challenge of lung tissue from asthmatics elicits bronchial contraction that correlates with the release of leukotrienes C_4, D_4 and E_4. Proc. Natl. Acad. Sci. USA 80: 1712, 1983.

2) G. C. Folco. Pharmacological studies on the release and effects of leukotrienes in human and guinea-pig lung tissue. Submitted Iuphar 9th International Congress of Pharmacology Macmillans Press. Ltd.

3) M. Griffin, J. Woodrow Weiss, A. Gordon Heitch, E.R. McFadden, E.J. Corey, K.F. Austen and J.M. Drazen. Effects of leukotriene D on the airways in asthma. New Eng. J. Med. 308 (8): 436, 1983.

4) B. Samuelsson. The leukotrienes: Mediators of Immediate Hypersensitivity Reactions and Inflammation. in: Leukotrienes and Prostacyclin. Ed: F. Berti, G. Folco and G.P. Velo. Plenum Press p. 15, 1983.

5) W. E. Brocklehurst: The release of histamine and formation of a slow reacting substance (SRS-A) during anaphylactic shock. J. Physiol (Lond) 151: 416, 1960.

6) P. J. Le Comte. Reactions anaphylactiques in vitro des arteres pulmonaires de lapin. Intern. Arch. Allergy. Appl. Immunol. 12: 339, 1958

7) P. Eyre. The Schultz-Dale reaction in bovine pulmonary smooth muscles. Br. J. Pharmacol 40: 166p, 1970.

8) J. H. Fleisch and K.D. Haisch. Release of slow reacting substance from various tissues by A23187. J. Pharm. Pharmacol. 34: 809, 1982

9) M. N. Samhoun and P.J. Piper. Actions and interactions of lipoxygenase and cyclooxygenase products in respiratory and vascular tissues. Prost. Leuk. Med. 13: 79, 1984.

10) J. M. Hand, J.A. Will and C.L. Buckner. Effects of leukotrienes on isolated guinea-pig pulmonary arteries. Eur. J. Pharmacol. 76: 439, 1981.

11) E. B. Weiss, S.G. Viswanath. Calcium hypersensitivity in airways smooth muscle. Isometric tension responses following anaphylaxis. Respiration 38: 266, 1979.

12) D. S. Dhillon, I.W. Rodger. Hyperreactivity of guinea-pig isolated airway smooth muscle. Br. J. Pharmacol. 74: 180P, 1981.

13) B. R. Creese and H.K. Bach. Hyperreactivity of airways smooth muscle produced in vitro by leukotrienes. Prost. Leuk. Med. 11: 161, 1983.

14) Sneidecor and Cochran. Factorial experiments in: "Statistical Methods VI" Ed. IOWA State University Press AMES. IOWA USA p. 339, 1967.

15) S. H. Ferreira and F.S. De Souza-Costa. A laminar flow superfusion technique with much increased sensitivity for the detection of smooth muscle stimulating substances. Eur. J. Pharmac. 39: 379, 1976.

16) P. Hedqvist, S.E. Dahlén, L. Gustafsson, S. Hammarström, B. Samuelsson. Biological profile of leukotrienes C_4 and D_4. Acta. Physiol. Scand. 110: 331, 1980.

17) R. R. Schellenberg and A. Foster. Differential activity of leukotrienes upon human pulmonary vein and artery. Prostaglandins 27 (3): 475, 1984.

18) T. Ahmed and W.Jr. Oliver. Does slow-reacting substance of anaphylaxis mediate hypoxic pulmonary vasoconstriction? Am. Rev. Respir. Dis. 127:566, 1983.

19) J. A. Burke, R. Levi, G. Zhao-gui and E.J. Corey. Leukotriene C_4, D_4 and E_4: effects on human and guinea pig cardiac preparations in vitro. J. Pharmac. Exp. Ther. 235: 241, 1982.

20) R. Levi and A. Burkej. Cardiac anaphylaxis: SRS-A potentiates and extends the effects of released histamine. Eur. J. Pharmacol. 62: 41, 1980.

21) G. Kito, H. Okuda, S. Ohkawa, S. Terzo and K. Kikuchi. Contractile activities of leukotrienes C_4 and D_4 on vascular strips from rabbits. <u>Life Science</u>. 29 (13): 1325, 1981.

22) D. J. McCaig, J.F. Sonbrada. Alteration of electrophysiological properties of airway smooth muscle from sensitized guinea-pigs. <u>Respir. Physiol.</u> 41: 49, 1980.

EVIDENCE FOR A THROMBOXANE ANTAGONIST IN

SELECTED <u>IN VITRO</u> AND <u>IN VIVO</u> SYSTEMS

P. E. Malo, M. A. Wasserman and R. R. Osborn

Department of Pharmacology
Smith Kline and French Laboratories
Philadelphia, PA 19101

INTRODUCTION

One of the identified products of enzyme action on prostaglandin endoperoxides is the highly unstable thromboxane A_2 (TXA_2) (Samuelsson et al., 1976). This substance, though short-lived biologically, has effects far exceeding that of either prostaglandin endoperoxide (PGH_2 or PGG_2) or $PGF_{2\alpha}$. As a product of cell membrane-derived arachidonic acid via the cyclooxygenase pathway, TXA_2 is produced in tissues and cells of vastly different origin (Table 1). As a result, TXA_2 has a number of characteristic actions (e.g., induction of platelet aggregation, contraction of vascular and respiratory smooth muscle and is pro-ulcerogenic/cytodestructive in the GI tract). Additionally, TXA_2 action has been shown to be mediated through a discrete class of thromboxane receptors (Jones et al., 1982).

Although the naturally occurring prostaglandin endoperoxides decompose rapidly (Figure 1), several stable structural analogs have been synthesized and are commercially available for biological examination. Derivatives of PGH_2 in which the 9,11-peroxide bridge has been replaced by either 9,11-epoxymethano or 11,9-epoxymethano (Bundy, 1975), azo (Corey et al., 1976a) or ethano (Corey et al., 1976b) groups have been shown to be thromboxane mimetics in a variety of systems. For example, we have previously reported that the epoxymethano analogs of PGH_2 known as U-44069 and U-46619 (Wasserman, 1976), produced potent dose-related alterations in pulmonary airway resistance (R_L) and dynamic lung compliance (C_{DYN}) in anesthetized dogs. Additionally, U-44069 has also been reported to induce a primary wave of human platelet aggregation (DiTullio et al., 1984).

Table 1. Sites of Thromboxane Biosynthesis

Platelets	Ocular tissues
Lung	Vascular tissues
Spleen	Urinary bladder
Kidney	Gastrointestinal tract
Brain	Endometrium
Polymorphonuclear leukocytes	Amniotic fluid
Macrophages	Human rheumatoid synovia
Lymphocytes	Fibroblasts
	Human burn blister fluid

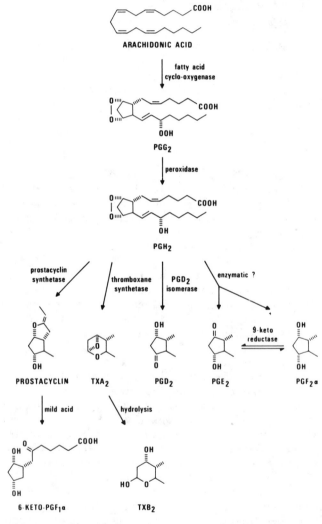

Fig. 1. The arachidonic acid cascade showing the generation of prostacyclin (PGI$_2$) and thromboxane (TXA$_2$).

THROMBOXANE ANTAGONISM IN RESPIRATORY TISSUES

In Vitro

With the advent of those previously mentioned stable, potent endoperoxide mimics of TXA_2 (e.g. U-44069 and U-46619), work has progressed fully to establish the presence of thromboxane receptors in various tissues and in what reactions TXA_2 may play a role. To aid·in these two fundamental avenues of research, the use of a thromboxane antagonist is critical.

SK&F 88046 [N N'-bis-7-(3-chlorobenzeneaminosulfonyl)-1,2,3,4-tetrahydroisoquinolyl disulfonylimide] (Figure 2) was originally developed as an SRS-A end-organ antagonist and, in fact, was shown to inhibit an LTD_4-induced contraction in the guinea pig lung parenchyma (Gleason et al., 1982). Subsequently, Weichman et al. (1982) demonstrated that, while LTD_4 contractile actions are directly mediated on the trachea, LTD_4 exerts its action both via a direct and, more importantly, an indirect (thromboxane-mediated) action on lung parenchyma. On this latter tissue, neither SK&F 88046 nor FPL 55712 affected resting base-line tension, but both compounds antagonized the LTD_4-induced contraction to a similar degree. On the trachea, however, SK&F 88046 failed to produce any significant antagonism of the direct, non-TXA_2 mediated, LTD_4-induced contraction, while FPL 55712 still shifted the LTD_4 concentration-response curve in a parallel fashion to the right. In addition, subsequent studies designed to differentiate the mechanism of action of SK&F 88046 showed it to differ clearly from that of FPL 55712, meclofenamic acid (cyclooxygenase inhibitor) and 1-benzylimidazole (thromboxane synthetase inhibitor) (Weichman et al., 1982; Muccitelli and Weichman, 1982). Therefore, while initially considered to be an SRS-A antagonist in the bronchopulmonary system, subsequent research actually proved it to be a thromboxane antagonist.

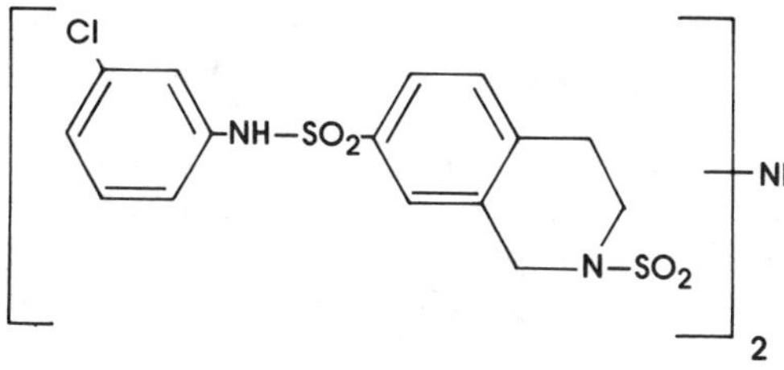

Fig. 2. SK&F 88046 [N N'-bis-(3-chlorobenzeneaminosulfonyl)-1,2,3,4-tetrahydroisoquinolyl disulfonylimide].

In the guinea pig trachea, a tissue very sensitive to the actions of TXA_2, SK&F 88046 preferentially antagonized the contractions elicited by U-44069 and U-46619 (Weichman et al., 1984). CTA_2, a stable analog of TXA_2 utilized in lung parenchyma, is 10-fold weaker in agonist activity relative to the endoperoxide analogs and may interact with a PG receptor; therefore, selection of the endoperoxide analogs was made. SK&F 88046 preferentially antagonized the contractions elicited by U-44069 and U-46619 in an apparently competitive manner with pA_2 values of 6.97 and 7.03, respectively.

In Vivo

Having established the action of SK&F 88046 in isolated guinea pig airway/lung tissues, the compound was, then, studied in whole animal systems utilizing anesthetized guinea pigs and dogs. Animals were anesthetized with urethane (2.0 g/kg, i.p.) or sodium pentobarbital (35 mg/kg, i.v.), respectively. Supplemental doses of anesthetic were administered as required to maintain a light level of anesthesia throughout the experiment. The animals were permitted to breathe room air spontaneously.

If the air passages decrease in diameter (as occurs in bronchoconstriction), then additional friction is encountered during ventilation (i.e. the same amount of air is required to go thru a tube of smaller diameter), hence resistance increases. Dynamic lung compliance is the measure of the elasticity or how compliant the lung is during ventilation, and is indicative of smaller airways (as well as other factors). During bronchoconstriction, the lung is less elastic and, therefore, a decrease in lung compliance is observed.

Pulmonary mechanics, i.e. resistance (R_L) and compliance (C_{DYN}), were estimated by the technique of Diamond (1972). This method for the anesthetized dog is a modification of the procedure introduced by Amdur and Mead (1958) for the unanesthetized guinea pig and has been described at length previously (Malo et al., 1982). Briefly, airflow rate, tidal volume and transpulmonary pressure were monitored simultaneously by established physiologic techniques. When there is no airflow and the airways are open, the pressure at the mouth equals the pressure in the alveoli. Resistance, then, is a measurement of the friction encountered by the passage of air thru the larger airways of the respiratory tract (i.e. trachea, bronchi).

Output signals were amplified and fed on-line into an analog Pulmonary Mechanics Computer Model 6 (Buxco Electronics, Sharon, CT.) (Figure 3). This device produced a continuous breath-by-breath analysis of the mechanical properties of the airways and lungs (Giles et al., 1971). The computer performed the necessary calculations at precisely the exact instant for measuring R_L and C_{DYN}; the output was displayed on a direct-writing Beckman R612 Dynograph. Between 5 and 10 consecutive breaths were analyzed and averaged before drug treat-

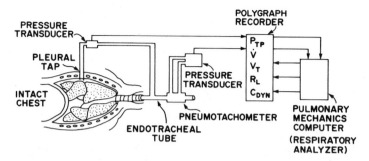

Fig. 3. Schematic representation of in vivo measurement of pulmonary parameters. Information from both the pleural space and trachea are delivered to a Pulmonary Mechanics Computer which then interprets the information and prints it in both tabular form and graphically on the polygraph. Transpulmonary pressure (P_{TP}), flow rate ($\dot{V}$), tidal volume (V_T) resistance (R_L) and compliance (C_{DYN}).

ment (baseline control) and again at the height of the response after treatment, using a Buxco Data Logger (Model DL-12) in conjunction with the Pulmonary Mechanics Computer.

In addition to the pulmonary functions, systemic blood pressure (as mean arterial pressure) was monitored continuously via a cannulated femoral artery coupled to a Gould Statham P23 ID pressure transducer. Heart rate was counted electronically from arterial pressure by the Buxco Computer. Tracings from all cardiovascular systems were recorded, likewise, on the direct writing polygraph.

In the anesthetized, instrumented guinea pig, the thromboxane mimic, U-44069, and arachidonic acid were infused separately in order to provoke bronchoconstriction. Alabaster (1980) reported that, in the guinea pig and rabbit, exogenously administered arachidonic acid is converted to TXA_2, while Frey and Dengjel (1980) reported that arachidonic acid produced a TXA_2- mediated contraction of cat bronchus in situ. Indeed, arachidonic acid (0.1 - 1.0 mg/kg) elicited a strong bronchoconstriction in our guinea pig model as reflected by a large increase in R_L and decrease in C_{DYN} (Figure 4). These responses were significantly reduced by pretreatment with SK&F 88046 (5 mg/kg) as well as by meclofenamic acid (2 mg/kg) and by the thromboxane synthetase inhibitor, UK 37, 248 (5 mg/kg) (Figure 4). In addition, SK&F 88046 was effective for > 120 min vs. arachidonic acid-induced provocations. SK&F 88046 was also able to shift to the right the in vivo response of varying doses of U-44069 as measured by changes in R_L and C_{DYN} (Figure 5).

Likewise, in the anesthetized dog, iv SK&F 88046 antagonized the airway effects of arachidonic acid and U-44069 (Figures 6 and 7);

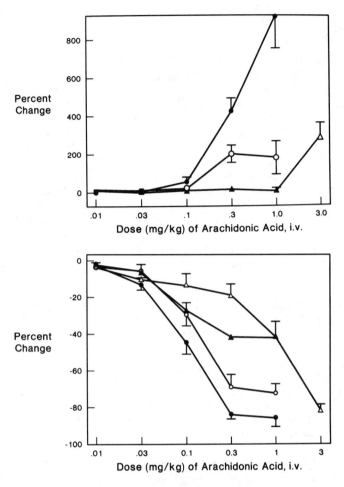

Fig. 4. Inhibition of R_L (top) and C_{DYN} (bottom) changes induced by arachidonic acid with either meclofenamic acid, UK37248 or SK&F 88046. Control arachidonic acid (·) is followed by a pretreatment with meclofenamic acid (2 mg/kg △) or UK37248 (5 mg/kg, ▲) or SK&F (88046 (5 mg/kg, 0) and then a repeat of arachidonic acid.

however, oral SK&F 88046 (50 mg/kg) was shown to be ineffective perhaps due to its poor absorption from the GI tract (data not shown).

Finally, specificity for thromboxane was demonstrated by a lack of antagonism of SK&F 88046 against histamine or cholinergic-induced bronchospasm in either the guinea pig or dog (Figure 8) and lack of inhibition of $PGF_{2\alpha}$ or PGD_2-induced bronchospasm in the dog (Figure 9 and Figure 10).

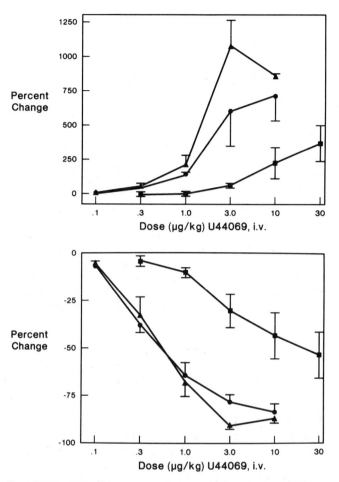

Fig. 5. U-44069 dose-response in anesthetized guinea pigs, R_L (top) and C_{DYN} (bottom). Control U-44069 ($\bullet$) is followed by a pretreatment with either meclofenamic acid (2 mg/kg $\blacktriangle$) or SK&F 88046 (5 mg/kg $\blacksquare$) and then a repeat of the U-44069 dose-response challenge.

THROMBOXANE ANTAGONISM IN CARDIOVASCULAR TISSUE

Platelets

Arachidonic acid metabolites, especially thromboxane A_2 and the endoperoxides, have been reported to induce platelet aggregation directly (Hamberg and Samuelsson, 1974; Hamberg et al., 1975), to be mediators of platelet aggregation induced by collagen (Best et al., 1980; Smith et al., 1974) and to be involved in mediation of the secondary wave of platelet aggregation induced by a widely diverse

255

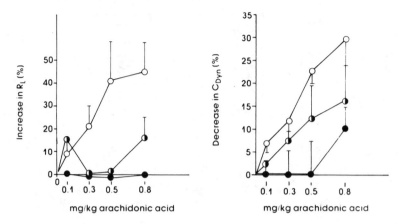

Fig. 6.   Effect of pretreatment with SK&F 88046 in anesthetized dogs
against arachidonic acid-induced bronchospasm as compared
with antagonism by dazoxiben.   Control response ○; SK&F
88046 (a thromboxane receptor antagonist) ◑; Dazoxiben (a
thromboxane synthetase antagonist) ●; (Reprinted with
permission from Churchill Livingston Publishers).

group of agents, such as epinephrine (Fitzpatrick et al., 1978),
adenosine (Fitzpatrick et al., 1978), a calcium ionophore A23187
(Oelz et al., 1978) and platelet activating factor (MacIntyre and
Shaw, 1983).

        Since SK&F 88046 apparently behaves as a TXA$_2$ receptor antagon-
ist (based on data from the previous section), the ability of SK&F
88046 to act as an antagonist of the human platelet TXA$_2$/PGH$_2$ receptor was investigated by testing for inhibition of platelet aggregation induced by the above agonists.   Indeed, a one min preincubation with SK&F 88046 (1-100 µM) inhibited platelet aggregation
induced by arachidonic acid, collagen and U-44069 (DiTullio et al.,
1984).   The secondary wave of platelet aggregation induced by epinephrine, adenosine, vasopressin, A23187 and platelet activating
factor were also all inhibited by similar concentrations of SK&F
88046 (DiTullio et al., 1984).   SK&F 88046 was, however, inactive
when tested as an inhibitor of cyclooxygenase or thromboxane synthetase (P. Needlam, personal communication); therefore, SK&F 88046
selectively inhibited either phase of human platelet aggregation,
depending upon the agonist employed (Table 2).

Cardiac Anaphylaxis

        In the whole animal, electrocardiographic changes which are
encountered during acute allergic reactions (i.e. rightward shifts in
the QRS axis, ischemic S-T segment changes and tachyarrhythmias)
could be secondary to pulmonary hypertension, systemic hypotension

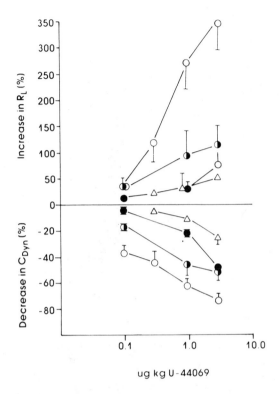

ug kg U-44069

Fig. 7. Effect of varying concentrations of SK&F 88046 against a thromboxane mimic (U-44069) induced change in R_L and C_{DYN}. Control response ○; 1 mg/kg SK&F 88046 ◑; 3 mg/kg SK&F 88046 ●; 5 mg/kg SK&F 88046 △. (Reprinted with permission from Churchill Livingston Publishers).

and reduced cardiac output (Halonen et al., 1980). A model of cardiac anaphylaxis was required in which myocardial dysfunction could be studied independently of systemic vascular platelet-mediated changes. The isolated, sensitized guinea pig heart provided such a model. Many of the cardiac abnormalities characteristic of systemic anaphylaxis are manifested in vitro when hearts from sensitized guinea pigs are challenged with specific antigen (Feigen et al., 1961). Sinus tachycardia, arrhythmias, decreased coronary blood flow and compromised left ventricular contractile failure are characteristic of cardiac anaphylaxis (Capurro and Leir, 1975). Currently, arachidonic acid metabolites which are released intra-cardially are among the endogenous substances known to mediate systemic anaphylaxis (Leir and Allan, 1980; Leir et al., 1982). Subsequently, SK&F 88046 was tested to determine efficacy in the above model of isolated guinea pig hearts. Indeed, SK&F 88046 was effective in preventing dose related decreases in myocardial contractile force and coronary

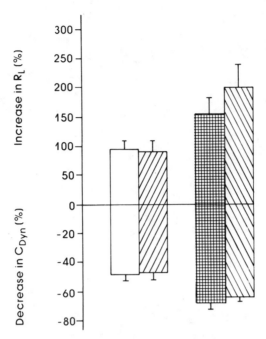

Fig. 8. Effect of SK&F 88046 on histamine (HIST) or acetylcholine
(ACH) - induced bronchospasm in the anesthetized dog.
Control response to HIST (□) or ACH (⊞) was followed by
pretreatment with SK&F 88046 with a repeat of either HIST
(▨) or ACH (▧). (Reprinted with permission from Churchill
Livingston Publishers).

blood flow rate; however, the mediator eliciting these biological
responses apparently was not TXA$_2$, but rather, LTC$_4$. Burke et al.
(1984) reported that, in fact, SK&F 88046 (4.8 x 10^{-7}M) and FPL 55712
(4.8 x 10^{-7}M) were equieffective in antagonizing the LTC$_4$-induced
decrease in coronary blood flow. In addition, SK&F 88046 was even
more potent than FPL 55712 in antagonizing the negative inotropic
effect on LTC$_4$.

Since the leukotrienes do not appear to release TXA$_2$ or prostaglandins from the challenged, sensitized guinea pig heart (Burke et
al., 1982), it remains questionable how SK&F 88046 is functioning in
the heart. Two possibilities remain: 1) low levels of thromboxane,
below the level of detection by available techniques, are released
following LT stimulation of the heart and account for at least part
of the observed effects on myocardial contractile force and coronary
blood flow rate, or 2) tissue differences in leukotriene receptors
may exist, such that SK&F 88046 does not interact with the airway LT
receptor, but does with the cardiac leukotriene receptor. In fact,
the latter seems to be the case. Hogaboom et al. (in press, 1984)

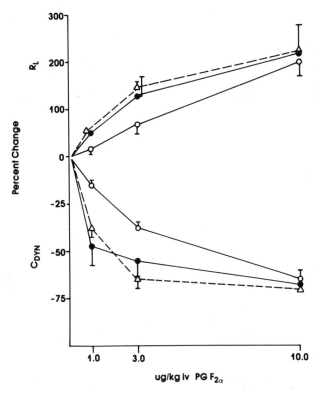

Fig. 9. Effect of SK&F 88046 on $PGF_{2\alpha}$-induced bronchospasm in the
anesthetized dog. Control prostaglandin response (o) is
followed by pretreatment with 1.0 mg/kg iv (·) or 5.0 mg/kg
iv (Δ) SK&F 88406. (Reprinted with permission from
Churchill Livingston Publishers).

reported direct biochemical evidence for specific $[^{3}H]$-LTC_4 binding
sites in the guinea pig heart membranes. The $[^{3}H]$-LTC_4 binding sites
appear to be modulated by divalent and monovalent cations and that
free sulfhydryl groups may be associated with the agonist binding
site. A monophasic Scatchard plot of saturation binding data yielded
a dissociation constant (Kd) of 27.5 ± 6.0 μM and a maximum number of
binding sites of 19.9 ± 5.23 pmol/mg of membrane protein. Competition binding studies of $[^{3}H]$-LTC_4, LTD_4, LTE_4, FPL 55712 and SK&F
88046 revealed an order of potency of LTC_4 >> SK&F 88046 > LTE_4 >
LTD_4 > FPL 55712. Therefore, it is indeed possible that myocardial
$[^{3}H]$-LTC_4 binding sites may be binding SK&F 88046; however, they may
also be pharmacologically distinct from LTC_4 binding sites identified
in other tissues. It is also possible that PAF may cause the release
of moderate amounts of TXA_2 thru which SK&F 88046 may exert some
action; however, additional research will be necessary to determine
if in actuality this is possible.

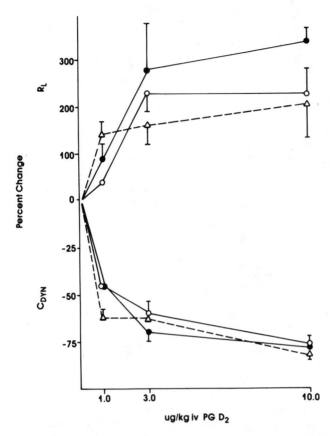

Fig. 10. Effect of SK&F 88046 on PGD_2-induced bronchospasm in the anesthetized dog. Control prostaglandin response (o) is followed by pretreatment with 1.0 mg/kg iv (·) or 5.0 mg/kg iv (Δ) SK&F 88046. (Reprinted with permission from Churchill Livingston Publishers).

CONCLUSIONS

The role of thromboxane as a putative mediator of disease is not limited to only the selected areas discussed above. In fact, TXA_2 has been recognized to be a possible mediator in adult respiratory distress syndrome (ARDS), a disease whose pathophysiology encompasses severe hypoxemia, pulmonary edema, increased pulmonary capillary permeability and increased pulmonary vascular resistance (Deby-Dupont et al., 1982; Gee et al., 1983). However, because no current pharmacotherapy exists, a specific thromboxane antagonist would prove valuable if, indeed, TXA_2 is the primary mediator involved. Other diseases in which thromboxane could play a role include: inflammatory states, (e.g. emphysema, rheumatoid arthritis), thrombogenic disorders (pulmonary embolism), coronary ischemic/myocardial infarc-

Table 2.   Inhibition of Human Platelet Aggregation In Vitro
by SK&F 88046

Agonist	IC_{50} (μM)
a) Inhibition of primary phase of platelet aggregation	
Arachidonic acid	19.0
Collagen	10.0
U-44069	2.5
b) Inhibition of secondary phase of platelet aggregation	
U-44069	1.7
A23187	12.0
Platelet Activating Factor (PAF)	4.5

tion, and even atherosclerosis. By careful modulation of this potent
mediator by a thromboxane end organ receptor antagonist, such as SK&F
88046, one could provide rational therapeutic intervention to many of
these debilitating diseases.

REFERENCES

Alabaster, V. A., 1980, Metabolism of arachidonic acid and its
    endoperoxide (PGH_2) to myotropic products in guinea pig and
    rabbit isolated lungs, Br.J.Pharmac., 69:479-89.
Amdur, M. O., and Mead, J., 1958, Mechanics of respiration in un-
    anesthetized guinea pigs, Am.J.Physiol., 192:364-368.
Best, L. C., Holland, T. K., Jones, P. B. B., and Russell, R. G. G.,
    1980, The interrelationship between thromboxane biosynthesis,
    aggregation and 5-hydroxytryptamine secretion in human plate-
    lets in vitro, Thromb.Haemostasis, 43:38-40.
Bundy, G. L., 1975, Synthesis of prostaglandin endoperoxide analogs,
    Tetra.Med.Lett., 24:1957-1960.
Burke, J. A., Levi, R., Guo, Z. G., and Corey, E. J., 1982, Leuko-
    trienes C_4, D_4 and E_4: Effects on human and guinea pig
    cardiac preparations in vitro, J.Pharmacol.Exp.Ther.,
    221:235-241.
Burke, J. A., Levi, R., and Gleason, J. G., 1984, Antagonism of the
    cardiac effects of leukotriene C_4 by compound SK&F 88046:
    Dissociation of effects on contractility and coronary flow,
    J.Card.Pharm., 6:122-125.
Capurro, N., and Levi, R., 1975, The heart as a target organ in
    systemic allergic reactions: Comparison of cardiac anaphyl-
    axis in vivo and in vitro, Cir.Res., 36:520-528.

Corey, E. J., Narasaka, K., and Shibazaki, M., 1976, A direct stereo-
controlled total synthesis of the 9,11-azo analogue of the
prostaglandin endoperoxide PGH$_2$, J.Am.Chem.Soc.,
98:6417-6418.

Corey, E. J., Shibazaki, M., Nicolaou, K. C., Malmsten, C., and
Samuelsson, B., 1976, Simple stereo-controlled total synthesis of a biologically active analogue of the prostaglandin
endoperoxide (PGG$_2$, PGH$_2$), Tetrahed.Lett., 737-741.

Deby-Dupont, G., Radoux, L., Haas, M., Larbuisson, R., Noel, F. X.,
and Lamy, M., 1982, Release of thromboxane B$_2$ during adult
respiratory distress syndrome and its inhibition by non
steroidal anti-inflammatory substances in man, Arch.Int.
Pharmacodyn., 259:317-319.

Diamond, L., 1972, Potentiation of bronchomotor responses by beta-
adrenergic antagonists, J.Pharmacol.Exp.Ther., 181:434-445.

Ditullio, N. W., Wasserman, M. A., and Storer, B. L., 1984, Effects
of SK&F 88046, a thromboxane A$_2$/prostaglandin H$_2$ antagonist,
on human platelet aggregation. Abstracts of Satellite
Symposium of IUPHAR on "Platelet Inhibition and Vascular
Occlusion in Man" London, 1984.

Feigen, G. A., Vurek, G. G., Irvin, W. S., and Peterson, J. K., 1981,
Quantitative absorption of antibody by the isolated heart and
the intensity of cardiac anaphylaxis, Cir.Res., 9:177-183.

Fitzpatrick, F. A., Bundy, G. L., Gorman, R. R., and Honoman, T.,
1978, 9, 11-epoxymethanoprosta- 5, 13-dienoic acid is a
thromboxane A$_2$ antagonist in human platelets, Nature,
275:764-766.

Frey, H. H., and Dengjel, C., 1980, Effects of inhibitors of thromboxane synthesis on reactions of the cat bronchus in situ to
prostaglandins, Prostaglandins, 20:87-93.

Gee, M. H., Perkowski, B. A., Havill, A. M., and Flynn, J. T., 1983,
Role of prostaglandins and leukotrienes in complement-
initiated lung vascular injury, Chest, 83:825-855.

Giles, R. E., Finkel, M. P., and Mazurowski, J., 1971, The use of an
analog on line computer for the evaluation of pulmonary
resistance and dynamic compliance in the anesthetized dog,
Arch.Int.Pharm.Ther., 194:213-222.

Gleason, J. G., Krell, R. D., Weichman, B. M., Ali, F. E., and
Berkowitz, B., 1982, Comparative pharmacology and antagonism
of synthetic leukotrienes on airway and vascular smooth
muscle, Adv.Prost.Thromb.Leuko.Res., 9:243-250.

Halonen, M., Palmer, J. D., Lohman, I. C., McManus, L. M., and
Pinckard, R. N., 1980, Respiratory and circulatory alter-
ations induced by acetyl glyceryl ether phosphorylcholine
(AGEPC), a mediator of IgE anaphylaxis in the rabbit,
Am.Rev.Resp.Dis., 122:915-924.

Hamberg, M., and Samuelsson, B., 1974, Prostaglandin endoperoxides.
Novel transformations of arachidonic acid in human platelets,
Proc.Natl.Acad.Sci., 71:3400-3404.

262

Hamberg, M., Svensson, J., and Samuelsson, B., 1975, Thromboxanes:
    A new group of biologically active compounds derived from
    prostaglandin endoperoxides, Proc.Natl.Acad.Sci.,
    72:2994-2998.
Hogaboom, G. K., Mong, S., Stadel, J. M., and Crooke, S. T., 1984,
    Characterization of myocardial leukotriene C_4 binding sites.
    Regulation by cations and sulfhydryl-directed reagents,
    Mol.Pharm. (in press).
Jones, R. L., Peesapati, V., and Wilson, N. H., 1982, Antagonism of
    the thromboxane-sensitive contractile systems of the rabbit
    aorta, dog saphenous vein and guinea pig trachea,
    Br.J.Pharmac., 76:423-438.
Levi, R., and Allan, G., 1980, Histamine-mediated cardiac effects,
    in: "Drug-induced Heart Disease," M. Bristow, ed., Elsevier-
    North Holland Biomedical Press, pp.377-395.
Levi, R., Burke, J. A., and Corey, E. J., 1982, SRS-A, leukotrienes
    and immediate hypersensitivity reaction of the heart,
    Ad.Prost.Thromb.Leuko.Res., 9:215-222.
MacIntyre, D. E., and Shaw, A. M., 1983, Phospholipid-induced
    platelet activation: Effects of calcium channel blockers and
    calcium chelators, Thromb.Res., 31:833-844.
Malo, P. E., Wasserman, M. A., and Griffin, R. L., 1982, The effects
    of lidocaine and hexamethonium on prostaglandin F_2 - and
    histamine-induced bronchoconstriction in normal and ascaris -
    sensitive dogs, Drug Develop.Res., 2:567-575.
Muccitelli, R. M., and Weichman, B. M., 1982, Effect of 1-benzyl-
    imidazole on the pulmonary activity of synthetic leukotriene
    D_4, The Pharmacologist, 24:571A.
Oelz, O., Knapp, H. R., Roberts, L. J., Oelz, R., Sweetman, B. J.,
    Oates, J. A., and Reed, P. W., 1978, Calcium - dependent
    stimulation of thromboxane and protaglandin biosynthesis by
    ionophores, Adv.Prostag.Thromb.Res., 3:147-158.
Samuelsson, B., Hamberg, M., Malmsten, E., and Svensson, J., 1976,
    The role of prostaglandin endoperoxides and thromboxanes in
    platelet aggregation, Adv.Prost.Thromb.Res., 2:737-746.
Smith, J. B., Ingerman, C., Kocsis, J. J., and Silver, J. J., 1974,
    Formation of an intermediate in prostaglandin biosynthesis
    and its association with the platelet release reaction,
    J.Clin.Invest., 53:1468-1472.
Wasserman, M. A., 1976, Bronchopulmonary pharmacology of some prosta-
    glandin endoperoxide analogs in the dog, Europ.J.Pharmacol.,
    36:103-108.
Weichman, B. M., Muccitelli, R. M., Osborn, R. R., Holden, D. A.,
    Gleason, J. G., and Wasserman, M. A., 1982, In vitro and in
    vivo mechanisms of leukotriene - mediated broncho-
    constriction in the guinea pig, J.Pharmacol.Exp.Ther.,
    222:202-208.
Weichman, B. M., Wasserman, M. A., and J. G. Gleason, 1984, SK&F
    88046: A unique pharmacologic antagonist of broncho-
    constriction induced by prostaglandins $F_{2\alpha}$ and D_2 in vitro,
    J.Pharmacol.Exp.Ther., 228:128-132.

PRECURSOR-PRODUCT RELATIONSHIP IN VASCULAR EICOSANOID FORMATION AFTER MANIPULATION OF DIETARY FATTY ACIDS IN EXPERIMENTAL ANIMALS

C. Galli, E. Giani and I. Masi

Institute of Pharmacology and Pharmacognosy
University of Milan
Via A. del Sarto 21, 20129 Milano

Introduction

The metabolic relationship between the long chain polyunsaturated fatty acid (PUFA), arachidonic acid (AA), and the prostaglandin system was discovered two decades ago. Although information on the eicosanoid family has considerably grown since then, our understanding of the complex relationships between the intake of the fatty acid precursors with the diet and the balance in the formation of various eicosanoids in a given tissue or district is still quite limited.

Arachidonic acid (20:4 Δ 5,8,11,14) in tissues is mainly derived from desaturation and elongation of the Essential Fatty Acid (EFA) precursor linoleic acid (LA, 18:2 Δ 9,12) of dietary origin, whereas the supply of AA by the diet is normally negligible. Other 20 carbon PUFA of the LA series such as 20:3 Δ8,11,14 which is the immediate precursor of AA through the Δ 5 desaturase, and of the α-linolenic acid series, such as 20:5 Δ 5,8,11,14,17 (eicosapentaenoic acid, EPA) have been shown to be precursors of prostaglandins in "in vitro" systems. The metabolic conversions of the 18 carbon EFA linoleic (18:2 Δ 9,12) and α linolenic (18:3 Δ 9,12,15) to the long chain PUFA, including the eicosanoid precursor Fatty Acids, are shown in the following scheme.

In the present paper the relationship between dietary fatty acids and tissue prostaglandin formation in the cardiovascular system will be discussed.

Essential fatty acid metabolism

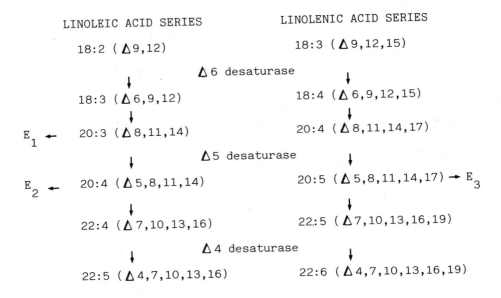

LINOLEIC ACID SERIES   LINOLENIC ACID SERIES

18:2 (Δ9,12)   18:3 (Δ9,12,15)

Δ6 desaturase

18:3 (Δ6,9,12)   18:4 (Δ6,9,12,15)

E_1 ← 20:3 (Δ8,11,14)   20:4 (Δ8,11,14,17)

Δ5 desaturase

E_2 ← 20:4 (Δ5,8,11,14)   20:5 (Δ5,8,11,14,17) → E_3

22:4 (Δ7,10,13,16)   22:5 (Δ7,10,13,16,19)

Δ4 desaturase

22:5 (Δ4,7,10,13,16) 22:6 (Δ4,7,10,13,16,19)

Dietary EFA and tissue PUFA accumulation

EFA metabolism occurs at the microsomal level and has been extensively studied especially in the liver (1,2). Investigations on LA metabolism have shown that the desaturating steps are limiting and that the first desaturating enzyme, which inserts a double bond in 6 position of LA (Δ6 desaturase) represents a key step in the entire process (3). This observation might explain the relatively high levels of LA found in tissue lipids in respect to those of AA. Several conditions and endogenous factors have been shown to modulate the Δ6 desaturase. Its activity, for instance, is enhanced by insulin and depressed by insulin deficiency (1). Limited information is available on the ability of different types of cells to produce AA from the precursor LA. In addition there seem to exist species differences in the overall conversion of EFA to PUFA.

The AA accumulated in tissues is mainly esterified in the 2 position of phospholipids, which are structural components of biological membranes.

From a biochemical point of view it would be expected that increasing dietary LA intake would result in elevation of AA levels in tissues. However, experimental data indicate that the correlation between dietary LA and phospholipid AA content in tissues are more complex, depending upon the animal species and the tissues under consideration. For instance, in rabbits fed for one month 11 percent of dietary calories (en%) LA, the levels of AA in platelet phospholipids were lower than in rabbits fed 2.5 en% LA. This reduction was associated with accumulation of LA in platelet phospholipids, thus resulting in replacement of AA by LA. The sum of PUFA in platelet phospholipids was the same in both animal groups, but the AA/LA ratio was double in the 2.5 en% LA fed group in respect of the 11 en% LA group of rabbits. In contrast, in liver phospholipids both levels of LA and AA were higher in the group fed 11 en% LA, as expected since conversion of LA to AA occurs in this tissue (table 1). In addition the sum of PUFA in liver phospholipids was higher in the 11 en% LA fed group of rabbits in respect to the 2.5 en% group, but the AA/LA ratio was the same in both experimental groups (4).

In other animal species such as the rat, however, in which PUFA metabolism is known to be very active, an increment of dietary LA content from 2.5 en% present in the standard diet up to 5 en% through supplementation of corn oil for one month, resulted in elevation of AA content of platelet phospholipids, with no change of LA content (table 2) (5).

Other fatty acids, such as 20:3 n-6 or 20:5 n-3 (EPA) may be directly administered through the diet and may be incorporated in tissue phospholipids thus resulting in accumulation of selected Eicosanoid precursors in membrane phospholipids (6,7). Studies carried out in humans have shown for instance, that administration of EPA or of EPA containing oils (fish oil) results in accumulation of this fatty acid in plasma and platelet phospholipids at the expenses of AA. We have also carried out investigations based on feeding fish oil (containing about 8% EPA), either alone or in association with an equal amount of corn oil, to growing rats and we have observed that when fish oil was fed alone, EPA accumulated in platelet phospholipids partially replacing AA (table 3). When the same amount of fish oil was given instead in association with an equal amount of the LA-rich oil no incorporation of EPA in platelet and aorta phospholipids occurred (table 4) (8), indicating that the presence of relatively high amounts of n-6 fatty acids in the diet prevented the incorporation of n-3 fatty acids in biological membranes.

Table 1: Levels of Linoleic Acid (LA) and Arachidonic Acid (AA) (% of total fatty acids) in platelet and liver Ethanolamine Phosphoglyceride (EPG) of rabbits fed 4 weeks with either 2.5 En% or 11 En% LA.

| | Platelets | | Liver | |
	Butter	Corn oil	Butter	Corn oil
LA	14.3+1.3	22.3+2.5*	25.0+1.6	30.2+2.4**
AA	34.6+2.9	26.9+1.3*	11.8+1.2	15.8+1.2**
LA+AA	48.9	49.2	36.8	46.0
AA/LA	2.42	1.21	0.47	0.52

Table 2: Levels of Linoleic Acid (LA) and Arachidonic Acid (AA) (% of total fatty acids) in platelet total phospholipids of rats fed a normal laboratory chow containing 2.5 en% LA (C) or a diet containing 5 en% LA (CO).

| | Platelet Phospholipids | |
	C	CO
LA	6	6.3
AA	9.7	20.0

Table 3: Levels of Linoleic Acid (LA), Arachidonic Acid (AA) and Eicosapentaenoic Acid (EPA) (% of total fatty acids) in platelet total phospholipids of rats fed diets containing either 5 en% corn oil (CO) or 5 en% fish oil (FO).

| | Platelet Phospholipids | |
	CO	FO
LA	2.5+0.1	1.9+0.2
AA	10.9+0.4	6.7+0.3
EPA	n.d.	2.4+0.2

Table 4: Levels of Linoleic Acid (LA), Arachidonic Acid (AA) and Eicosapentaenoic Acid (EPA) (% of total fatty acids) in platelet total phospholipids of rats fed 10 en% corn oil (10 en% CO) or 5 en% fish oil plus 5 en% corn oil (5 en% CO + 5 en% FO).

	Platelet Phospholipids	
	10 En% CO	5 En% CO + 5 En% FO
LA	3.8+0.3	4.5+0.1
AA	10.2+0.5	7.0+0.4
EPA	n.d.	n.d.

Platelet fatty acids and thromboxane formation

Several studies have shown that modifications of dietary LA levels, in experimental animals, result in changes of the thromboxane generating capacity of platelets (9). We have observed more generally, that dietary induced changes of platelet thromboxane formation are related to modifications of platelet AA content. Elevation of AA levels in platelet phospholipids, induced by dietary manipulations, results in a greater thromboxane B_2 (TxB_2) production by stimulated platelets, and in particular a significant correlation was found between the AA/LA ratio in platelet phospholipids and the levels of TxB_2 in collagen and thrombin stimulated platelet rich plasma (PRP) in the rat.

The correlation between AA/LA ratio in platelet phospholipids and TxB_2 levels in PRP 5 minutes after thrombin stimulation in rats fed various dietary fats is shown in fig. 1.

This correlation (r = 0.89) was found in platelets at different AA/LA ratios, but in the absence of EPA.

In the presence of EPA in platelet phospholipids, instead, although the AA/LA ratio was similar to that found in platelets of animals fed a diet containing 5 en% corn oil, which is rich in LA (5 en% corn oil), TxB_2 production by stimulated PRP was 70% lower. These results indicate that the presence of EPA in platelet membrane phospholipids interferes directly with the formation of TxB_2. It is possible, in our experimental conditions, that also an inactive thromboxane A_3, which was not detected by us, was formed. Formation of thromboxane B_3 after stimulation of platelets obtained from subjects fed EPA has been recently demonstrated (10).

In the collagen stimulated platelets from animals (rats) fed different dietary fatty acids, the correlation between AA/LA ratios and TxB_2 formation was also highly significant. In contrast with the above findings, the previously mentioned studies carried out in rabbits (4), have shown that elevation of dietary LA content, not only resulted in reduced AA levels in platelet phospholipids, but also in reduced conversion of AA to TxB_2 in stimulated PRP.

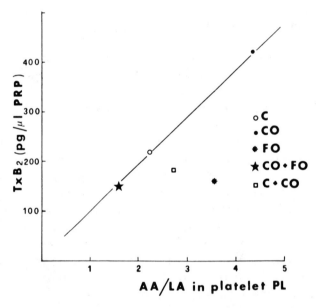

Fig. 1. Relationship between the Arachidonic Acid/Linoleic Acid (AA/LA) ratios in platelet phospholipids (PL) and TxB_2 levels (pg/ ul) in thrombin stimulated (5 I.U. 2 min. after stimulation) PRP, in the rat. Correlation coefficient of the line drawn excluding the FO value, was 0.89. C, control diet; CO, diet containing corn oil (60% LA); FO, diet containing Fish oil (8% EPA); CO+FO, diet containing the combination corn oil + fish oil; C+CO, control diet supplemented with corn-oil.

In summary, thus, as far as the effects of dietary fatty acids on platelet eicosanoid production are concerned, it appears that elevation of dietary levels of LA, resulted in both reduction of the eicosanoid precursor AA in platelet phospholipids and in depression of TxB_2 generation in rabbits (4), whereas, in the rat, resulted in the opposite effects of elevation of AA content and enhanced formation of cycloxygenase products (5). All the effects of dietary manipulation on platelet TxB_2 production appeared to be mediated by corresponding changes of the fatty acid precursor levels.

Not only species differences appear to influence the effects of dietary LA, but also sex differences, since TxB_2 formation in platelet from female rats (5) and humans (11) are not equally affected as those in males, by elevation of dietary LA.

Another factor which contributes to modulate the effects of dietary LA on eicosanoid production in the vascular compartment appears to be the exact level of this fatty acid in the diet, since it has been shown in rats fed increasing amounts of LA, that a linear correlation between the two parameters is present only in a given range of dietary concentrations (9).

Finally, the effects of high dietary levels of LA on platelet TxB_2 formation in humans have been investigated in a limited number of studies. In an investigation carried out in an international project on normal volunteers in North Karelia, Finland and South Italy, we have observed that elevation of dietary LA resulted in reduced TxB_2 formation in collagen-stimulated PRP of male subjects only (11). An opposite effect was observed when dietary LA levels were reduced.

The observed modifications of platelet TxB_2 formation were not associated with significant changes of the fatty acid composition of platelet phospholipids. These results confirmed the sex- related differences previously reported in the response of the platelet thromboxane system to dietary fatty acids, and suggest that other factors, in addition to changes of the precursor fatty acid concentrations, may be responsible of these effects.

Dietary fatty acids and prostacyclin production
by vascular tissue

In vitro studies on the effects of PUFA, such as 18:2 n-6, and 20:5 n-3, on prostacyclin formation have shown that these fatty acids are able to reduce the release of the eicosanoid, measured as its stable non enzymatic metabolite 6 keto PGF$_{1\alpha}$, by cultured human umbelical vein endothelial cells (12,13).

We have studied the effects of diets containing different LA (4,5) and EPA levels (8), on PGI$_2$ formation by aortic tissue. More specifically PRP samples obtained from animals under the various dietary conditions were perfused through isolated segments of thoracic aorta, and both the levels of 6 keto PGF$_{1\alpha}$

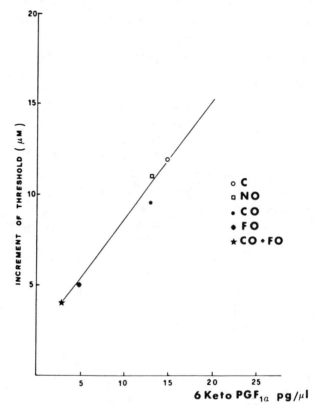

Fig. 2. Relationship between the concentration (pg/ul) of 6 keto PGF$_{1\alpha}$ in PRP perfused through isolated segments of thoracic aorta and the increment in the threshold concentration (ADP, uM) for PRP aggregation after perfusion, in respect of the values for non-perfused PRP, in the rat. Correlation coefficient = 0.97°C, standard diet, NO, standard diet supplemented with Naudicelle oil (73% LA, 7.6% Linolenic Acid).

CO, standard diet supplemented with corn oil (60% LA); FO, diet containing fish oil (8% EPA); CO+FO, diet containing the combination corn oil + fish oil.

272

in the perfusate and the inhibition of platelet aggregation following perfusion were evaluated. The elevation of PUFA levels of the n-6 series in the diets for periods of 4 to 8 weeks resulted in reduction of 6 keto $PGF_{1\alpha}$ levels in the PRP samples perfused through the isolated vessel. The inhibition of platelet aggregation, measured as the increase of the threshold concentration for ADP-induced aggregation after perfusion, was also lower in animals fed diets with high LA content.

The correlations between levels of 6 keto $PGF_{1\alpha}$ in PRP and the inhibition of PRP aggregation after perfusion, measured as increment of threshold concentration of the aggregant (ADP, μM) in the perfused PRP in respect of the values in non perfused PRP, are shown in fig. 2.

A highly significant correlation ($r = 0.97$) in animal groups under different dietary conditions was found.

The presence of fish oil (8% EPA) alone or of a combination of fish oil plus corn oil in the diet resulted also in a marked reduction of the above parameters. These effects, however, in contrast to the results described in platelets, could not be correlated with concomitant changes of the composition of aorta phospholipids, suggesting that the prostacyclin producing capacity of aortic tissue is regulated not only by the levels of the fatty acid precursors of prostaglandins in the tissue but also by other factors possibly present in plasma.

The observed correlation between changes of prostacyclin release by aortic tissue and the antiaggregatory activity of the vessel wall, in "ex vivo" preparations obtained from animals fed different n-6 and n-3 fatty acids, indicates, anyway, that dietary induced changes of the antiaggregatory activity of the arterial walls are mediated by corresponding changes in the production of the antiaggregatory eicosanoid.

Conclusions

In conclusion, dietary fatty acids contribute to modulate the fatty acid composition of tissue phospholipids and the levels of 20 carbon eicosanoid precursors fatty acids by modulating the availability of the 18 carbon precursor (e.g. dietary LA as precursor of tissue AA) or by their direct incorporation following supplementation of the preformed fatty acid with the diet, such as in the case of EPA.

However changes of fatty acid precursor levels do not appear to be the only mechanisms responsible of dietary induced changes of vascular prostaglandin production, since other factors may also be involved.

References

1. R.R. Brenner, Nutritional and hormonal factors influencing desaturation of Essential Fatty Acids, in: "Progress in Lipid Research" vol. 20, R.T. Holman Ed. Pergamon Press (1981).

2. H. Sprecher, Biochemistry of Essential Fatty Acids, in: "Progress in Lipid Research" vol. 20, R.T. Holman Ed., Pergamon Press (1981).

3. J.J. Bernert and H. Sprecher, Studies to determine the role rates of chain elongation and desaturation play in regulating the unsaturated fatty acid composition of rat liver lipids, Biochim Biophys. Acta, 398:354 (1975).

4. C. Galli, E. Agradi, A. Petroni and E. Tremoli, Differential effects of dietary fatty acids on the accumulation of arachidonic acid and its metabolic conversion through the cycloxygenase and the lipoxygenase in platelets and vascular tissue, Lipids 16:165 (1981).

5. E. Giani, E. Masi, C. Colombo and C. Galli, Sex differences in platelet thromboxane and arterial prostacyclin production in control n-6 fatty acid supplemented rats, Prostaglandins 28:573 (1984).

6. W. Siess, B. Scherer, B. Bohlig, P. Roth, I. Kurzman and P.C. Weber, Platelet membrane fatty acids, platelet aggregation and thromboxane formation during mackerel diet, Lancet i:441 (1980).

7. T. Terano, A. Hirai, T. Hamazaki, S. Kobayashi, T. Fujuta, Y. Tamura and A. Kumagai. Effect of oral administration of highly purified eicosapentaenoic acid on platelet function, blood viscosity and red-cell deformability in healthy human subjects, Atheroscl. 46(3):321 (1983).

8. A. Socini, C. Galli, C. Colombo and E. Tremoli, Fish oil administration as a supplement to a Corn Oil containing diet affects arterial prostacyclin production more than platelet thromboxane formation in the rat, Prostaglandins 25:693 (1983).

9. M.M. Mathias and J. Dupont, The relationship of dietary fats to prostaglandin biosynthesis, Lipids 14:124 (1979).

10. S. Fischer and P.C. Weber, Thromboxane A_3 (TxA$_3$) is formed in human platelets after dietary eicosapentaenoic acid (C 20:5 omega 3), Biochim. Biophys. Res. Comm. 16(3):1091 (1983).

11. E. Tremoli, A. Petroni, C. Galli, R. Paoletti, P. Puska, R. Dougherty and J. Iacono, North Karelian Study: Changes in

dietary fat reduce Thromboxane B_2 formation by platelets only in male subjects - Preliminary report, Adv. Prostag. Thromb. Leuko. Res. 12:203 (1983).

12. A.A. Spector, J.C. Hoak, G.L. Fry, G.M. Denning, L.L. Stall and J.B. Smith, Effect of fatty acid modification on prosta-cyclin production by cultured human endothelial cells, J. Clin. Invest. 65:1003 (1980).

13. A.A. Spector, T.L. Kaduce, P.H. Figard, K.C. Norton, J.C. Hoak and R.L. Czervionke, Eicosapentaenoic acid and prostacy-clin production by cultured human endothelial cells, J. Lipid Res. 24(12):1595 (1983).

FORMATION OF LEUKOTRIENES AND OTHER EICOSANOIDS IN THE GASTROINTESTINAL TRACT AND EFFECT OF DRUGS

Brigitta M. Peskar[+], Karl W. Dreyling[+++],
Klaus Schaarschmidt[++] and Harald Goebell[+]

[+]Department of Gastroenterology, Medical Clinic
and [++]Department of General Surgery
University of Essen
D-43oo Essen
[+++]Department of Pharmacology
Ruhr-University of Bochum
D-463o Bochum

BIOSYNTHESIS AND METABOLISM OF CYCLOOXYGENASE PRODUCTS

The gastrointestinal tract has a high capacity to synthesize eicosanoids from endogenous substrate. A great number of studies has shown the formation of cyclooxygenase-derived products of arachidonic acid metabolism by the tissues of the gastrointestinal tract of many species including man (for ref. 1). The amount and pattern of prostaglandins (PG) synthesized is species-specific and shows regional variations. Thus, in rat, guinea-pig and rabbit, gastric mucosal formation of PGI_2 exceeds formation of PGE_2 (2). Tissue of rat small intestine synthesizes considerably more PG than rat gastric tissue, PGD_2 being the most prominant PG formed in this region (3, 4). In the human gastrointestinal tract we found mucosal PG generation to be most abundant in the stomach and duodenum, while mucosa of the small intestine and large bowel had lower PG synthesizing capacity (Fig. 1). In all regions of the human gastrointestinal tract PGE_2 was the predominant mucosal PG synthesized (Fig. 1).

In addition to the various PG gastrointestinal mucosa and muscle synthesize considerable amounts of thromboxane (TX) (5, 6, 7, 8, 9). In man, release of TXB_2 by gastric mucosal biopsy specimens incubated in vitro equals formation of PGE_2 (9). While PG, particularly PGE_2 and PGI_2, exert gastric prtection (10) and are vasodilating (11,12), TXA_2, the biologically

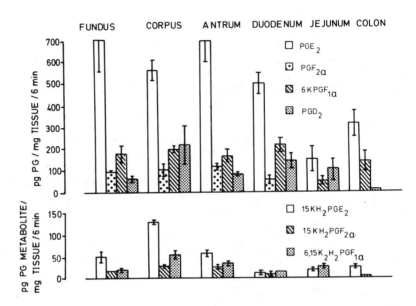

Fig. 1.   Release of PG and PG metabolites by mucosal
           tissue of the various regions of the human
           gastrointestinal tract. Mucosal biopsy speci-
           mens obtained by endoscopy or suction biopsy
           were incubated in 1 ml Krebs-Henseleit-bicar-
           bonate buffer at 37°C as described previously
           (31). The release of PG and PG metabolites
           into the incubation medium was measured using
           radioimmunoassays. Values represent the means
           + S.E.M. of 6 experiments.

active precursor of TXB_2, has recently been found to
induce severe gastric mucosal damage in the canine stomach in the presence of acidified taurocholate, probably
due to its potent vasoconstrictor action (13). The
balance between vasodilating and vasoconstricting cyclo-
oxygenase products formed in the gastrointestinal tissues
may play a crucial role for the regulation of blood flow
and may influence the capacity of the mucosa to resist
injury.

The cytoplasmic fractions of human gastric and duo-
denal mucosal homogenates contain high activities of the
enzymes 15-hydroxy-PG-dehydrogenase and Δ^{13}-PG reductase
and lower activities of Δ^9-PG-reductase (14, 15). 15-
hydroxy-PG-dehydrogenase and Δ^{13}PG-reductase metabolize
PG to the 15-keto-13,14-dihydro-derivatives that are virtually devoid of biological activity. Δ^9-PG-reductase
catalyzes a reaction converting PGE_2 to $PGF_{2\alpha}$ which
differs from PGE_2 in its biological actions. As shown
in Fig. 1 mucosal biopsies of all regions of the human
gastrointestinal tract release the 15-keto-13,14-dihydro-
metabolites of PGE_2, PGI_2 and $PGF_{2\alpha}$ during incubation in
vitro indicating that PG formed from endogenous substrate
within the mucosal tissues are degraded via the 15-hydro-
xy-PG-dehydrogenase pathway. Similar results have been
found for human gastrointestinal muscle as well as mucosal and muscular tissue of various animal species (unpublished results). In addition, large amounts of 15-
keto-13,14-dihydro-metabolites exceeding the amounts of
unmetabolized PG are released into human gastric juice
(16) as well as into luminal perfusates of the rat stomach (Fig.2). This indicates that in vivo local enzymatic metabolism contributes significantly to the inactivation of PG formed within the stomach wall.

INHIBITION OF GASTRIC PROSTAGLANDIN FORMATION BY NON-STEROIDAL ANTI-INFLAMMATORY DRUGS

Both gastrointestinal PG biosynthesis and metabolism
can be influenced by drugs. In the upper gastrointestinal
tract inhibition of mucosal PG formation obviously interferes with the capacity of the mucosa to maintain its
integrity. Thus, non-steroidal anti-inflammatory drugs
that reduce gastric mucosal PG synthesis usually are
ulcerogenic, while agents that do not affect the gastric
PG system do not cause mucosal damage. We have
shown previously that indomethacin in a dose-dependent
manner inhibits conversion of arachidonic acid to PGE_2
and $PGF_{2\alpha}$ by a microsomal fraction of human gastric
mucosal homogenates, while paracetamol even in concentrations above 10^{-3} moles/l had no inhibitory activity
on PG synthesis in this tissue (17). Contrary to indomethacin, which exhibits high gastric toxicity in experimental animals (18) and man (19), paracetamol has no
gastrointestinal side-effects. Similarly, the non-
steroidal anti-inflammatory compounds salicylic acid (18),
BW755C (18) and carprofen (2o) did not cause gastric
mucosal damage and simultaneously did not inhibit gastric
PG synthesis ex vivo. The lack of inhibition of gastric
PG formation observed with paracetamol, salicylic acid

and BW755C has been attributed to an organ-selective inhibitory activity on cyclooxygenase by these compounds.
Thus, paracetamol has been found to effectively inhibit

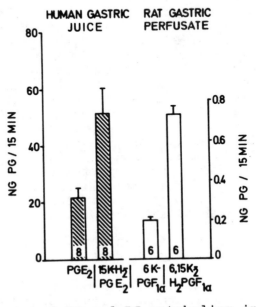

Fig. 2.   Release of PG and PG metabolism into the gastric
           lumen in vivo in man and rat. Human gastric
           juice was collected under basal conditions.
           Aliquots of the gastric juice were extracted
           using a 3:3:1 mixture of ethylacetate, iso-
           propanol, HCl (o.1 N). The dried-down residues
           were resuspended in buffer and analysed for the
           content on PGE_2 and 15-keto-13,14-dihydro-PGE_2
           (15K-H_2PGE_2) using radioimmunoassays as des-
           cribed previously (16). The gastric lumen of
           urethan-anesthetized rats was perfused with
           NaCl (o.9%, 1 ml/min). The perfusate was
           collected and analysed for the content of
           6-keto-$PGF_{1\alpha}$ (6K-$PGF_{1\alpha}$) and 6,15-diketo-
           13,14-dihydro-$PGF_{1\alpha}$ (6,15K_2-$H_2PGF_{1\alpha}$ using
           radioimmunoassays without prior extraction.
           The values represent the means $\pm$ S.E.M. of
           (n) experiments.

a PG-synthetase prepared from rabbit and dog brain but not dog spleen (21), while salicylic acid and BW755C significantly reduced PG formation in inflammatory exudates but not gastric mucosa in rats (18).

ROLE OF PHARMACOKINETIC FACTORS FOR DRUG-INDUCED INHIBITION OF GASTRIC PROSTAGLANDIN FORMATION

In addition to the lack of sensitivity of gastric mucosal cyclooxygenase against the inhibitory action of certain non-steroidal anti-inflammatory drugs pharmacokinetic properties may contribute to a low gastric toxicity of some of these agents. Patients treated with proquazone were found to have fewer gastrointestinal side-effects than patients treated with indomethacin in doses of comparable anti-inflammatory and analgesic activity (19). Similarly, in rats proquazone was less ulcerogenic than indomethacin (22, 23). However, if biopsies of human gastric mucosa were incubated in the presence of indomethacin or proquazone in vitro proquazone much more effectively inhibited release of PGE_2 and $6\text{-keto-PGF}_{1\alpha}$. Furthermore, conversion of arachidonic acid to PGE_2 by a microsomal fraction of human gastric mucosal homogenates was more effectively reduced by proquazone than by indomethacin (25) indicating a high affinity of proquazone to gastric mucosal cyclooxygenase. As in human gastric mucosa, during incubation in vitro proquazone exhibited higher inhibitory activity on the release of $6\text{-keto-PGF}_{1\alpha}$ (IC_{50} 2.2/umoles/l) than indomethacin (IC_{50} 41.5/umoles/l) by fragments of rat gastric corpus mucosa. Three hours after oral administration, however, both proquazone and indomethacin induced equal inhibition of rat gastric PG formation ex vivo (25). This finding is in agreement with work of Brune et al. (26). Using autoradiography these authors demonstrated that acidic agents such as indomethacin are readily absorbed from the stomach and reach high concentrations in the stomach wall while non-acidic compounds such as proquazone are mainly absorbed from the intestine and do not accumulate in the gastric tissues.

As indomethacin has higher gastric toxicity than proquazone the equal reduction of gastric mucosal PG formation observed after oral administration of the drugs may indicate that other factors in addition to the gastric PG system contribute to or modify gastric lesion production by non-steroidal anti-inflammatory compounds. Thus, various agents may differ in their inhibitory actions on gastric mucosal TXA2 formation and/or their effects on gastric mucosal arachidonic acid metabolism via the lipoxygenase pathway. Further studies are necessary to fully elucidate the role of fatty acid metabolites in the gastric toxicity of non-steroidal anti-inflammatory compounds.

BW755C, a dual inhibitor of cyclooxygenase and lipoxygenase, did not induce gastric mucosal damage in rats. Simultaneously, BW755C given orally did not inhibit gastric PG synthesis of the gastric corpus mucosa ex vivo (18). During incubation in vitro low concentrations of BW755C (below 1oo/umoles/l) stimulated (27), while higher concentrations inhibited (28) rat gastric corpus mucosal PG synthesis indicating that the compound has inhibitory affinity to the cyclooxygenase of this tissue. The concentration of BW755C necessary to induce a 5o% inhibition of the release of 6-keto-PGF$_1\alpha$ by rat gastric corpus and antrum mucosa (2o8 $\pm$ 47 and 18o $\pm$ 47 /umoles/l, respectively) was approximately tenfold higher than the concentration of indomethacin necessary to induce the same inhibition of PG formation by these tissues (28). After oral administration, however, BW755C in a dose of 1oo mg/kg did not reduce 6-keto-PGF$_1\alpha$ formation of rat corpus mucosa, while indomethacin in a dose of 2.5 mg/kg significantly reduced PG synthesis (28) confirming results of Whittle et al. (18). As BW755C is a basic compound lower amounts of the drug can be expected to accumulate in the gastric corpus mucosa as compared to the acidic indomethacin after oral administration. This may explain the difference in the inhibitory activities of the two agents on gastric PG formation in vitro and in vivo.

Interestingly, BW755C (1oo mg/kg) given orally effectively inhibited 6-keto-PGF$_1\alpha$ formation by tissues of the rat forestomach and antrum mucosa (28). As during incubation in vitro the inhibitory activity of the compound was identical in corpus and antrum mucosa this again points to the importance of pharmacokinetic parameters for the inhibitory action of drugs on gastric PG synthesis in vivo. Similarly, oral indomethacin (2.5 mg/kg) significantly reduced PG synthesis in the forestomach and antrum mucosa of rats (28). However, neither indomethacin nor BW755C induce mucosal damage in these regions of the rat stomach. Thus, BW755C does not produce lesions in any part of the stomach and, under the experimental conditions used, indomethacin-induced lesions are confined to the corpus region. In the forestomach and antrum mucosa of rats the endogenous PG system seems, therefore, to be less crucial for the maintenance of mucosal integrity than in the corpus region.

EFFECTS OF ULCER-HEALING DRUGS ON THE GASTRIC MUCOSAL PROSTAGLANDIN and THROMBOXANE SYSTEM

Carbenoxolone was the first drug shown to accelerate peptic ulcer healing (29). Contrary to compounds such as H_2-receptor blockers, carbenoxolone does not inhibit gastric acid secretion (3o), but seems to strengthen mucosal defense reactions. Thus, the compound has been found to stimulate gastric mucus biosynthesis, increase the half-life of mucosal cells, reduce the rate of gastric mucosal cell turnover and increase mucosal blood flow (for ref. 31). Some of these effects have also been observed with certain PG. It was, therefore, of interest that we could show that carbenoxolone inhibits the PG metabolizing enzymes 15-hydroxy-PG-dehydrogenase and Δ^{13}PG-reductase partially purified from guinea-pig lung and human gastric mucosal homogenates (32) without affecting PG synthesis by a microsomal fraction of human gastric mucosa (17). Carbenoxolone-induced inhibition of PG inactivation can also be observed in intact mucosal cells. Thus, formation of the metabolite 15-keto-13,14-dihydro-PGE_2 is dose-dependently reduced if biopsy specimens of human gastric mucosa are incubated in the presence of carbenoxolone. Simultaneously, mucosal release of PGE_2 is significantly increased (9, 31) indicating that inhibition of PG degradation results in enhanced release of biologically active PGE_2. In addition to the inhibitory action on PG metabolizing enzymes carbenoxolone in a dose-dependent manner inhibits synthesis of TXB_2 by biopsies of human gastric mucosa (9. 31). As PGE_2 and TXB_2 are derived from the same cyclic endoperoxide intermediates inhibition of TX synthesis could possibly contribute to the enhanced formation of PGE_2 in the presence of carbenoxolone by diverting the metabolism of the endoperoxides to the PG pathway. PGE_2 has vasodilating (11) and protective (1o) properties, while TXA_2 is a potent vasoconstrictor and ulcerogenic compound (13). Both effects of carbenoxolone on mucosal arachidonate metabolism could, therefore, combine in assisting the gastroduodenal mucosa to resist injury and to promote ulcer healing.

Similar to carbenoxolone sucralfate accelerates peptic ulcer healing by a mechanism not involving inhibition of acid secretion. Recently, Hollander et al. (33) have shown that sucralfate increases the release of PGE_2 into gastric secretions in rats. Similar observations have been made for some antacids (34). Stimulation of the endogenous PG system and/or inhibition of TX formation in the gastroduodenal mucosa may thus be an interesting approach for the development of new ulcer healing drugs. As the mode of action of this type of agents does not depend on inhibition of acid secretion they may favourably combine with antisecretory drugs in their therapeutic efficacy on promotion of healing and/or prevention of recurrences of gastroduodenal ulcerations.

DRUG-INDUCED MODULATION OF COLONIC ARACHIDONIC ACID METABOLISM

Contrary to the upper gastrointestinal tract in colonic mucosa the correlation of clinical effectiveness and actions of drugs on the PG system is less clear. Sulphasalazine (SASP) and its colonic metabolite 5-aminosalicylic acid (5-ASA) have been found to affect both PG synthesis and metabolism. Several groups have shown that SASP and 5-ASA inhibit conversion of arachidonic acid to PGE_2 by microsomal fractions prepared from various animal organs and human colonic mucosa (35, 36). However, results from our laboratory have demonstrated that SASP can inhibit as well as stimulate the activity of human colonic mucosal PG synthetase depending on the concentration of the substrate arachidonic acid present in the incubation mixtures. Thus, SASP-induced inhibition of PG synthetase occurred in the presence of low concentrations of arachidonic acid only, while at high substrate concentrations the drug stimulated PG synthesis (37, 38). 5-ASA, on the other hand, inhibited the enzyme reaction at low as well as at high substrate concentrations (37, 38).

Hoult and Moore (39) first reported inhibition of the initial PG metabolizing enzyme 15-hydroxy-PG-dehydrogenase of various animal tissues by SASP but not 5-ASA. This effect was confirmed for human colonic 15-hydroxy-PG-dehydrogenase (4o). Furthermore, work from our laboratory could demonstrate an additional inhibitory activity of SASP on Δ^{13}-PG-reductase and of 5-ASA on 15-hydroxy-PG-dehydrogenase of human colonic mucosa (37, 38). Thus, SASP and 5-ASA exert complex and divergent effects on the enzymes of both PG synthesis and metabolism. From this one should expect that the modulatory action of the compounds on arachidonic acid metabolism may vary in different cells of the gastrointestinal tract and in different physiological or pathophysiological conditions. This view is supported by the conflicting results on the effects of SASP and 5-ASA on PG formation by intact mucosal cells incubated under various experimental conditions. Thus, we found stimulation of the release of PGE_2 and 15-keto-13,14-dihydro-PGE_2 by fragments of human colonic mucosa incubated in the presence of SASP for up to two hours, while 5-ASA inhibited eicosanoid formation (37, 38). Ligumsky et al. (41), on the other hand, prolonging mucosal incubations up to 24 hours, observed parallel inhibition of eicosanoid formation in the presence of both SASP and 5-ASA. This discrepancy could be due to differences in the activation state of mucosal phospholipases. Thus, during the initial period of an in vitro incubation phospholipase stimulation may result in high concentrations of arachidonic acid at the site of cyclooxygenase resulting in a stimulatory action of SASP, while during long time incubation phospholipase activity may decrease with only small amounts of arachidonic acid liberated from the phospholipids. In this situation the inhibitory activity of SASP may predominate. The divergent modulatory actions of SASP and 5-ASA on the PG system may also explain the lack of effect of SASP withdrawal on the net secretion of PGE_2 by colonic mucosa in vivo in patients with quiescent ulcerative colitis (42).

Colonic mucosa from patients with active ulcerative colitis synthesizes more PG, particularly PGE_2 and PGI_2, than normal tissue (37, 41). As PGE_2 and PGI_2 are pro-inflammatory and PGE_2 stimulates intestinal secretion enhanced formation of these eicosanoids could possibly contribute to the maintenance of the inflammatory process and the clinical symptoms in these patients. On the other hand, PGE_2 and PGI_2 are cytoprotective (1o) and PGE_2 has been found to inhibit the activity of chronic inflammatory cells (43). Thus, both inhibition and stimulation of mucosal PG formation could possibly explain the beneficial effects of SASP therapy. However, to further complicate the issue administration of classical cyclooxygenase inhibitors such as flurbiprofen (44) as well as of 15(R),15-methyl-PGE_2 (45) induced clinical deterioration in patients with quiescent ulcerative colitis. Recently, inhibition of various lipoxygenase enzymes by SASP and 5-ASA in vitro has been described (46, 47, 48). However, the concentrations of SASP and 5-ASA necessary to inhibit formation of lipoxygenase-derived

products of arachidonic acid metatbolism by human polymorphonuclear cells and human colonic mucosa are much
higher than the concentrations necessary to affect the
PG system in these tissues. It remains, therefore, to
be established, if modulation of the lipoxygenase pathway of fatty acid metabolism occurs in vivo and mediates the beneficial effect of SASP therapy in patients
with chronic inflammatory bowel disease.

BIOSYNTHESIS OF LEUKOTRIENES

While much information has accumulated on synthesis
and metabolism of cyclooxygenase products in the gastrointestinal tract,only few data are available on the formation of lipoxygenase-derived metabolites of arachidonic acid in this organ. Bennett et al. (7) and Hawkey
et al. (49) have shown that human colonic mucosa can
convert exogenous arachidonic acid to various hydroxy
fatty acids. Sharon and Stenson (47) recently reported
increased synthesis of leukotriene (LT) B4 by colonic
mucosa of patients with chronic inflammatory bowel
disease as compared to normal colonic mucosa. We have
studied the formation of LTC_4-like immunoreactivity by
gastrointestinal tissues of guinea-pig and man.

Table 1 shows the release of immunoreactive LTC_4
and of biologically active slow reacting substance (SRS)
by human intestinal mucosa. The tissue was obtained from
patients with active Crohn's disease undergoing surgery.
Histological examination showed severe inflammatory reactions in all tissues used for the experiments. Mucosal
fragments incubated in the presence of the divalent
cation ionophore A23187 released significant amounts
of immunoreactive LTC_4 into the incubation medium. The
selective lipoxygenase inhibitor nordihydroguaiaretic
acid and the dual inhibitor of lipoxygenase and cyclo-
oxygenase BW755C significantly reduced mucosal formation of immunoreactive LTC_4. Furthermore, the mucosal
tissues generated biologically active material that
contracted the isolated guinea-pig ileum. The release
of biologically active material was significantly reduced, if the mucosa was incubated in the presence of
BW755C. Furthermore, the contractions of the guinea-pig
ileum elicited by addition of mucosal incubates were
antagonized by FPL 55712, a selective inhibitor of LT
action.

Gastrointestinal formation of LTC_4-like immunoreactivity differs from synthesis of PG in several aspects.
If colonic tissue of guinea-pigs that had been sensitized

286

Table 1. Release of immunoreactive leukotriene C_4 and biologically active slow
reacting substance by ileal mucosa of patients with Crohn's disease

	Immunoreactivity (ng/g wet weight)	Contractile response (histamine equivalents/g wet weight)	
		without FPL 55712	with FPL 55712
Mucosa incubated in the presence of ionophore only	33.8 ± 7.9	12.2 ± 4.4	4.4 ± 2.0***
Mucosa incubated in the presence of ionophore and NDGA	3.3 ± 1.3§***	4.2 ± 1.4§	—
Mucosa incubated in the presence of ionophore and BW755C	7.3 ± 2.8**	3.2 ± 2.3*	—

Fragments of ileal mucosa (600 mg) were incubated in 3 ml modified Tyrode solution
at 37ºC. After 20 min the medium was removed and replaced by 3 ml Tyrode solution
containing the divalent cation ionophore A23187 (5/ug/ml). Incubations were continued for 20 min. In additional experiments nordihydroguaiaretic acid (NDGA,
10/ug/ml) or BW755C (10/ug/ml) were added to the incubates. Release of immunoreactive LTC_4 into the incubation medium was measured as described previously (50).
Formation of SRS was determined by the contractile response of the isolated
guinea-pig ileum to addition of mucosal incubates in the absence or presence of
FPL 55712 (200 ng/ml) as described elsewhere (50). Results are expressed as
means ± S.E.M. of 5 experiments: (§) n = 3, *p < 0.01, **p < 0.025, ***p < 0.05
compared with control incubates.

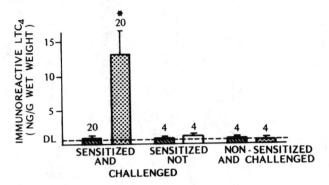

Fig. 3.   Effect of antigen-challenge in vitro on the
release of immunoreactive LTC_4 of guinea-pig
colonic mucosa. Guinea-pigs were sensitized
against ovalbumin. Three weeks after the immu-
nization procedure the colon was removed and
the mucosal tissue separated from the underlying muscular layer. The chopped tissue was
preincubated in 3.o ml modified Tyrode solution at 37°C. After 5 min ovalbumin (1 mg/ml
final concentration) was added to the incubates and incubations were continued for 2o
min. Additional experiments were performed in
which colonic mucosa of sensitized guinea-pigs
was incubated without addition of antigen.
Furthermore, incubation experiments in the presence of antigen were performed using colonic
mucosa of non-sensitized guinea-pigs. Release
of LTC_4 into the incubation medium during the
preincubation period (▨), incubation with
antigen (▨) and incubation period without
antigen (□) was determined using radioimmunoassay as described previously (5o). Statistical
analysis was calculated using the Student's t-
test for paired values. The results represent the
means ± S.E.M. of (n) experiments.*p < o.oo5.

against ovalbumin was incubated in vitro, addition of antigen to the incubation mixture significantly stimulated release of immunoreactive LTC$_4$ as well as biologi-

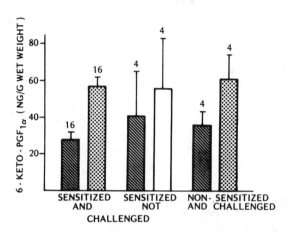

Fig. 4. Effect of antigen-challenge on the release of 6-keto-PGF$_{1\alpha}$ by guinea-pig colonic mucosa. Colonic mucosa of guinea-pigs sensitized against ovalbumin was incubated as described in Fig. 3. Release of 6-keto-PGF$_{1\alpha}$ during a 5 min preincubation (▨) and 2o min incubation in the presence (▨) or absence (□) of antigen was determined using radioimmunoassay as described previously (5o). In additional experiments mucosa of non-sensitized guinea-pigs was incubated in the presence of antigen. The results show the means ± S.E.M. of (n) experiments.

cally active SRS (5o). The antigen-induced release of LTC$_4$ was confined almost exclusively to the mucosal layer and was negligible in the muscular and subserosal layer (5o). Colonic formation of PG, on the other hand, was most abundant in the serosal and lowest in the mucosal tissue. Furthermore, as shown in Fig. 3 and Fig. 4, significant mucosal release of immunoreactive LTC$_4$

occurs in the presence of an antigen-antibody reaction only indicating that a specific trigger mechanism is necessary for effective conversion of arachidonic acid to LTC_4 whereas PG formation is identical in the presence or absence of antigen (5o). Antigen-induced immunoreactive and biologically active release of LTC_4 could also be demonstrated in the gastric mucosa of ovalbumin-sensitized guinea-pigs challenged with antigen in vitro (24).

ACKNOWLEDGEMENTS

We thank Miss B. Schlüter, Miss G. Knaup and Mr. K.H. Ehrlich for excellent technical assistance. The work was supported by the Deutsche Forschungsgemeinschaft.

REFERENCES

1. C. Johansson, and S. Bergström, Prostaglandins and protection of the gastroduodenal mucosa, Scand. J. Gastroenterol. Suppl. 77: 21 (1982).
2. B. J. R. Whittle, Role of prostaglandins in the defense of the gastric mucosa, In: "Brain Research Bulletin", vol. 5, Suppl. 1, p. 7, ANKHO International Inc. (198o).
3. H. R. Knapp, O. Oelz, B. J. Sweetman, and J. A. Oates, Synthesis and metabolism of prostaglandins E_2, $F_{2\alpha}$ and D_2 by the rat gastrointestinal tract. Stimulation by a hypertonic environment in vitro, Prostaglandins 15: 751 (1978).
4. B. M. Peskar, H. Weiler, E. E. Kröner, and B.A. Peskar, Release of prostaglandins by small intestinal tissue of man and rat in vitro and the effect of endotoxin in the rat in vivo, Prostaglandins 21, Suppl.: 9 (1981).
5. M. Ali, and J. W. D. McDonalds, Synthesis of thromboxane B_2 and 6-keto-prostaglandin-$F_{1\alpha}$ by bovine gastric mucosal and muscle microsomes, Prostaglandins 2o: 245 (198o).
6. L. I. LeDuc, and P. Needleman, Regional localisation of prostacyclin and thromboxane synthesis in dog stomach and intestinal tract, J. Pharmacol. Exp. Ther. 211: 181 (1979).
7. A. Bennett, C. N. Hensby, G. J. Sanger, and I. F. Stamford, Metabolites of arachidonic acid formed by human gastrointestinal tissues and their actions on the muscle layers, Br. J. Pharmac. 74: 435 (1981).

8. P. Sharon, S. Cohen. A. Zifroni, F. Carmeli,
    L. Ligumsky, and D. Rachmilewitz, Prostanoid
    synthesis by cultured gastric and duodenal
    mucosa: possible role in pathogenesis of duo-
    denal ulcer, Scand. J. Gastroenterol. 18: 1o45
    (1983).

9. B. M. Peskar, and H. Weiler, Carbenoxolone inhibits
    thromboxane B_2 synthesis by human gastric
    mucosa, Gut 24: A48o (1983).

1o. A. Robert, Cytoprotection by prostaglandins,
    Gastroenterology 77: 761 (1979).

11. I. H. M. Main, and B. J. R. Whittle, The effects
    of E and A prostaglandins on gastric mucosal
    blood flow and acid secretion in the rat, Br.
    J. Pharmac. 49:428 (1973).

12. B. J. R. Whittle, K. Boughton-Smith, S. Moncada,
    and J. R. Vane, Actions of prostacyclin (PGI$_2$)
    and its product, 6-oxo-PGF$_{1\alpha}$ on the rat gastric
    mucosa in vivo and in vitro, Prostaglandins,
    15: 955 (1978).

13. B. J. R. Whittle, G.L. Kauffman, and S. Moncada,
    Vasoconstriction with thromboxane A$_2$ induces
    ulceration of the gastric mucosa, Nature 292:
    472 (1981).

14. B. M. Peskar, and B. A. Peskar, On the metabolism
    of prostaglandins by human gastric mucosa,
    Biochim. Biophys. Acta 424: 43o (1976).

15. B. M. Peskar, Regional distribution of prostaglan-
    din metabolizing enzymes in the mucosa of the
    human upper gastrointestinal tract, Acta hepato-
    gastroent. 25: 49 (1978).

16. B. M. Peskar, B. Günter, and B. A. Peskar, Prosta-
    glandins and prostaglandin metabolites in human
    gastric juice, Prostaglandins 2o: 419 (198o).

17. B. M. Peskar, On the synthesis of prostaglandins
    by human gastric mucosa and its modification
    by drugs, Biochim. Biophys. Acta 487: 3o7 (1977).

18. B. J. R. Whittle, G. A. Higgs, K. E. Eakins,
    S. Moncada, and J. R. Vane, Selective inhibition
    of prostaglandin production in inflammatory exu-
    dates and gastric mucosa, Nature 284: 371 (198o).

19. R. Allen, and M. Bleicher, Die Behandlung degenera-
    tiver Gelenkerkrankungen mit Biarison[R], Schweiz.
    Rundschau Med. 46: 1481 (1977).

2o. S. J. Konturek, N. Kwiecién, W. Obtulowics, A. Kiéc-
    Dembinska, M. Polański, B. Kopp, E. Sito, and
    J. Olesky, Effect of carprofen and indomethacin
    on gastric functions, mucosal integrity and ge-
    neration of prostaglandins in man, Hepato-
    gastroenterol. 29: 267 (1982).

21. R. J. Flower, and J. R. Vane, Inhibition of prosta-
     glandin synthetase in brain explains the anti-
     paretic activity of paracetamol (4-acetamidophe-
     nol), Nature 24o: 41o (1972).
22. E. I. Takesne, J.W. Perrine, and J. H. Trapold,
     The anti-inflammatory profile of proquazone,
     Arch. int. Pharmacodyn. 221: 122 (1976).
23. H. U. Gubler, and M. Baggiolini, Pharmacological
     properties of proquazone, Scand. J. Rheumatol.
     21: 8 (1978).
24. U. Aehringhaus, H. Weiler, B. A. Peskar, and
     B. M. Peskar, Molecular mechanisms of the gastric
     toxicity of anti-rheumatic drugs, Arch. Toxicol.,
     im Druck.
25. B. M. Peskar, H. Weiler, and Ch. Meyer, Inhibition
     of prostaglandin production in the gastrointesti-
     nal tract by antiinflammatory drugs, in: "Ad-
     vances in Inflammation Research", vol. 6,
     K. D. Rainsford, G. D. Velo ed., Raven Press,
     New York, p. 39 (1984).
26. K. Brune, H. Gubler, and A. Schweitzer, Autoradio-
     graphic methods for the evaluation of anti-
     inflammatory drugs, Pharmacol. Ther. 5: 199 (1979).
27. N. K. Boughton-Smith, and B. J. R. Whittle, Stimula-
     tion and inhibition of prostacyclin formation in
     the gastric mucosa and ileum in vitro by anti-
     inflammatory agents, Br. J. Pharmac. 78: 173 (1983)
28. B. M. Peskar, H. Weiler, and B. A. Peskar, Effect of
     BW755C on prostaglandin synthesis in the rat
     stomach, Biochem. Pharmacol. 31: 1652 (1982).
29. R. Doll, I. D. Hill, and C.F. Hutton, Treatment of
     gastric ulcer with carbenoxolone sodium and
     oestrogens, Gut 6: 19 (1965).
3o. J. H. Baron, Effect of carbenoxolone sodium on human
     gastric acid secretion, Gut 18: 721 (1977).
31. B. M. Peskar, Effects of carbenoxolone on the gastric
     mucosal prostaglandin and thromboxane system,
     Acta gastroent. Belg. 46: 429 (1983).
32. B. M. Peskar, A. Holland, and B.A. Peskar, Effect
     of carbenoxolone on prostaglandin synthesis
     and degradation, J. Pharm. Pharmacol. 28: 146
     (1976).
33. W. Hollander, A. Tarnawski, H. Gergeley, and
     R. D. Zipser, Sucralfate protection of the
     gastric mucosa against ethanol-induced injury:
     a prostaglandin-mediated process? Scand. J.
     Gastroenterol. 19, Suppl. 1o1: 97 (1984).

34. W. Hollander, A. Tarnawsky, D. Cummings, W. J. Krause, H. Gergeley, and R.B. Zipser, Cytoprotective action of antacids against alcohol-induced gastric mucosal injury. Morphologic, ultrastructural and functional time sequence analysis, Gastroenterology 86: 1114 (1984).

35. S. R. Gould, and J. E. Lennard-Jones, Production of prostaglandins in ulcerative colitis and their inhibition by sulphasalazine, Gut 17: 828 (1976).

36. P. R. Smith, D. J. Dawson, and C. H. J. Swan, Prostaglandin synthetase activity in acute ulcerative colitis: effects of treatment with sulphasalazine, codein phosphate and prednisolone, Gut 2o: 8o2 (1978).

37. B. M. Peskar, T. Schlenker, and H. Weiler, Effect of sulphasalazine (SASP) and 5-aminosalicylic acid (5-ASA) on the human colonic prostaglandin (PG) system, Gut 23: A444 (1982).

38. B. M. Peskar, Effect of sulphasalazine and 5-aminosalicylic acid on the human colonic prostaglandin system, in: "New Trends in Pathophysiology and Therapy of the Large Bowel",L. Barbara, M. Miglioli, and S. F. Phillips, eds., Elsevier Science Publish., Amsterdam, p. 185 (1983).

39. J. R. S. Hoult, and P.K. Moore, Sulphasalazine is a potent inhibitor of prostaglandin 15-hydroxy-dehydrogenase: possible basis for therapeutic action in ulcerative colitis, Br. J. Pharmac. 64: 6 (1978).

4o. K. Hillier, P. G. Mason, and C. L. Smith, Ulcerative colitis: prostaglandin metabolism and the effect of sulphasalazine, 5-amino salicylic acid and indomethacin in human colonic mucosa, Br. J. Pharmac. 73: 217P (1981).

41. P. Sharon, M. Ligumsky, D. Rachmilewitz, and U. Zor, Role of prostaglandins in ulcerative colitis. Enhanced production during active disease and inhibition by sulfasalazine, Gastroenterology 75: 638 (1978).

42. W. S. Rampton, and G.E. Sladen, The effect of sulphasalazine withdrawal on rectal mucosal function and prostaglandin E_2 release in inactive ulcerative colitis, Scand. J. Gastroent. 16: 157 (1981).

43. J. Morley, Prostaglandins and lymphokines in arthritis, Prostaglandins 8: 315 (1974).

44. D. S. Rampton, and G. E. Sladen, Prostaglandin
    synthesis inhibitors in ulcerative colitis:
    flurbiprofen compared with conventional treat-
    ment, Prostaglandins 21: 417 (1981).
45. E. Goldin, and D. Rachmilewitz, Prostanoid cyto-
    protection for maintaining remission in ulcera-
    tive colitis. Failure of 15(R),15-methylprosta-
    glandin E$_2$, Dig. Dis. Sci. 28: 8o7 (1983).
46. W. F. Stenson, and E. Lobos, Sulfasalazine inhibits
    the synthesis of chemotactic lipids by neutro-
    phils, J. Clin. Invest. 69: 494 (1982).
47. P. Sharon, and W. F. Stenson, Enhanced synthesis of
    leukotriene B$_4$ by colonic mucosa in inflammatory
    bowel disease, Gastroenterology 86: 453 (1984).
48. J. C. Sircar, C. F. Schwender, and M. E. Carethers,
    Inhibition of soybean lipoxygenase by sulphasa-
    lazine and 5-aminosalicylic acid: a possible
    mode of action in ulcerative colitis, Biochem.
    Pharmacol. 32: 17o (1983).
49. C. J. Hawkey, N. K. Boughton-Smith, and B. J. R.
    Whittle, In: "Proceedings of the V. International
    Conference on Prostaglandins", Florence, Raven
    Press, New York, p. 87 (1982).
5o. R. H. Wölbling, U. Aehringhaus, B. A. Peskar,
    K. Morgenroth, and B. M. Peskar, Release of slow-
    reacting substance of anaphylaxis and leukotriene
    C$_4$-like immunoreactivity from guinea-pig colonic
    tissue, Prostaglandins 25: 8o9 (1983).

ROLE OF EICOSANOIDS IN THE PATHOGENESIS

OF INFLAMMATORY BOWEL DISEASES

Brendan J.R. Whittle, Nigel K. Boughton-Smith and Christopher J. Hawkey*

Department of Prostaglandin Research, Wellcome Research Laboratories, Langley Court, Beckenham, Kent BR3 3BS and *Department of Therapeutics, University Hospital Nottingham, U.K.

The eicosanoids are metabolites of the essential fatty acid arachidonic acid formed via the cyclo-oxygenase and lipoxygenase enzyme pathways. The cyclo-oxygenase metabolites characterized as prostanoids have been implicated in the aetiology of inflammatory bowel diseases. Several of these long-chain unsaturated fatty acids, notably prostaglandin E_2 (PGE_2), have potent pro-inflammatory properties and can alter intestinal motility, fluid secretion and electrolyte transport[1]. These arachidonate metabolites could thus be involved in inflammatory diseases of the intestine and underlie the associated diarrhoea in diseases such as ulcerative colitis. In patients with active ulcerative colitis, higher levels of prostaglandin-like material could be detected in the stools[2], with increased cyclo-oxygenase activity in vitro in rectal biopsies[3]. In other studies using radioimmunoassay techniques, elevated accumulation of PGE_2 as well as thromboxane B_2 (TXB_2) and the prostacyclin breakdown product, 6-oxo-$PGF_{1\alpha}$ in 24 h cultures of rectal mucosa biopsies were determined[4,5] while studies in vivo using rectal dialysis procedures likewise indicated enhanced formation of PGE_2 in patients with active ulcerative colitis[6].

Although these findings can be taken to imply that local elevated prostaglandin levels are associated with active disease, it is not known whether this is the cause or the result of the inflammatory disease. Certain prostaglandins could contribute to the inflammatory process by enhancing local vasodilation and subsequent oedema formation. However, they have limited effects on the movement of inflammatory cells, and thus could not account for the tissue infiltration of leucocytes characteristic of inflammatory bowel diseases.

295

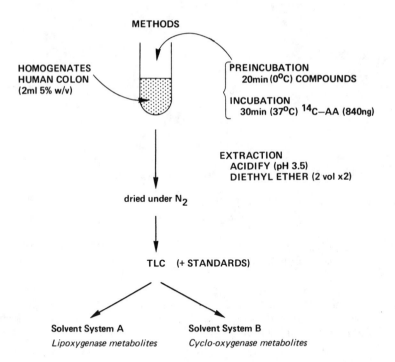

METHODS

HOMOGENATES
HUMAN COLON
(2ml 5% w/v)

PREINCUBATION
20min (0°C) COMPOUNDS

INCUBATION
30min (37°C) ^{14}C–AA (840ng)

EXTRACTION
ACIDIFY (pH 3.5)
DIETHYL ETHER (2 vol x2)

dried under N$_2$

TLC   (+ STANDARDS)

Solvent System A   Solvent System B
Lipoxygenase metabolites   *Cyclo-oxygenase metabolites*

<u>Fig. 1</u> Incubation, extraction and separation of radiolabelled metabolites following incubation of homogenates of human colon with ^{14}C-arachidonic acid.

The biosynthesis of arachidonate metabolites via the lipoxygenase enzymes have been described in platelets[7] and more recently in leucocytes[8,9]. The products formed include the leukotrienes and 5-hydroxy-eicosatetraenoic acid (5-HETE) from the 5-lipoxygenase pathway, and 12- and 15-HETE formed by the 12-and 15-lipoxygenase enzymes respectively. In addition, non-prostaglandin products of the cyclo-oxygenase pathway such as 11-HETE and 12-hydroxy-heptadecatrienoic acid (HHT) can be formed. In contrast to prostaglandins, some of these lipoxygenase products have been demonstrated to stimulate locomotion, lysosomal enzyme release and superoxide production by human leucocytes[10,11,12].

Since such arachidonate products thus have potential importance as mediators of inflammatory disease, we have investigated the metabolism of radiolabelled arachidonic acid ([^{14}C]-AA) via both cyclo-oxygenase and lipoxygenase enzymes present in human colonic mucosa. In addition, the actions of sulphasalazine, the drug known to decrease the incidence of relapse in ulcerative colitis, has been evaluated on arachidonate metabolism in the human colon <u>in vitro</u> and compared to the effects of specific pharmacological agents known to selectively inhibit the enzymic pathways.

296

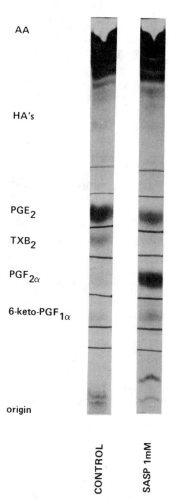

AA

HA's

PGE$_2$

TXB$_2$

PGF$_{2\alpha}$

6-keto-PGF$_{1\alpha}$

origin

CONTROL

SASP 1mM

Fig. 2 Autoradiogram of radiolabelled metabolites of [^{14}C]-arachidonic acid formed by homogenates of human colon mucosa and separated by TLC using solvent system B. The profile shows separation of cyclo-oxygenase metabolites of arachidonic acid and the inhibition of TXB$_2$ formation and the enhancement of PGF$_{2\alpha}$ formation by sulphasalazine (1 mM).

Methods

Histologically-normal sections of human colon were obtained at operation from patients undergoing resection of carcinomas. Mucosal tissue, stripped from the resected human colon and stored at -70°C, was manually homogenized in 50 mM Tris buffer (pH 8.0). Aliquots (50-85 mg ml^{-1} w/v final suspension; 2 ml) were incubated for 20 mins at 37°C with 840 ng (160 nCi) of [^{14}C]-AA[13].

After acidification to pH 3.5 with citric acid (2.3 M), the products were extracted twice into 2 volumes of diethyl ether (8 ml total volume). Extracted samples were dried under nitrogen, redissolved in 75 µl of chloroform : methanol (2:1) and applied to multi-lane TLC plates (Whatman LK 5D). In each experiment, duplicate TLC plates were prepared and were developed using two separate solvent systems (Fig. 1). Solvents system "A" consisted of ether:hexane:acetic acid (60:40:1, v/v/v) which separated TXB_2 and prostaglandins from the lipoxygenase products. Solvent system "B" was the organic phase of ethyl acetate:trimethyl pentane:water:acetic acid (110:50:100:20, v/v/v/v) which separated the individual prostaglandins and TXB_2. In an additional study, a further solvent system (consisting of chloroform-methanol-acetic acid-H_2O (90:8:1:0.8; v/v/v/v) was used to separate the individual prostanoids.

The radioactive products were localised using autoradiography (3 days contact with Kodak NS2T film), the silica gel zone corresponding to each radioactive band was scraped off, and the radioactivity was determined by liquid scintillation counting. A typical autoradiograph of the products separated using solvent system "B" is shown in Fig. 2.

In further experiments, the effect of sulphasalazine on the metabolism of $[^{14}C]$-AA by the homogenates of human colonic mucosa was compared to that of the selective thromboxane (TX) synthetase inhibitor, 1-benzyl imidazole[14,15] as the fumarate salt. Sulphasalazine was used at a low concentration (50 µM) corresponding to serum concentrations of unchanged drug and at a higher concentration (1 mM) in the range reported for the faecal concentration found in subjects taking sulphasalazine[16,17].

Results

The homogenates of human colonic mucosa converted 6.4 ± 0.9% (mean ± s.e.m., n=5) of the added $[^{14}C]$-AA to radioactive products. The predominant cyclo-oxygenase products formed, as characterised by their chromatographic mobility using solvent system "B" were PGE_2, $PGF_{2\alpha}$, PGD_2, TXB_2, 6-oxo-$PGF_{1\alpha}$, as shown in Fig. 3.

To further characterise these products as cyclo-oxygenase metabolites, homogenates were pre-incubated with indomethacin, the potent cyclo-oxygenase inhibitor. As shown in Fig. 3, preincubation (20 min at $0^{\circ}C$) with indomethacin (1 µg ml^{-1}, 3 µM) significantly reduced the formation of these products. The dual inhibitor of both cyclo-oxygenase and lipoxygenase enzymes[18], BW755C (5 µg ml^{-1}, 19 µM) also significantly reduced their formation (Fig. 3). In studies employing solvent system "A" in which the cyclo-oxygenase products run as a single band, indomethacin (3 µM) and BW755C (19 µM) likewise significantly reduced their formation (Fig. 4).

Sulphasalazine (50 µM and 1 mM), at both concentrations used, significantly inhibited the formation of the product having

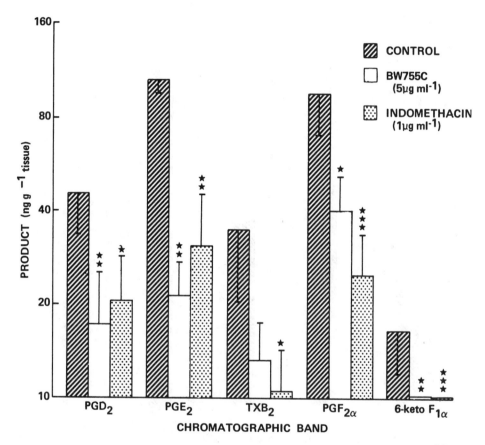

Fig. 3 Formation of radiolabelled cyclo-oxygenase products from [^{14}C]-arachidonic acid by homogenates of human colonic mucosa and their inhibition by indomethacin (3 µM) and BW755C (19 µM). The level of prostanoids separated on TLC by solvent system B are shown as formation ng g^{-1} tissue from [^{14}C]-AA (8.4 µg g^{-1} tissue). The results are expressed as mean ± s.e.m. of 5 experiments, where * P < 0.05, ** P < 0.01, *** P < 0.001.

chromatographic mobility of TXB$_2$ (Table 1).   This inhibition was
accompanied by a dose-related enhancement of PGF$_{2\alpha}$ formation (Fig. 2)

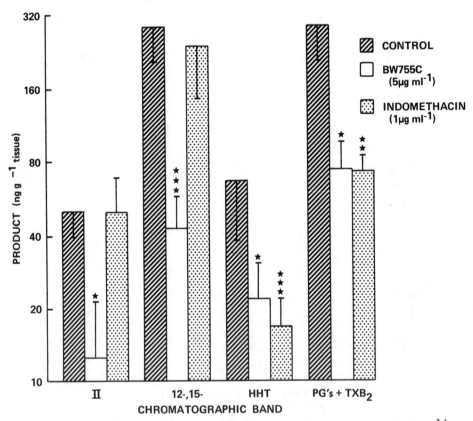

Fig. 4 Formation of radiolabelled lipoxygense products from [^{14}C]-arachidonic acid by homogenates of human colonic mucosa and their selective inhibition by BW755C (19 μM). The level of product formation, separated on TLC by solvent system A, are shown as formation ng g^{-1} tissue from [^{14}C]-AA (8.4 μg g^{-1} tissue). The results are expressed as mean ± s.e.m. of 5 experiments, where * P < 0.05, ** P < 0.01, *** P < 0.001.

whilst the synthesis of the other cyclo-oxygenase products was unchanged (Table 1). Benzyl imidazole (15, 75 and 370 μM) significantly inhibited TXB_2 formation, whereas the synthesis of the other cyclo-oxygenase products was not significantly changed (Table 1).

To confirm the selective effects of sulphasalazine and benzyl imidazole and the identity of the radiolabelled products, an additional solvent system was used to separate by TLC, the cyclo-oxygenase products formed from ^{14}C-AA by the colonic mucosal homogenates. Products from duplicate incubations were separated using solvent system "B" for one incubate and the chloroform:methanol:acetic acid:H_2O solvent system[19] for the second incubate. As shown in Fig. 5, comparable results for the inhibition of TXB_2 were obtained using these two different solvent systems. Thus, the arachidonate product with the chromatographic mobility of TXB_2 was inhibited by both sulphasalazine (1 mM) and benzyl imidazole (30, 150 and 750 μM) in each TLC system. In addition, in this experiment, sulphasalazine increased the synthesis of products with the chromatographic mobility of PGE_2 and $PGF_{2\alpha}$, while benzyl imidazole had little effect on these cyclo-oxygenase products.

The predominant lipoxygenase products, characterised using solvent system "A" had a chromatographic mobility corresponding with 11-,12- or 15-HETE (which ran together) as shown in Fig. 4. Previous studies, using HPLC techniques to separate these products, have shown these products to be a mixture of 12- and 15-HETE. Whereas indomethacin (3 μM) failed to reduce significantly the formation of these products, BW755C (19 μM) inhibited their production by 75 ± 9%, n=5, (P < 0.001; Fig. 4) thereby further characterizing these metabolites as lipoxygenase products. Smaller amounts of other radiolabelled products were also separated using this solvent system. The synthesis of product II was inhibited by BW755C (19 μM) but not by indomethacin (2.8 μM) suggesting that it was also a lipoxygenase product, but its identification requires further study. A product corresponding to HHT (a cyclo-oxygenase product) whose synthesis was inhibited by both indomethacin and BW755C was also detected. A radiolabelled product having the chromatographic mobility of 5-HETE was also detected[13], but its formation was inhibited by both indomethacin (by 64 ± 2%) and BW755C (by 89 ± 3%). Although the inhibition by BW755C was significantly greater than that for indomethacin, the identification of this product as a lipoxygenase product thus requires further clarification. Likewise, a further radiolabelled product with the chromatographic mobility of LTB_4 were detected (Fig. 6), but its formation was inhibited by indomethacin as well as by BW755C[13] and thus its characterization requires additional investigation.

Incubations with ^{14}C]-AA were also performed on homogenates of inflamed colonic mucosa from two patients who were free of drug treatment but had undergone colectomy for ulcerative colitis. A similar profile of radiolabelled products, separated by thin layer chromatography,

TABLE 1

% Control Formation

	PGE_2	TXB_2	$PGF_{2\alpha}$	$6\text{-k-F}_{1\alpha}$
[SASP]				
$5 \times 10^{-5}M$	+14 ± 18	-55 ± 9**	+37 ± 16	+1 ± 9
$10^{-3}M$	+38 ± 14	-83 ± 5***	+104 ± 36*	-8 ± 7
[BZI]				
$1.5 \times 10^{-5}M$	-15 ± 70	-76 ± 6**	+23 ± 22	+8 ± 8
$7.5 \times 10^{-5}M$	-42 ± 18	-84 ± 4**	+8 ± 12	-17 ± 21
$3.7 \times 10^{-4}M$	-53 ± 18	-87 ± 5**	+1 ± 42	-51 ± 11

The effect of sulphasalazine (SASP) and benzyl imidazole (BZI) on the synthesis of the major cyclo-oxygenase metabolites formed from [^{14}C]-arachidonic acid by homogenates of human colonic mucosa. The results are the mean ± s.e.m. of 3 and 6 experiments for BZI and SASP respectively, and are expressed as a % of the paired control metabolite formation. The level of statistical significance from control, using the paired data t-test is shown as *P < 0.05; ** P < 0.01; *** P < 0.001.

was synthesized by the inflamed colonic tissue compared to that from control tissue. However, there was an increase in conversion of [^{14}C]-AA by the inflamed mucosa to both cyclo-oxygenase and lipoxygenase products separated using solvent system "A" and to the cyclo-oxygenase products separated using solvent system "B" (Fig. 6).

Discussion

The current study confirms that arachidonate metabolites of both lipoxygenase and cyclo-oxygense enzyme pathways can be formed by homogenates of human colonic mucosa incubated in vitro. The formation by the colonic mucosa of the products separated on TLC using solvent system "B" was inhibited by the cyclo-oxygenase inhibitor indomethacin and by the dual cyclo-oxygenase-lipoxygenase inhibitor BW755C confirming the identity of these products as metabolites of the cyclo-oxygenase pathway of arachidonic acid.

In contrast to the effect of the potent inhibitors of cyclo-oxygenase, sulphasalazine whilst inhibiting the formation by the colonic mucosal homogenates of a radiolabelled product having the chromatographic mobility of TXB_2, either enhanced or had no effect on the other cyclo-oxygenase products. A similar inhibitory profile was also seen with the selective thromboxane synthetase inhibitor, benzyl imidazole. The inhibitory effects of sulphasalazine and benzyl imidazole on TXB_2 formation by human colonic mucosa was confirmed using two TLC systems, thereby supporting both the identity of the product with the chromatographic mobility of TXB_2 and the selectivity of inhibition by the two compounds. Sulphasalazine has also been reported to inhibit selectively the synthesis of TXB_2 by both platelets and peripheral blood mononuclear cells in culture[20,21]. Inhibition of colonic mucosal TXB_2 formation may be of importance since in a small study on the colonic formation of prostanoids in Crohn's disease[22], an imbalance in the synthesis of TXB_2 and prostacyclin (determined as 6-keto $PGF_{1\alpha}$) has been reported. In addition, TXA_2, which is a potent vasoconstrictor and aggregator of platelets[23], is cytolytic in myocardial and hepatic tissue[24,25] and its local generation can lead to gastric mucosal ulceration[15]. Conversely, certain prostaglandins could have a local protective effect on the colonic mucosa, as proposed for the gastric mucosa[1,26,27], perhaps by effects on colonic blood flow, mucus or fluid secretion or immune responsiveness. In a study to determine whether exogenous prostaglandins could alter the course of colonic disease in man, the (15R)-15-methyl PGE_2 analogue, was administered orally to patients with ulcerative colitis in remission[28]. A high relapse rate (42%) was noted within one month of therapy, whereas with patients receiving sulphasalazine, only a 16% relapse rate was seen over the 6 months trial period. However, the findings of this study are complicated by the high incidence of diarrhoea in patients receiving this prostaglandin analogue, which may have masked any potential beneficial action[28]. Whether other prostanoids which have fewer effects on gastrointestinal motility or fluid secretion would be useful to maintain remission requires further evaluation.

It has been postulated that the therapeutic action of sulphasalazine results from its ability to enhance colonic levels of prostaglandins which could exert a protective function in the colonic mucosa. This suggestion arises from the observations that sulphasalazine can prevent the

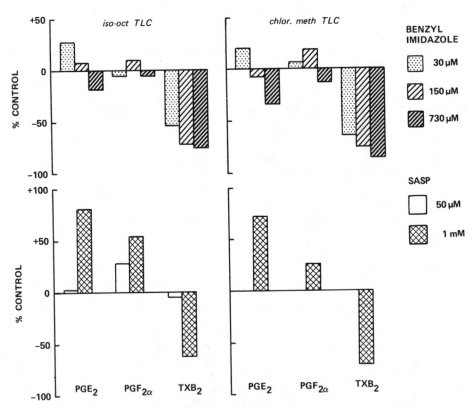

Fig. 5 The effect of benzyl imidazole (30,150 and 730 µM) and sulphasalazine (50 mM and 1 mM) on the formation by homogenates of human colonic mucosa of PGE_2, $PGF_{2\alpha}$ and TXB_2 from $[^{14}C]$-arachidonic acid. The radiolabelled metabolites were separated using either solvent system "B" (iso-oct TLC) or chloroform : methanol : acetic acid : H_2O (Chlor-meth TLC). The results are expressed as percentage conversion of $[^{14}C]$ AA.

degradation of prostaglandins by inhibiting the enzyme, prostaglandin dehydrogenase[29]. In addition, sulphasalazine and its main colonic metabolite 5-amino-salicylic acid (5-ASA) can increase the activity of the cyclo-oxygenase (or of the endoperoxide-metabolising enzymes), leading to an increased prostaglandin formation[24,30]. However, this "co-factor" effect of sulphasalazine, is apparently dependent on the substrate (arachidonate acid) concentration, at least in vitro[31]. From the present data, we suggest that rather than by enhancing overall levels of colonic prostaglandins, sulphasalazine modulates the biosynthesis of cyclo-oxygenase products in such a way as to establish a profile of products in which the balance of prostanoids of opposing actions renders the mucosa more resistant to damage.

The biosynthesis of lipoxygenase products has been characterised both by their chromatographic mobility and by the selective inhibition with the dual lipoxygenase-cyclo-oxygenase inhibitor BW755C while indomethacin, the selective cyclo-oxygenase inhibitor, failed to inhibit their formation. In our further studies, resolution of the 11-,12- and 15-HETE band by HPLC techniques has shown 12-HETE and 15-HETE (with little or no 11-HETE) to be the predominant identifiable monohydroxy lipoxygenase products formed in homogenates of both normal and inflamed human colonic mucosa[13]. More recent studies on the conversion of [^{14}C]-AA by mucosal scrapings of both normal colon and inflamed colonic tissue have confirmed that 12 and 15-HETE are the predominant products formed[32]. The synthesis of 12-HETE from endogenous substrate in homogenates of human colon has also been detected by GC-MS techniques[33].

Although in the present study using homogenates of human colonic mucosa, products with the chromatographic mobility of 5-HETE and leukotriene B_4 (LTB$_4$) were formed, their identity remains in question since their biosynthesis was inhibited by the cyclo-oxygenase inhibitor, indomethacin. The formation of metabolites via the 5-lipoxygenase pathway of arachidonic acid may require intact cells rather than the broken cell preparations used in the present study. Indeed, the biosynthesis of LTB$_4$-like material from scrapings of human colonic mucosa incubated with either [^{14}C]-AA or unlabelled arachidonic acid and stimulated with calcium ionohpore has recently been determined using both TLC[32] and HPLC chromatography and supported by GC-MS techniques[32]. Studies on the biosynthesis of this product using inhibitors of cyclo-oxygenase and lipoxygenase will provide further confirmation of the enzymatic route of synthesis of the colonic LTB$_4$.

Although less potent than 5-HETE or LTB$_4$, 12-HETE and 15-HETE have chemotactic and chemokinetic activity and can induce degranulation of polymorphonuclear leucocytes[7,11,12]. The biological properties of the trihydroxytetraenes or lipoxins derived from the transformation of 15-HPETE by human leucocytes remains to be explored[34]. However, both

305

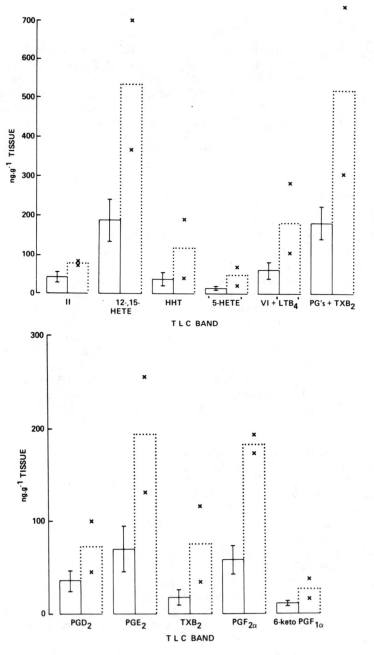

Fig. 6 Comparison of the profile of radiolabelled metabolites from [^{14}C]-arachidonic acid, separated on TLC using solvent system "A" and "B" formed by homogenates of human colonic mucosa from control tissue and from inflamed tissue from patients with ulcerative colitis. Results expressed as product formation, ng g^{-1} of colonic mucosal tissue, are mean ± s.e. mean (n=5) for control tissue and mean (of the two values shown) for inflamed tissue.

the 12- and 15-HETE, as well as the corresponding HPETE's may be involved in the modulation of leukotriene biosynthesis and lipoxygenase activity in inflammatory cells[35,36]. Such lipoxygenase metabolites of arachidonic acid thus have the potential to contribute to the inflammatory processes in the intestine. Indeed, as well as showing an increased capacity of inflamed colonic mucosa to form prostaglandins and TXB_2, which has been previously described[2-6], we have demonstrated an increase in the formation of radiolabelled lipoxygenase products by homogenates of inflamed colonic mucosa from patients with active ulcerative colitis[13]. In recent studies, Sharon and Stenson have also demonstrated a raised level of LTB_4 in scrapings of inflamed colonic mucosa from patients with inflammatory bowel diseases (including ulcerative colitis). The colonic synthesis of LTB_4 stimulated by calcium ionophore and exogenous arachidonic acid was also significantly increased in these patients[32].

The cellular source of the lipoxygenase enzymes is as yet unknown. The 12-HETE may be derived from entrapped platelets in the mucosal microcirculation, while 15-HETE and LTB_4 biosynthesis may reflect the presence of leucocytes which have infiltrated the mucosa. The contribution of other colonic tissue cells to lipoxygenase-product generation should not, however, be excluded.

The biosynthesis of lipoxygenase arachidonate metabolites by the human colon and their potential role as mediators of the inflammatory process has important implications for the therapy of inflammatory bowel disease. The synthesis of LTB_4 by human isolated neutrophils stimulated with calcium ionophore is inhibited by the clinically-useful drug sulphasalazine (IC_{50}, 900 µM) and at higher concentrations by the proposed active moeity 5-ASA (IC_{50}, 4000 µM)[37]. The isolated lipoxygenase enzyme from soybean is also inhibited by sulphasalazine (IC_{50}, 60 µM)[38] and at higher concentrations by 5-ASA (170 µM) and its major metabolite N-acetyl amino salicylic acid (250 µM) whereas sulphapyridine was inactive[39]. Furthermore, in our recent studies using homogenates of human colonic mucosa, sulphasalazine inhibited the formation from [^{14}C]-AA of radiolabelled 12-, 15-HETE lipoxygenase products (by 40% at 1 mM)[40] at a concentration found in the faeces of patients receiving sulphasalazine therapy. In addition, sulphasalazine at higher concentrations (2.5 mM) has been shown to inhibit LTB_4 formation (by 62%) as well as -12, -15-HETE formation (by 59%) in human colonic mucosa[32].

Potent, specific inhibitors of cyclo-oxygenase such as indomethacin or flurbiprofen have not been demonstrated to be of clinical benefit in the treatment of ulcerative colitis[41,42]. It is therefore unlikely that the therapeutic benefit of sulphasalazine or 5-amino-salicylic acid is the result of direct inhibition of cyclo-oxygenase in the colonic tissue or inflammatory cells. A more subtle change in the ratio of cyclo-oxygenase products, perhaps resulting in part from inhibition of thromboxane formation may be an underlying pharmacological mechanism. Studies with selective inhibitors of thromboxane synthase could therefore be of interest to explore such a possibility. Furthermore, sulphasalazine may bring about a change in the balance of cyclo-oxygnase and lipoxygenase products of arachidonate metabolism. Thus, the development of anti-inflammatory agents which can inhibit the biosynthesis of such lipoxygenase products may offer a novel approach to the clinical treatment of inflammatory disorders of the intestine.

References

1. Whittle BJR, Vane JR. Prostacyclin, thromboxanes and prostaglandins. Actions and roles in the gastro-intestinal tract. In: Progress in Gastroenterology, eds. G.B. Jerzy-Glass, P. Sherlock, Grune & Stratton, New York, pp. 3-30 (1983).
2. Gould SR. Assay of prostaglandin-like substances in faeces and their measurement in ulcerative colitis. Prostaglandins, 11: 489 (1976).
3. Harris AW, Smith PR, Swan CHI. Determination of prostaglandin synthetase activity in rectal biopsy material and its significance in colonic disease. Gut, 19:875 (1978).
4. Ligumsky M, Karmeli F, Sharon P, Zor U, Cohen F, Rachmilewitz D. Enhanced thromboxane A_2 and prostacyclin production by cultured rectal mucosa in ulcerative colitis and its inhibition by steroids and sulfasalazine. Gastroenterology, 81: 444 (1981).
5. Hawkey CJ, Truelove SC. Effect of prednisolone on prostaglandin synthesis by rectal mucosa in ulcerative colitis: investigation by laminar flow bioassay and radio-immunoassay. Gut, 22: 190 (1981).
6. Rampton DS, Sladen GE, Youlten LJF. Rectal mucosal prostaglandin E_2 release and its relation to disease activity, electrical potential difference, and treatment in ulcerative colitis. Gut, 21:591 (1980).
7. Turner, SR, Tainer, JA, Lynn WS. Biogenesis of chemotactic molecules by the arachidonate lipoxygenase system of platelets. Nature, 257:680 (1975).
8. Borgeat P, Hamberg M, Samuelsson B. Transformation of arachidonic acid and di-homo-γ-linoleic acid by rabbit polymorphonuclear leukocytes. J Biol Chem 251: 7816 (1976).
9. Borgeat P, Samuelsson B. Arachidonic acid metabolism in polymorphonuclear leukocytes: effect of ionohpore A23187. Proc Natl Acad Sci 76: 2148 (1979).
10. Ford-Hutchinson AW, Bray MA, Doig MV, Shipley ME, Smith MJH. Leukotriene B_4, a potent chemokinetic and aggregating substance released from polymorphonuclear leukocytes. Nature, 286: 264 (1980).
11. Palmer RMJ, Stepney R, Higgs GA, Eakins KE Chemokinetic activity of arachidonic acid lipoxygenase products on leukocytes from different species. Prostaglandins 20: 411 (1980).
12. Stenson WF, Parker CW Monohydroxy-eicosatetraenoic acids (HETEs) induce degranulation of human neutrophils. J Immunol 124: 2100 (1980).

13. Boughton-Smith NK, Hawkey CJ, Whittle BJR. Biosynthesis of lipoxygenase and cyclo-oxygenase products from [^{14}C]-arachidonic acid by human colonic mucosa. Gut 24: 1176 (1983).

14. Tai H, Yuan B. On the inhibitory potency of imidazole and its derivatives on thromboxane synthetase. Biochem Biophys Res Comm 80: 236 (1978).

15. Whittle BJR, Kauffman GL, Moncada S. Vasoconstriction and thromboxane A_2 induces ulceration of the gastric mucosa. Nature 292:472 (1980.

16. Peppercorn MA, Goldman P. Distribution studies of salicylazosulfapyridine and its metabolites. Gastroenterology, 64: 240 (1973).

17. Azad Khan AK, Truelove SC, Aronson JK. The disposition and metabolism of sulphasalazine (salicylazosulphapyridine) in man. Br J Clin Pharmac. 13:532 (1982).

18. Higgs GA, Flower RJ, Vane JR. A new approach to anti-inflammatory drugs. Biochem. Pharmacol. 28: 1959 (1979).

19. Salmon JA, Flower RJ. Prostaglandins and related compounds, in "Hormones in Blood", Gray, C.H. and James, V.H.T. ed., Academic Press, New York (1979).

20. Stenson WF, Lobos E. Inhibition of platelet thromboxane synthetase by sulfasalazine. Biochem. Pharmac. 32: 2205 (1983).

21. Rachmilewitz D, Ligumsky M, Haimaritz A, Treves A. Prostanoid synthesis by cultured peripheral blood mononuclear cells in inflammatory disease of the bowel. Gastroenterology, 82: 673 (1982).

22. Hawkey CJ, Karmeli F, Rachmilewitz D. Imbalance of prostacyclin and thromboxane synthesis in Crohn's disease. Gut 24: 881 (1983).

23. Whittle BJR, Moncada S. The pharmacological interactions between prostacyclin and thromboxanes. Brit Med Bull. 39: 232 (1983).

24. Lefer AM, Ogletree ML, Smith JB, Silver MJ, Nicolaou KC, Barnette WE, Gasic GP. Prostacyclin: A potentially valuable agent for preserving myocardial tissue in acute myocardial ischemia. Science 200: 52 (1978).

25. Stachura J, Tarnawski A, Ivey K, Mach T, Bogdal J, Szczudrawa J, Klimczyk B. Prostaglandin protection of carbon tetrachloride-induced liver cell necrosis in the rat. Gastroenterology 81: 211 (1981).

26. Robert A, Nezamis J, Lancaster C, Hanchar AJ. Cytoprotection by prostaglandins in rats - prevention of gastric necrosis produced by alcohol, HCL, NaOH, hypertonic NaCl and thermal injury. Gastroenterology, 77: 433 (1979).

27. Miller TA, Jacobson ED. Gastrointestinal cytoprotection by prostaglandins. Gut 20:75 (1979).

28. Hoult JRS, Moore PK. Sulphasalazine, a potent inhibitor of prostaglandin 15-hydroxy dehydrogenase: possible basis for therapeutic action in ulcerative colitis. Br J Pharmac. 64: 6 (1978).

29. Goldin E, Rachmilewitz D. Prostanoids cytoprotection for maintaining remission in ulcerative colitis. Failure of 15(R), 15-methyl-prostaglandin E_2. Dig. Dis. Sci., 28:807 (1983).

30. Hoult JRS, Page H. 5-amino salicylic acid, a co-factor for colonic prostacyclin synthesis? Lancet 2: 255 (1981).
31. Schlenker T, Peskar BM. Dual effect of sulphasalazine on colonic prostaglandin synthetase. Lancet ii: 815 (1981).
32. Sharon P, Stenson WF. Enhanced synthesis of leukotriene B_4 by colonic mucosa in inflammatory bowel disease. Gastroenterology 86: 453 (1984).
33. Bennett A, Hensby CN, Sanger GJ, Stamford IF. Metabolites of arachidonic acid formed by human gastrointestinal tissues and their actions on the muscle layers. Br J Pharmac. 74: 435 (1981).
34. Sherhan CN, Hamberg M, Samuelsson B. Trihydroxytetraenes: a novel series of compounds formed from arachidonic acid in human leukocytes. Bioch Biophys Res Comm 118: 943 (1984).
35. Vanderhoek JY, Bryant RW, Bailey JM. Regulation of leukocyte and platelet lipoxygenases by hydroxy eicosanoids. Biochem Pharmac 31:3463 (1982).
36. Borgeat P, de Lacos BF, Maclouf J. New concepts in the modulation of leukotriene synthesis. Biochem Pharmacol 32: 381 (1983).
37. Stenson WF, Lobos E. Sulfasalazine inhibits the synthesis of chemotactic lipids by neutrophils. J Clin Invest 69: 494 (1982).
38. Sircar JC, Schwender CF, Carethers ME. Inhibition of soybean lipoxygenase by sulfasalazine and 5-amino salicylic acid: a possible mode of action in ulcerative colitis. Biochem Pharmacol 32: 170 (1983).
39. Allgayer H, Eisenburg J, Paumgartner G. Soybean lipoxygenase inhibition: Studies with the sulphasalazine metabolites N-acetyl amino salicylic acid, 5-amino salicylic acid and sulphapyridine. Eur J Clin Pharmacol. 265: 449 (1984).
40. Boughton-Smith NK, Hawkey CJ, Whittle BJR. Sulphasalazine and the inhibition of thromboxane synthesis in human colonic mucosa. Br J Pharmac. 80: 604P (1983).
41. Gilat T, Ratan J, Rosen P, Peled Y. Prostaglandins and ulcerative colitis. Gastroenterology, 76: 1083 (1979).
42. Rampton DS, Sladen GE. Prostaglandin synthesis inhibitors in ulcerative colitis. Flurbiprofen compared with conventional treatment. Prostaglandins 21: 417 (1981).

INHIBITION OF 5'LIPOXYGENASE: RELEVANCE TO INFLAMMATION

R.M.J. Palmer and J.A. Salmon

Department of Pharmacology and Prostaglandin Research
The Wellcome Research Laboratories
Langley Court, Beckenham, Kent, BR3 3BS, U.K.

INTRODUCTION

The mechanism by which non-steroidal anti-inflammatory drugs (NSAID), such as aspirin and indomethacin, provide symptomatic relief for patients with inflammatory disease is generally recognised to be by inhibition of the formation of prostaglandins (PG's) from arachidonic acid (AA). The evidence for the involvement of PG's in inflammation is that elevated levels of PG's have been detected in inflamed tissues and that PG's, particularly PGE_2, have properties which suggest that they could mediate oedema, erythema and hyperalgesia. In addition, therapeutic doses of NSAID reduce the concentrations of PG's in inflamed tissues (for review see 1).

However, the value of NSAID therapy in chronic inflammatory diseases is limited since they do not reduce tissue damage. Leukocytes accumulate at sites of inflammation and are believed to contribute to tissue damage by releasing lysosomal enzymes and toxic oxygen radicals. Some NSAID potentiate leukocyte influx into inflammatory exudates in an animal model (2), suggesting that this class of compound could indirectly exacerbate deterioration of, for example, joint tissues in rheumatoid arthritis.

In contrast, anti-inflammatory steroids produce clinical improvement in patients by reducing cell infiltration as well as providing symptomatic relief (3). Whereas NSAID inhibit the fatty acid cyclooxygenase, anti-inflammatory steroids prevent the release of free AA from the phospholipid stores where most of this acid is located. Since only free AA can be metabolised by cyclooxygenase (4,5), it follows that anti-inflammatory steroids effectively block the formation of PG's. Recent work has indicated that the glucocorticoids affect phospholipase activity

311

indirectly; they induce the synthesis of a polypeptide which inhibits phospholipase (for review see 6). These compounds would be the drugs of choice for the treatment of chronic inflammation were it not for their severe side-effects.

In recent years another pathway of AA metabolism has been elucidated which may also be involved in the inflammatory response. AA can be converted by lipoxygenases to non-cyclised hydroperoxy derivatives (hydroperoxy-eicostetraenoic acids; HPETEs) which can be reduced to the corresponding hydroxy-acids (HETEs) either enzymically by glutathione peroxidase or non-enzymically. One lipoxygenase pathway, the 5' lipoxygenase pathway, is of particular interest since its initial product (5-HPETE) is the precursor of a novel group of compounds known as leukotrienes (7). These compounds are formed in leukocytes and have potent biological activities which suggest that they could also have pathophysiological roles.

BIOLOGICAL ACTIVITIES OF PRODUCTS OF 5' LIPOXYGENASE

The mono-substituted 5' lipoxygenase products are weak chemotactic, chemokinetic and aggregatory agents in vitro for human and rabbit neutrophils (PMN), but not for rat PMN (8,9,10). Furthermore they are very weak stimuli for other PMN functions such as degranulation (11). These compounds do not induce PMN accumulation in vivo following intradermal or intracameral administration (12,13) and have no direct effect on vascular permeability, although high doses of 5-HPETE potentiate bradykinin induced plasma exudation (12).

Leukotriene B_4 (LTB$_4$) has more powerful effects on PMN function; it is a potent chemotactic, chemokinetic and degranulating agent for PMN of several species in vitro and causes PMN accumulation in vivo (for review see 14). In the presence of a vasodilator PG, this compound also increases plasma exudation (12,15,16) which is probably mediated by its effects on PMN (15). Other chemoattractants such as the complement fragment C5a and the synthetic peptide F-Met-Leu-Phe (FMLP) exhibit similar indirect activity on plasma exudation (15). The actions of LTB$_4$ on PMN are stereospecific (16-19), are not shared by other leukotrienes (20) and receptors on PMN for LTB$_4$ have recently been demonstrated which are distinct from those for C5a and FMLP (21,22).

PRODUCTS OF 5' LIPOXYGENASE AS INFLAMMATORY MEDIATORS

Clearly LTB$_4$ fulfils the first of the classic criteria used to define a physiological mediator i.e. the suspected mediator must possess the appropriate biological activity at relevant concentrations. Additional criteria as modified from those of Sir Henry Dale are: (ii) the mediator must be recoverable from sites of inflammation (iii) the mediator should be identified by various pharmacological and physico-chemical tests (iv) antagonists of the action or inhibitors of the release of the suspected mediator must also reduce the inflammatory response thought to be due to that substance and (v) inhibition of the destruction (metabolism) of the suspected mediator should increase the magnitude and duration of the inflammatory response attributable to the substance.

The second and third criteria were satisfied in an animal model of inflammation. LTB_4 was detected by specific radioimmunoassay (RIA) in inflammatory exudates produced by the subcutaneous implantation in rats of 0.5% carrageenan-soaked polyester sponges (23). LTB_4 was not detected up to 2h post implantation but then the concentration increased and reached a maximum 6h after implantation; thereafter the level declined and was undetectable after 16-24h. The peak of LTB_4 concentration correlated with the maximum rate of PMN influx into the exudate, but the cell number continued to increase even after 6h (Fig 1). The identity of the immunoreactive material was established by extraction and high pressure liquid chromatography (HPLC) of the exudate; peaks of immunoreactivity and U.V. absorbance (at 270 nm) eluted at the same retention time as authentic LTB_4. Additionally the material caused aggregation of rat PMN in vitro indicating that the concentrations attained were biologically relevant. In experiments in which the animals were pre-dosed with colchicine (1 mg/kg) the concentration of LTB_4 in the exudate, as well as the PMN count, was decreased. These findings suggest that PMN were the source of LTB_4 and probably, therefore, that LTB_4 is not the initial signal for PMN infiltration, but may contribute to an amplification of the response.

Experiments using zymosan as well as carrageenan-soaked sponges have confirmed the above findings (20). Synovial fluids from patients with rheumatoid arthritis (24) and gout (25) and fluids from involved skin of psoriatics (26) contain elevated levels of LTB_4. These data have been generated using a variety of analytical techniques e.g. U.V. detection after HPLC and bioassay. Unfortunately the reported levels of LTB_4 vary considerably implying that careful attention to the procedures for collection and handling of samples, as well as the accuracy and precision of the final assay, are essential (29).

Thus, LTB_4 could be an important mediator of leukocyte influx at sites of inflammation and it follows that inhibition of LTB_4 synthesis represents an attractive therapeutic goal. Inhibitors of LTB_4 synthesis would also be invaluable experimental tools for establishing the pathophysiological roles of LTB_4.

The peptido-lipid leukotrienes, LTC_4, LTD_4 and LTE_4 are the major components of slow-reacting substance of anaphylaxis. These leukotrienes have pronounced inflammatory actions in the skin, causing wheal and flare responses and vasodilatation (28,29) and increased vascular permeability (30,31). There are as yet no reports of the detection of peptido-lipid leukotrienes in inflammatory exudates, although these compounds are synthesised by PMN in vitro (32,33). However the lack of activity of LTC_4, LTD_4 and LTE_4 in mediating cell accumulation (20) suggests that they are not mediators of the cellular phase of inflammation. The finding that

313

these leukotrienes are present in sputum of asthmatics (34), together with their potent spasmogenic activity on airway smooth muscle, suggests that these compounds should be considered as potential mediators of asthma and other hypersensitivity responses.

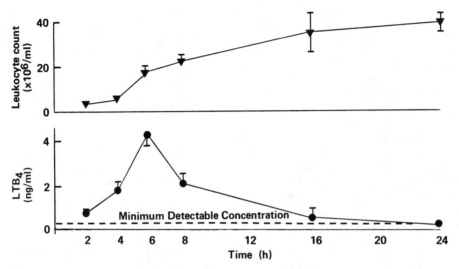

Fig 1.   Leukocyte count (▼) and concentration of LTB_4 (●) in inflammatory exudate obtained by implanting 0.5% carageenan soaked sponges subcutaneously in rats. Each point is the mean ± s.e. of at least five observations.

INHIBITION OF 5' LIPOXYGENASE

Leukotriene B_4 is synthesised from AA via three separate enzymic reactions (i) 5' lipoxygenase which converts AA to 5-HPETE (ii) a dehydrase which metabolises 5-HPETE to an unstable 5,6 epoxide (LTA_4) and (iii) a hydrolase which transforms LTA_4 into LTB_4. Thus, reduction of LTB_4 synthesis could be achieved by inhibiting any of the above reactions. However, inhibition of 5' lipoxygenase has received most attention (and will be the only approach discussed in this review) because it could reduce the synthesis of other 5' lipoxygenase pathway products (see above) which may be involved in pathological events.

A.   In vitro

Several in vitro procedures for assessing inhibition of 5' lipoxygenase have been reported: most involve monitoring the conversion of exogenous [^{14}C]-AA to 5-HETE and/or LTB$_4$ by cells stimulated with the calcium ionophore A23187 (Fig 2). PMN from different species and also various cell-lines (e.g. RBL-1 and HL-60) have been employed. Purification of the enzyme has been attempted; several putative inhibitors have been evaluated using a partially purified enzyme from human PMN (35). Detection of LTB$_4$ by U.V. absorption after HPLC separation has also been employed, but is limited by poor sensitivity and through-put of samples.

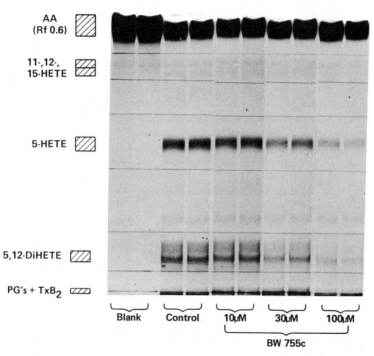

Fig 2. The effect of BW755C on the metabolism of [^{14}C]-AA by rabbit peritoneal leukocytes. Rabbit peritoneal cells were incubated with 0.1 μCi [^{14}C]-AA and 1μg/ml A23187 for 10 min and the products separated and detected by autoradiography as described (36). The 5, 12-DiHETE band comprises LTB$_4$ and isomers of 5, 12-DiHETE.

315

A specific RIA for LTB_4 (37) permits rapid assessment of low levels of the compound without prior extraction or chromatography, and consquently we consider it to be the method of choice for evaluating inhibitors of 5' lipoxygenase. The sensitivity of the RIA allows more physiologically relevant stimuli than A23187 (e.g. opsonised zymosan) to be used to induce the metabolism of endogenous AA by 5' lipoxygenase. This could be crucial as A23187 may produce some misleading inhibitory data (see below).

The standard protocol for assessing inhibitors of 5' lipoxygenase in our laboratories is as follows:

Human PMN are purified from heparinised (20 u/ml) venous blood from healthy volunteers on Ficoll-Paque gradients followed by ammonium chloride lysis of erythrocytes, giving a final purity of >95% (10). The final concentration of PMN is 5×10^6 cells/ml in indicator-free Hanks' balanced salts solution buffered to pH 7.4 with 30 mM HEPES.

The cell suspension is equilibrated at 37°C for at least 30 min prior to the addition of test compound (dissolved in DMSO) or medium control. After 10 min incubation at 37°C, A23187 (1.0 µg/ml in ethanol) is added and incubation continued for a further 5 min. The final concentration of DMSO and ethanol in incubations is not greater than 0.25 and 0.2% respectively. Incubations are terminated by centrifugation at 12000g for 30 sec, and the supernatants are decanted for determination of LTB_4 by specific RIA (37).

The formation of thromboxane B_2 (TXB_2) and/or PGE_2 can also be monitored by specific RIA in the above incubations thereby allowing the assessment of the inhibition of cyclooxygenase as well as lipoxygenase under identical conditions. This should provide more reliable comparative data than using several different enzyme systems (e.g. plant, platelet and PMN lipoxygenases; platelet, PMN and seminal vesicle cyclooxygenases). A summary of the IC_{50} values of a number of compounds against 5' lipoxygenase and cyclooxygenase obtained using the above protocol is shown in Table 1. It should be noted that reduced formation of LTB_4 in this system does not necessarily reflect an inhibition of 5' lipoxygenase; it could also result from inhibition of phospholipase, 5-HPETE dehydrase or LTA_4-hydrolase. Similarly, lower TXB_2 synthesis could reflect inhibition of phospholipase, cyclooxygenase or thromboxane synthetase. Consequently further experiments are required to establish the site(s) of action of the inhibitors.

The substrate analogue 5,8,11,14-eicosatetraynoic acid (ETYA) inhibits both cyclooxygenase and 12' lipoxygenase approximately equally (38) but is less effective against 5' lipoxygenase. However, ETYA does reduce enzymic formation of LTA_4 from 5-HPETE (39) so that the concentration of LTB_4 is reduced (see Table 1). 5,8,11-eicosatriynoic acid (40), 4,7,10,13-eicosatetraynoic acid (41), 5,8,11,14-henicosatetraynoic acid and 4,7,10,13, henicosatetraynoic acid (42) also have differential effects on cyclooxygenase, 5' lipoxygenase and other enzymes in the cascade.

The anti-oxidant nordihyroguaiaretic acid (NDGA; 43) has been used by several investigators as a selective inhibitor of 5' lipoxygenase although it inhibits other lipoxygenases and also thromboxane synthesis at higher concentrations (see Table 1).

Metabolites of AA can themselves inhibit 5' lipoxygenase; Vanderhoek et al (44,45) demonstrated that 15-HPETE and 15-HETE inhibit 12-HETE synthesis by platelets and 5-HETE and LTB_4 production by rabbit PMN. Prostaglandin E_2 and I_2 (or stable analogues of the latter) inhibit LTB_4 synthesis by A23187 and opsonised-zymosan stimulated PMN (46,47; Table 1). These interactions of AA metabolites suggest the possibility of complicated feedback mechanisms in the formation of other products. These data may explain the finding that low doses of indomethacin reduce the concentration of PGE_2 but potentiate PMN accumulation in the sponge implant model (2); cell influx could be mediated by increased synthesis of a lipoxygenase product (e.g. LTB_4).

Natural products, such as flavonoids, exhibit potent and relatively selective activity against 5' lipoxygenase; baicalein and cirsilol inhibit 5' and 12' lipoxygenase but not cyclooxygenase (48,49). Quercetin and some of its derivatives and esculetin also inhibit the 5' and 12' lipoxygenases without affecting cyclooxygenase (50,51; Table 1). Some of these compounds are present in plant extracts which have been used for centuries in oriental medicine for treatment of inflammatory ailments; it is tempting to speculate that the benefits of these remedies could, in part, be due to inhibition of 5' lipoxygenase. Some retinoids, in particular retinol (Vitamin A), are also effective inhibitors of LTB_4-synthesis (52; Table 1) and these have been used in the treatment of psoriasis. Caffeic acid also reduces AA metabolism via 5' lipoxygenase (53).

The potential therapeutic benefits of inhibitors of 5' lipoxygenase have prompted considerable research activity in the pharmaceutical industry. The limitations of present anti-inflammatory agents indicate that a selective inhibitor of 5' lipoxygenase or a dual-inhibitor of both 5' lipoxygenase and cyclooxygenase could produce significant improvements in therapy. BW755C (3-amino-1-[m-trifluoromethyl)-phenyl]-2-pyrazoline) has been extensively investigated; it blocks lipoxygenase of platelets (54) and PMN (36,55; Table 1) at similar concentrations to those required to inhibit cyclooxygenase. Interestingly, Radmark et al (55) demonstrated that the 5' lipoxygenase pathway was more vulnerable to inhibition by BW755C than was the synthesis of 15-HETE.

Benoxaprofen was claimed to be a selective inhibitor of 5' lipoxygenase when it was evaluated by monitoring the conversion of exogenous [^{14}C]-AA to 5-HETE and LTB_4 in PMN stimulated with A23187 (56). Inhibition of LTB_4 synthesis from endogenous substrate in A23187-stimulated human PMN has been confirmed, although this compound was a more effective inhibitor of TXB_2 synthesis (57; Table 1). However, benoxaprofen was a less effective inhibitor of opsonised zymosan-induced LTB_4 synthesis by PMN, leading these authors to speculate that this

317

compound may affect A23187-stimulation directly (58). Support for this hypothesis comes from reports that benoxaprofen does not inhibit LTC_4 synthesis by zymosan-stimulated macrophages at doses up to $10^{-4}M$ (59) and 5-HETE or LTB_4 synthesis in a cell-free system derived from human PMN (35).

Table I Inhibition of A23187-induced synthesis of LTB_4 and TXB_2 by human PMN

Compound	(n)	IC_{50} (μM)	
		$v\,LTB_4$	$v\,TXB_2$
Indomethacin	3	27.0	0.0016
Phenylbutazone	3	85.0	5.4
ETYA	3	1.9	0.63
NDGA	3	0.52	7.9
PGE_2	2	0.09	>100
Quercetin	4	1.5	10.0
Baicalein	4	2.4	28.0
Esculetin	3	24.0	95.0
Esculin	4	>100	>100
Retinol	2	18.0	>100
Retinyl acetate	2	93.0	>100
BW755C	7	5.4	4.7
Nafazatrom	3	1.6	>100
Benoxaprofen	4	36.0	4.7
Piroprost	3	3.7	24.0

The compounds were preincubated with cells for 10 min prior to addition of A23187 (1 $\mu g/ml$). Incubation was continued for a further 5 min and the concentrations of LTB_4 and TXB_2 determined by specific radioimmunoassay (37,73). The effects of the compounds are expressed as the mean IC_{50} from (n) experiments performed in duplicate.

Nafazatrom (BAY G 6576), originally developed as an anti-thrombotic agent, is a relatively selective inhibitor of 5' lipoxygenase (60; Table 1). Since nafazatrom is believed to be a co-factor for peroxidase, it could act by increasing 15-HETE synthesis (61) which in turn inhibits 5' lipoxygenase (45); however as 15-HPETE also limits the activity of the latter enzyme this seems an unlikely explanation.

Analogues of LTA_4, such as 5,6-methano-LTA_4 and carbanalogues of LTA_4 block 5' lipoxygenase and 12' lipoxygenase (62,63). Recently some N-hydroxyamide derivatives of AA have also been shown to inhibit 5' lipoxygenase (64). A derivative of benzoquinone, AA861, selectively inhibits 5' lipoxygenase (65).

Piroprost (6,9-deepoxy-6,9-phenylimino)-6,8-prostaglandin I$_1$ U60257) is reported to inhibit the generation of leukotrienes but not the formation of 12-HETE or cyclooxygenase products (66), although as indicated in Table 1, it may reduce cyclooxygenase product synthesis at higher concentrations in some systems. Piroprost is being evaluated primarily as an inhibitor of peptido-lipid leukotriene synthesis and therefore as a potential anti-asthmatic drug.

Eicosapentaenoic acid (EPA) is a poor substrate for cyclooxygenase (67,68) but is a competitive inhibitor of this enzyme, which may account for its anti-thrombotic activity through inhibition of pro-thrombotic TXA$_2$ synthesis. However EPA is a good substrate for lipoxygenase enzymes and can be converted to leukotrienes and other lipoxygenase products (69-72). The actions of lipoxygenase products of EPA and the influence of EPA on AA metabolism will be discussed later.

B.   In vivo

Although there are many compounds which inhibit 5' lipoxygenase in vitro, there are few reports of in vivo activity. Investigators have used some of the compounds cited in the previous section in animal models and have drawn conclusions as to the involvement of lipoxygenase products in these models. Many of the compounds which are active in vitro have very short half-lives in vivo; for example the potent inhibitory activities exhibited in vitro by ETYA, NDGA and nafazatrom have not been confirmed in vivo. In addition, the specificity of some of the compounds is questionable and therefore assignment of biological activities in vivo to inhibition of 5'-lipoxygenase should be considered cautiously.

Salmon et al (74) have studied the effects of several compounds on the synthesis of LTB$_4$ and cyclooxygenase products and PMN accumulation 6h after implantation of carrageenin-soaked sponges (23). BW755C reduced the concentration of LTB$_4$ and the cell count (Fig 3). Although inhibition of LTB$_4$ synthesis and cell accumulation were both dose related, the two dose-response curves were not parallel; cell influx still occurred at doses of BW775C that completely inhibited the synthesis of LTB$_4$. Administration of dexamethasone produced comparable data, presumably because it prevented the release of AA from phospholipids. Leukocyte accumulation was also inhibited by the NSAIDs indomethacin and flurbiprofen. In addition, the latter drugs reduced the concentration of both PGE$_2$ and TXB$_2$ in the exudate but did not affect LTB$_4$ levels. Similar data was also reported for benoxaprofen (58) suggesting that this drug has a mechanism of action identical to conventional NSAID. These data suggest that reduction of PMN accumulation by NSAID is mediated by a mechanism other than inhibition of LTB$_4$ synthesis. However, the mechanism by which both BW755C and dexamethazone reduce cell accumulation could be attributable in part to inhibition of the synthesis of chemotactic principles formed via 5' lipoxygenase (e.g. LTB$_4$). Although LTB$_4$ may have a chemotactic role, it does not appear to be the only mediator of cell accumulation in vivo in this model.

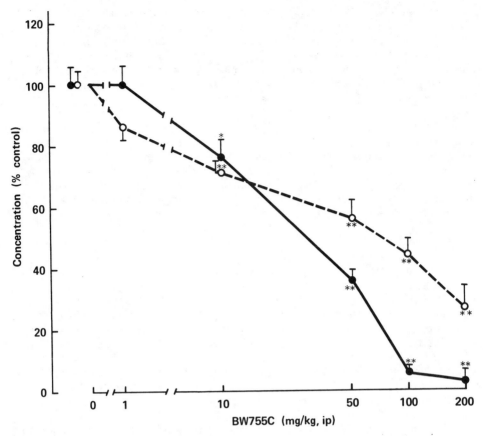

Fig 3.   Effect of BW755C on leukocyte count (○) and LTB$_4$
concentration (●) in inflammatory exudate obtained from s.c.
implantation in rats of sponges impregnated with 0.5%
carageenan. Each point is the mean ± s.e. (n=10). *p < 0.05; **
p < 0.01.

INHIBITORS OF THE METABOLISM OF LTB$_4$

      As yet no inhibitors of the ω-oxidation of LTB$_4$ have been
described.   The products of ω-oxidation, namely 20-OH-LTB$_4$ and 20-
COOH-LTB$_4$, are at least five times less active than LTB$_4$ in vitro (75,76).
We have recently examined the effect of a number of compounds including:
ETYA, NDGA, BW755C, indomethacin and nafazatrom on ω-oxidation of
LTB$_4$ using a specific RIA for LTB$_4$ to monitor the disappearance of added
LTB$_4$ from incubations of human PMN (77).   None of these compounds
affected the rate of disappearance of immunoreactive LTB$_4$ at
concentrations up to 100µM.   These data indicate that the action of
BW755C and the other compounds on LTB$_4$ synthesis is probably not as non-
specific anti-oxidants.   Since no inhibitors of LTB$_4$ destruction exist, it is

320

not possible to evaluate whether administration of such a compound potentiates the inflammatory response.

EFFECTS OF EPA ON AA METABOLISM

Although EPA is a good substrate for 5' lipoxygenase and subsequent enzymic transformations, the product LTB_5 was shown to be approximately 30 times less active than LTB_4 in affecting PMN function <u>in vitro</u> (aggregation, degranulation and chemokinesis; 71). Furthermore the potency of LTB_5 in potentiating bradykinin-induced plasma exudation was at least ten times lower than that of LTB_4. Oral administration of EPA also reduced the formation of LTB_4 by rat leukocytes stimulated with A23187 <u>in vitro</u> (78). These authors found that the ratio of LTB_4 to LTB_5 produced was directly correlated with the AA:EPA ratio in leukocyte phospholipids. The effect of an EPA-rich diet on leukocyte accumulation and LTB_4 and PGE_2 levels in inflammatory exudates induced by implanting carageenan-soaked sponges has also been evaluated (79). Supplementation of the diet for 4 weeks with 240 mg/kg/day EPA significantly decreased the concentration of PGE_2 and TXB_2 in the exudate, indicating the inhibition of cyclooxygenase by EPA. The concentration of LTB_4 and the total leukocyte count was also suppressed, but not significantly. In another model of acute inflammation, the rat-foot carageenan model, an EPA-rich diet caused significant reduction of oedema (79). Thus supplementation of the diet with EPA could, by reducing the synthesis of metabolites of AA and by antagonising the biological activity of LTB_4, be beneficial in the prevention and/or treatment of inflammatory diseases.

THE ROLE OF LIPOXYGENASE PRODUCTS IN STIMULUS-RESPONSE COUPLING IN PMN

Inhibition of leukocyte accumulation at sites of inflammation could be the result of inhibition of either (i) the generation of a chemoattractant or (ii) the response of PMN to a chemoattractant. A role for lipoxygenase products in stimulus-response coupling in PMN has been suggested by observations that dual-inhibitors of AA metabolism, but not selective cyclooxygenase inhibitors, abrogate responses of these cells to chemoattractants in vitro. For example NDGA inhibits rabbit PMN degranulation and chemotaxis (80), ETYA inhibits human PMN degranulation and superoxide generation (81,82) and rabbit PMN aggregation (83). However, Smith et al (84) concluded that 5-HETE was not the mediator since acetylenic analogues of AA enhanced 5-HETE synthesis at concentrations that inhibited A23187-induced degranulation. Furthermore, these authors showed that certain phenylhydrazone derivatives inhibited 5-HETE synthesis without affecting degranulation in this system and that these inhibitors abrogated FMLP-induced degranulation even though FMLP failed to elicit 5-HETE synthesis.

Similar studies in our laboratory have shown that LTB_4 synthesis is neither quantitatively nor qualitatively related to degranulation induced by A23187, opsonised zymosan or FMLP (85). We have recently extended these findings (77) by studying the effects of some compounds on A23187-induced degranulation and LTB_4 synthesis and on FMLP-induced degranulation (Table 2). These data indicate that LTB_4 does not mediate PMN degranulation, and probably not other PMN responses, since inhibition of degranulation and LTB_4 synthesis are not quantitatively related. This is illustrated by the effect of BW755C (Fig 4) which inhibits both LTB_4 and TXB_2 (data not shown) generation but not degranulation. Furthermore, FMLP does not stimulate LTB_4 synthesis in the absence of exogenous AA (85). These data indicate that products of the 5' lipoxygenase pathway do not mediate stimulus-response coupling in PMN.

Table II Inhibition of A23187-induced release of LTB_4 and β-glucuronidase and FMLP induced β-glucuronidase release from human PMN

Compound	IC_{50} (µM)		
	v A23187 induced release of		*v* FMLP induced release of
	LTB_4	β-glucuronidase	β-glucuronidase
Indomethacin	27.0	*	59.0
Phenylbutazone	85.0	78.0	9.4
ETYA	1.9	16.0	11.0
NDGA	0.52	1.5	6.5
BW755C	2.8	N.E.	89.0

N.E. = Inactive at 100µM. * 30% inhibition at 100µM.

The compounds, together with cytochalasin B (5 µg/ml) in experiments with FMLP, were pre-incubated with the cells for 10 min prior to stimulation with A23187 (1 µg/ml) or FMLP (0.1 µM). Incubation was continued for a further 5 min and the concentration of LTB_4 and β-glucuronidase released were determined by specific RIA and by colourimetric assay respectively. The effects of the compounds are expressed as the mean IC_{50} from three experiments performed in duplicate.

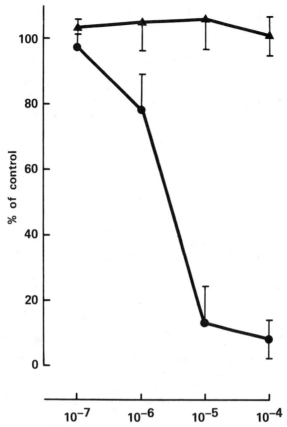

Fig 4.   Effect of BW755C on A23187-induced LTB_4 (●) and β-glucuronidase (▲) release. The effects of this compound were studied as described in the legend to Table I. Each point is the mean ± s.e. of three experiments performed in duplicate.

SUMMARY

In this paper, the 5' lipoxygenase pathway of AA metabolism and its inhibition has been briefly reviewed together with the biological activity of those products which may mediate inflammatory responses.   Present evidence indicates that LTB_4 is not the initial mediator of cell accumulation at sites of inflammation but may represent an important mechanism for amplifying this response.   The importance of LTB_4 in inflammatory diseases will not be clarified until selective inhibitors of the 5' lipoxygenase pathway, that have activity in vivo, become available and are studied clinically.   Such compounds will also be very useful tools for elucidating the importance of the peptido-lipid leukotrienes as mediators of asthma and other hypersensitivity diseaes.

Steroids are potent anti-inflammatory compounds, and their mode of action can be explained by their ability to interfere with both pathways of AA metabolism by limiting substrate availability. It is possible that dual-inhibitors of cyclooxygenase and lipoxygenase (e.g. BW755C) may exhibit a 'steroid-like' anti-inflammatory activity without the toxicity and thus lead to more effective therapy. The recent description of more selective lipoxygenase inhibitors suggests that there may be exciting new developments in the treatment of inflammatory disease in the next few years.

REFERENCES

1.   R.J. Flower, S. Moncada and J.R. Vane, Analgesic-antipyretics and anti-inflammatory agents: Drugs employed in the treatment of gout. In: Pharmacological Basis of Therapeutics Ed. A.G. Gilman, L.S. Goodman and A. Gilman, 682-728 (1980).

2.   G.A. Higgs, K.E. Muggeridge, S. Moncada and J.R. Vane, The effects of non-steroid anti-inflammatory drugs on leukocyte accumulation in carrageenin-induced inflammation. Eur. J. Pharmacol. 66: 81-86 (1980).

3.   R.C. Haynes and F. Murad, Adrenocorticotrophic hormone; adrenocortical steroids and their synthetic analogues; inhibitors of adrenocortical steroid biosynthesis. In: Pharmacological Basis of Therapeutics. Ed. A.G. Gilman, L.S. Goodman and A. Gilman, 1466-1496 (1980).

4.   H. Kunze and W. Vogt, Significance of phospholipase A for prostaglandin formation. Ann. N.Y. Acad. Sci. 180: 123-125 (1971).

5.   H. Vonkeman and D.A. Van Dorp, The action of prostaglandin synthetase on 2-arachidonyl lecithin. Biochim. Biophys. Acta. 164: 430-432 (1968).

6.   R.J. Flower, G.J. Blackwell, M. Di Rosa and L. Parente, Mechanism of steroid-induced inhibition of arachidonate oxygenation. In: Mechanisms of steroid action. Ed. Lewis G.P. and Ginsberg, M. MacMillan Press. 97-114 (1981).

7.   B. Samuelsson, S. Hammarstrom, R.C. Murphy and P. Borgeat, Leukotrienes and slow reacting substance of anaphylaxis (SRS-A). Allergy. 35: 375-381 (1980).

8.   E.J. Goetzl and F.F. Sun, Generation of unique mono-hydroxy-eicosatetraenoic acids from arachidonic acid by human neutrophils. J. Exp. Med. 150: 406-411 (1979).

9.   .J.T. O'Flaherty, M.J. Thomas, C.J. Lees and C.E. McCall, Neutrophil-aggregating activity of monohydroxy-eicosatetraenoic acids. Am. J. Pathol. 104: 55-62 (1981).

10. R.M.J. Palmer, R.J. Stepney, G.A. Higgs and K.E. Eakins, Chemokinetic activity of arachidonic acid lipoxygenase products on leukocytes from different species. Prostaglandins. 20: 411-418 (1980).

11. W.F. Stenson and C.W. Parker, Monohydroxy-eicosatetraenoic acids (HETEs) induce degranulation of human neutrophils. J. Immunol. 124: 2100-2104 (1980).

12. G.A. Higgs, J.A. Salmon and J.A. Spayne, The inflammatory effects of hydroperoxy and hydroxy- acid products of arachidonate lipoxygenase in rabbit skin. Br. J. Pharmacol. 74: 429-433 (1981).

13. P. Bhattacherjee, B. Hammond, J.A. Salmon, R.J. Stepney and K.E. Eakins, Chemotactic response to some arachidonic acid lipoxygenase products in the rabbit eye. Eur. J. Pharmacol. 73: 21-28 (1981).

14. M.A. Bray, Pharmacology and pathophysiological of leukotriene B_4. Brit. Med. Bull. 39: 249-254 (1983).

15. C.V. Wedmore and T.J. Williams, Control of vascular permeability by polymorphonuclear leukocytes in inflammation. Nature (Lond). 289: 646-650 (1981).

16. M.A. Bray, F.M. Cunningham, A.W. Ford-Hutchinson and M.J.H. Smith, Leukotriene B_4: a mediator of vascular permeability. Br. J. Pharmacol. 72: 483-486 (1981).

17. C.L. Malmsten, J. Palmblad, A.M. Uden, O. Radmark, L. Engstedt and B. Samuelsson, Leukotriene B_4: a highly potent and stereospecific factor stimulating migration of polymorphonuclear leukocytes. Acta. Physiol. Scand. 110: 449-451 (1980).

18. I. Hafstrom, J. Palmblad, C.L. Malmsten, O. Radmark and B. Samuelsson, Leukotriene B_4- a stereospecific stimulator for release of lysosomal enzymes from neutrophils. FEBS Lett. 130: 146-148 (1981).

19. A.W. Ford-Hutchinson, M.A. Bray, F.M. Cunningham, E.M. Davidson and M.J.H. Smith, Isomers of leukotriene B_4 possess different biological potencies. Prostaglandins. 21: 143-151 (1981).

20. A.W. Ford-Hutchinson, G. Brunet, P. Savard and S. Charleson, Leukotriene B_4, polymorphonuclear leukocytes and inflammatory exudates in the rat. Prostaglandins. 28: 13-37 (1984).

21. D.W. Goldman and E.J. Goetzl, Specific binding of leukotriene B_4 to receptors on human polymorphonuclear leukocytes. J. Immunol. 129: 1600-1604 (1982).

22. R.A. Kreisle and C.W. Parker, Specific binding of leukotriene B_4 to a receptor on human polymorphonuclear leukocytes. J. Exp. Med. 157: 628-641 (1983).

23. P.M. Simmons, J.A. Salmon and S. Moncada, The release of leukotriene B_4 during experimental inflammation. Biochem. Pharmacol. 32: 1353-1359 (1983).

24. L.B. Klickstein, J. Shapleigh and E.J. Goetzl, Unique products of the oxygenation of arachidonic acid in synovial fluid in rheumatoid arthritis and spondylarthritis. Arth. Rheum. 23: 704-708 (1980).

25. S.A. Rae, E.M. Davidson and M.J.H. Smith, Leukotriene B_4, an inflammatory mediator in gout. Lancet. 2: 1122-1123 (1982).

26.   S.D. Brain, R.D.R. Camp, P.M. Dowd, A.K. Black, P.M. Woollard, A.I. Mallet and M.W. Greaves, Psoriasis and Leukotriene B_4. Lancet. 2: 762 (1982).

27.   J.A. Salmon, Bioassay and radioimmunoassay of eicosanoids. Brit. Med. Bull. 39: 227-231 (1983).

28.   R.D.R. Camp, A.A. Coutts, M.W. Greaves, A.B. Kay and M.J. Walport, Responses of human skin to intradermal injections of leukotrienes C_4, D_4 and B_4. Br. J. Pharmacol. 75: 168P (1982).

29.   J. Bisgaard, J. Kristensen and J. Sondergaard, The effect of leukotriene C_4 and D_4 on cutaneous blood flow in humans. Prostaglandins. 23: 797-801 (1982).

30.   S-E., Dahlen, J. Bjork, P. Hedqvist, K-E, Arfors, S. Hammarstrom, J.A. Lindgren and B. Samuelsson, Leukotrienes promote plasma leakage and leukocyte adhesion in post capillary venules: In vivo effects with reference to the acute inflammatory response. Proc. Natl. Acad. Sci. U.S.A. 78: 3887-3891 (1981).

31.   A.W. Ford-Hutchinson and A. Rackman, Leukotrienes as mediators of skin inflammation. Brit. J. Dermatol. 109: 26-29 (1983).

32.   G. Hansson and O. Radmark, Leukotriene C_4: isolation from human polymorphonuclear leukocytes. FEBS Lett. 127: 87-90 (1980).

33.   U. Aehringhaus, R.H. Wobling, W. Konig, C. Patrono, B.M. Peskar and B.A. Peskar, Release of leukotriene C_4 from human polymorphonuclear leukocytes as determined by radioimmunoassay. FEBS Lett. 146: 111-114 (1982).

34.   J.T. Zakrewski, N.C. Barnes, P.J. Piper and J.F. Coslello, Quantitation of leukotrienes in asthmatic sputum. Brit. J. Pharmacol. Proceedings of Dec. 1984 Meeting.

35.   D.J. Masters and R.M. McMillan, 5-lipoxygenase from human leukocytes. Brit. J. Pharmacol. 81: 70P (1984).

36.   R.W. Randall, K.E. Eakins, G.A. Higgs, J.A. Salmon and J.E. Tateson, Inhibition of arachidonic acid cyclooxygenase and lipoxygenase activities of leukocytes by indomethacin and compound BW755C. Agents and Actions. 10: 553-555 (1980).

37.   J.A. Salmon, P.M. Simmons and R.M.J. Palmer, A radioimmunoassay for leukotriene B_4. Prostaglandins. 24: 255-265 (1982).

38.   M. Hamberg and B. Samuelsson, Prostaglandin endoperoxides. Novel transformations of arachidonic acid in human platelets. Proc. Natl. Acad. Sci. U.S.A. 71: 3400-3404 (1974).

39.   G.M. Bokoch and P.M. Reed, Evidence for inhibition of leukotriene A_4 synthesis by 5,8,11,14-eicosatetraynoic acid in guinea pig polymorphonuclear leukocytes. J. Biol. Chem. 256, 4156-4159 (1981).

40.   S. Hammarstrom, Selective inhibition of platelet n-8 lipoxygenase by 5,8,11-eicosatriynoic acid. Biochim. Biophys. Acta. 487: 517-519 (1977).

41. F.F. Sun, J.C. McGuire, D.R. Morton, J.E. Pike, H. Sprecher and W.H. Kuman, Inhibition of platelet arachidonic acid 12-lipoxygenase by acetylenic acid compounds. Prostaglandins. 21: 333-343 (1981).

42. J.E. Wilhelm, S.K. Sankarappa, M. Van Rollins and H. Sprecher, Selective inhibitors of platelet lipoxygenase: 4,7,10,13-icosatetraynoic acid and 5,8,11,14-henicosatetraynoic acid. Prostaglandins. 21: 323-332 (1981).

43. M. Hamberg, On the formation of thromboxane B_2 and 12L-hydroxy 5,8,10,14-eicosatetraenoic acid (12-ho-20:4) in tissues from the guinea pig. Biochim. Biophys Acta. 431: 651-654 (1976).

44. J.Y. Vanderhoek, R.W. Bryant and J.M. Bailey, 15-hydroxy-5,8,11,13-eicosatetraenoic acid. A potent and selective inhibitor of platelet lipoxygenase. J. Biol. Chem. 255: 5996-5998 (1980).

45. J.Y. Vanderhoek, R.W. Bryant and J.M. Bailey, Inhibition of leukotriene biosynthesis by the leukocyte product 15-hydroxy-5,8,11,13-eicosatetraenoic acid. J. Biol. Chem. 10064-10066 (1980).

46. E.A. Ham, D.D. Soderman, M.E. Zanetti, M.W., H.W. Dougherty, E. McCauley and F.A. Kuehl, Inhibition by prostaglandins of leukotriene B_4 release from activated neutrophils. Proc. Natl. Acad. Sci. U.S.A. 80: 4349-4353 (1983).

47. H-E, Claesson, U. Lundberg and C. Malmsten, Serum-coated zymosan stimulates the synthesis of leukotriene B_4 in human polymorphonuclear leukocytes. Inhibition by cyclic AMP. Biochem. Biophys. Res. Commun. 99: 1230-1237. (1981).

48. K. Sekiya and H. Okuda, Selective inhibition of platelet lipoxygenase by baicalein. Biochem. Biophys. Res Commun. 105: 1090-1095 (1982).

49. J. Baumann, F.V. Bruchhausen and G. Wurm, Flavonoids and related compounds as inhibitors of arachidonic acid peroxidation. Prostaglandins. 20: 627-639 (1980).

50. W.C. Hope, A.F. Welton, C. Fiedler-Nagy, C. Batula-Bernardo and J.W. Coffey, In vitro inhibition of the biosynthesis of slow reacting substance of anaphylaxis (SRS-A) and lipoxygenase activity by quercetin. Biochem. Pharmacol. 32: 367-371 (1983).

51. T. Neichi, Y. Koshihara and S. Murota, Inhibitory effect of esculetin on 5-lipoxygenase and leukotriene biosynthesis. Biochim. Biophys. Acta. 753: 130-132 (1983).

52. M.A. Bray, Retinoids are potent inhibitors of the generation of rat leukocyte leukotriene B_4-like activity in vitro. Eur. J. Pharmacol. 98: 61-67 (1984).

53. Y. Koshihara, T. Neichi, S. Murota, A. Lao, Y. Fujimoto and T. Tatsuno, Caffeic acid as a selective inhibitor for leukotriene biosynthesis. Biochim. Biophys. Acta. 792: 92-97 (1984).

54. G.A. Higgs, R.J. Flower and J.R. Vane, A new approach to anti-inflammatory drugs. Biochem. Pharmacol. 28: 1959-1961 (1979).

55. O. Radmark, C. Malmsten and B. Samuelsson, The inhibitory effects of BW755C on arachidonic acid metabolism in human polymorphonuclear leukocytes. FEBS Lett. 110: 213-215 (1980).

56. J.R. Walker and W. Dawson, Inhibition of rabbit PMN lipoxygenase activity by benoxaprofen. J. Pharm. Pharmacol. 31: 778-780 (1979).

57. J.A. Salmon, L.C. Tilling and S. Moncada, Benoxaprofen does not inhibit formation of leukotriene B_4 in a model of acute inflammation. Biochem. Pharmacol. 23: 2928-2930 (1984).

58. J.A. Salmon, L.C. Tilling and S. Moncada, Evaluation of inhibitors of eicosanoid synthesis in leukocytes: possible pitfall of using calcium ionophore A23187 to stimulate 5'-lipoxygenase. Sumbitted.

59. J.L. Humes, S. Sadowski, M. Galavage, M. Goldenberg, E. Subers, F.A. Kuehl and R. Bonney, Pharmacological effects of non-steroidal anti-inflammatory agents on prostaglandin and leukotriene synthesis in mouse peritoneal macrophages. Biochem. Pharmacol. 32: 2319-2322 (1983).

60. S. Fischer, M. Struppler and P.C. Weber, In vivo and in vitro effects of nafazatrom (BAY G 6576), an anti-thrombotic compound, on arachidonic acid metabolism in platelets and vascular tissue. Biochem. Pharmacol. 32: 2231-2236 (1983).

61. W.D. Busse, M. Mardin, R. Grutzmann, L.J. Marnett and T.E. Eling, Effect of nafazatrom and other lipoxygenase inhibitors on guaiacol peroxidation and arachidonic acid metabolism in microsomes and blood cells. V. Int. Conf. Prostaglandins Florence. p147 (1982).

62. Y. Koshihara, S. Murota, N. Petasis and K.C. Nicolaou, Selective inhibition of 5-lipoxygenase by 5,6-methano leukotriene A_4, a stable analogue of leukotriene A_4. FEBS Lett. 143: 13-16 (1982).

63. Y. Arai, M. Toda and M. Hayashi, Synthesis of ($\pm$)-carbanalogues of 5-HPETE and leukotrene A_4. Adv. Prostaglandin, Thromboxane and Leukotriene Res. 11: 169-172 (1983).

64. E.J. Corey, J.R. Cashman, S.S. Kantner and S.W. Wright, Rationally designed potent competitive inhibitors of leukotriene biosynthesis. J. Am. Chem. Soc. 106: 1503-1504 (1984).

65. T. Yoshimoto, C. Yokoyama, K. Ochi, S. Yamamoto, Y. Maki, Y. Ashida, S. Terao and M. Shiraishi, 2,3,5-trimethyl-6-(12-hydroxy-5, 10-dodecadinyl)-1,4-benzoquinone (AA 861), a selective inhibitor of the 5-lipoxygenase reaction and the biosynthesis of slow reacting substance of anaphylaxis. Biochim. Biophys. Acta. 713: 470-473 (1982).

66. M.K. Bach, J.R. Brashler, H.W Smith, F.A. Fitzpatrick, F.F. Sun and J.C. McGuire, 6,9-deepoxy-6,9-(phenylimimo)-Δ6,8-prostaglandin I_1 (U60257), a new inhibitor of leukotriene C and D synthesis: in vitro studies. Prostaglandins. 23: 759-771 (1982).

67. P. Needleman, A. Raz, M. Minkes, J.A. Ferrendelli and H. Sprecher, Triene prostanglandins:prostacyclin and thromboxane biosynthesis and unique biological properties. Proc. Natl. Acad. Sci. 76: 944-948 (1979).

68. D.A. Van Dorp, Aspects of the biosynthesis of prostaglandins. Progr. Biochem. Pharmacol. 3: 71-75 (1967).

69. B.A. Jakschik, A.R. Sams, H. Sprecher and P. Needleman, Fatty acid structural requirement for leukotriene biosynthesis. Prostaglandins. 23: 401-410 (1980).

70. R.C. Murphy, W.C. Pickett, B.R. Culp and W.E.M. Lands, Tetraene and pentaene leukotrienes: selective production from murine mastocytoma cells after dietary manipulation. Prostaglandins. 22: 613-622 (1981).

71. T. Terano, J.A. Salmon and S. Moncada, Biosynthesis and biological activity of leukotriene B_5. Prostaglandins. 27: 217-232 (1984).

72. C. Yokoyama, K. Mizuno, H. Mitachi, T. Yoshimoto, S. Yamamoto and C.R. Pace-Asciak, Partial purification and characterisation of arachidonate 12-lipoxygenase from rat lung. Biochim. Biophys. Acta. 750: 237-241 (1983).

73. J.A. Salmon, A radioimmunoassay for 6-keto-PGF$_{1\alpha}$. Prostaglandins. 15: 383-397 (1978).

74. J.A. Salmon, P.M. Simmons and S. Moncada, The effects of BW755C and other anti-inflammatory drugs on eicosanoid concentrations and leukocyte accumulation in experimentally-induced acute inflammation. J. Pharm. Pharmacol. 35: 808-813 (1983).

75. J. Palmblad, A.M. Uden, J-A, Lindgren, O. Radmark, G. Hansson and C. Malmsten, Effects of novel leukotrienes on neutrophil migration. FEBS Lett. 144: 81-84 (1982).

76. R.D.R. Camp, P.M. Woollard, A.I. Mallet, N.J. Fincham, A.W. Ford-Hutchinson and M.A. Bray, Neutrophil aggregating and chemokinetic properties of a 5,12,20-trihydroxy-6,8,10,14-eicostetraenoic acid isolated from human leukocytes. Prostaglandins. 23: 631-641 (1982).

77. R.M.J. Palmer and J.A. Salmon, Comparison of the effects of some compounds on human neutrophil degranulation and leukotriene B_4 and thromboxane B_2 synthesis. Biochem. Pharmacol. In Press (1985).

78. T. Terano, J.A. Salmon and S. Moncada, Effect of orally administered eicosapentaenoic acid (EPA) on the formation of leukotriene B_4 and leukotriene B_5 by rat leukocytes. Biochem. Pharmacol. 33: 3071-3076 (1984).

79. T. Terano, J.A. Salmon, G.A. Higgs and S. Moncada, Anti-inflammatory activity of eicosapentaenoic acid. Submitted.

80. H.J. Showell, P.H. Naccache, R.I. Sha'afi and E.L. Becker, Inhibition of rabbit neutrophil lysosomal enzyme secretion, non-stimulated and chemotactic factor stimulated locomotion by nordihydroguaiaretic acid. Life Sci. 27: 421-426 (1980).

81. G.M. Bokoch and P.W. Reed, Inhibition of the neutrophil oxidative response to a chemotactic peptide by inhibitors of arachidonic acid oxygenation. Biochem. Biophys. Res. Commun. 90: 481-487 (1979).

82. J.E. Smolen and G. Weissmann, Effects of indomethacin, 5,8,11,14-eicosatetraynoic acid and p-bromophenacyl bromide on lysosomal enzyme release and superoxide anion generation by human polymorphonuclear leukocytes. Biochem. Pharmacol. 29: 533-538 (1980).

83. J.T. O'Flaherty, H.J. Showell, P.A. Ward and E.L. Becker, A possible role of arachidonic acid in human neutrophil aggregation and degranulation. Am. J. Pathol. 96: 799-809 (1979).

84. R.J. Smith, F.F. Sun, S.S. Iden, B.J. Bowman, H. Specher and J.C. McGuire, An evaluation of the relationship between arachidonic acid lipoxygenation and human neutrophil degranulation. Clin. Immunol. Immunophathol. 20: 157-169 (1981).

85. R.M.J. Palmer and J.A. Salmon, Stimulation of leukotriene B_4 (LTB$_4$) release from human neutrophils by N-formyl-L-methionyl L-leucyl-L-phenylalanine (FMLP), serum-treated zymosan (STZ) and A23187 and its relationship to degranulation. Immunology. 50: 65-74 (1983).

THE ROLE OF GLUCOCORTICOID-INDUCED PHOSPHOLIPASE

INHIBITORY PROTEINS

Massimo Di Rosa

Department of Experimental Pharmacology

University of Naples, Italy

INTRODUCTION

Glucocorticoids are powerful anti-inflammatory agents. Although their chief clinical utility in the treatment of acute and chronic inflammatory processes the knowledge of the mode of action of gluco – corticoids is still fragmentary. However at least some anti-inflam – matory effects of glucocorticoids depend on their ability to prevent the formation of arachidonic acid oxidation products, i.e. the prostaglandins and leukotrienes which are important mediators of the inflammatory response. Glucocorticoids although do not inhibit cyclo-oxygenase or lipoxygenase are able to prevent phospholipid deacylation from occurring in intact cells by inhibiting phospholi-pase A_2 thereby causing a shortage of precursor arachidonic acid.

This inhibition is not due to a direct effect of glucocorticoids on the enzyme but depends on their ability to induce the formation of phospholipase inhibitory proteins.

The discovery of phospholipase inhibitory proteins which act as 'second messengers' of steroid action has represented a key step for disclosing the mechanism of action of glucocorticoids since this finding seems to drive the 'pharmacology' of these hormones toward their 'physiology'.

The current view is that corticosteroids, like other steroid hormones, act by controlling the rate of synthesis of regulatory proteins. Such a control is mediated by specific glucocorticoid receptors and represents the final step of an intricate chain of events[1,2,3]. The hormone freely diffuses through the membrane of the target cell and then binds non-covalently to a cytoplasmic soluble protein (steroid receptor) to from the hormone-receptor complex. The receptors have high specificity and affinity for

steroids with glucocorticoid activity while they exhibit little or
no affinity for androgens or oestrogens. Receptor affinities for
glucocorticoids are correlated to their biological activities.
Once formed the cytoplasmic hormone-receptor complex enters the
nucleus where it binds to chromatin and directs the genetic apparatus to transcribe specificl messenger ribonucleic acid (mRNA)which
translocates to the ribosomes and codes for newly synthetized proteins which are responsible for the biological effect of the
hormone.

DISCOVERY AND BIOCHEMISTRY

The first indication that the inhibitory effect of corticosteroids on prostaglandin formation depends on gene expression was
given by Danon and Assouline[4] in a study on the effect of cortisol
on prostaglandin synthesis by rat renal papillae in vitro. It was
observed that cortisol was able to reduce prostaglandin formation
only after a latency period and the steroid effect on prostaglandin
formation was prevented by RNA/protein synthesis inhibitors.
One year later it was proved[5] that a similar mechanism involving RNA and protein synthesis underlay the inhibitory effect of
hydrocortisone on prostaglandin synthesis by phagocytosing rat
leukocytes, the first observation in cells directly involved in the
inflammatory process.
Moreover the presence of a soluble factor capable of reducing
phospholipase activity was demonstrated[6] in the effluent from lungs
treated with dexamethasone.
It was also reported[7] that unstimulated rat peritoneal leukocytes incubated with hydrocortisone released a nondialyzable factor
which inhibited prostaglandin formation by phagocytosing leukocytes.
Cyclohexamide blocked the synthesis of the factor but was unable to
modify the effect exhibited by the preformed inhibitor.
The first evidence that corticosteroids inhibit prostaglandin
formation by inducing the synthesis of proteinaceous 'second messengers' came in 1980 with the preliminary identification of glucocorticoid-induced proteins which inhibit phospholipase A_2 activity.
The synthesis and the secretion of such proteins under anti-inflammatory steroid treatment has been demonstrated in rat macrophages
(macrocortin)[8] and in rabbit neutrophils[9] (lipomodulin).
Recently it has been also shown[10] that rat renomedullary interstitial cells in culture when treated with dexamethasone synthesize
and release anti-phospholipase proteins (renocortins). The mol wt.
of these proteins have been estimated as follows: macrocortin, 15k;
lipomodulin, 40k; renocortins, 15 and 30k. Further studies have
demonstrate[11,12]that the peritoneal lavage fluids from rats treated
with dexamethasone contain three species of phospholipase inhibitory
proteins with mol wt. of 15k, 30k and 40k.

Since preparation of phospholipase inhibitory proteins are carried out in the presence of various proteases secreted by macrophage or neutrophils it is conceivable that the 40k species is cleaved to the smaller species by these proteases. Thus omission of protease inibitors from buffers used for purification resulted in poor recovery of the 40k species.

The three species hitherto described might all derive from a high mol wt. (200k) precursor which has been recently partially purified from rat peritoneal macrophages[13]. Further evidence that macrocortin, lipomodulin and renocortins are mutually related proteins is supported by the immunological cross reactivity which occurs between macrocortin and monoclonal anti-lipomodulin antibody[12] as well as between renocortins and monoclonal anti-macrocortin antibody[14].

It has been shown[15] that macrocortin secretion by rat peritoneal macrophages is specific for glucocorticoids and is inhibited by agents which interfere with microtubule assembly (colchicine, vinbastine) as well as prostacyclin and dibutyryl adenosine 3':5'-cyclic monophosphate.

It has been also shown[16] that phosphorylation of lipomodulin by a cyclic AMP-dependent protein kinase causes a decrease of its ability to inhibit phospholipase A_2. Therefore it is conceivable that elevation of intracellular cyclic AMP may cause phosphorylation of macrocortin with concomitant loss of its anti-phospholipase activity. Phosphorylation - dephosphorylation of phospholipase inhibitory proteins may represent a mechanism which modulates arachidonic acid release from membrane phospholipids.

ANTI-INFLAMMATORY EFFECT

The anti-inflammatory effect of glucocorticoids seems to be associated with the induction of phospholipase inhibitory proteins since these are able to suppress rat carrageenin edema[17,18].

Arachidonate metabolites play a major role in carrageenin edema[19] which explains the sensitivity of this model to both glucocorticoids and nonsteroidal anti-inflammatory drugs.

In contrast, dextran edema, which mainly depends on the release of histamine and 5-hydroxytryptamine[19], is suppressed by glucocorticoids but is insensitive to aspirin-like drugs.

We have investigated[18] the anti-inflammatory effect of both dexamethasone and phospholipase inhibitory proteins in dextran edema. This edema is inhibited by dexamethasone but is not affected by indomethacin (a cyclo-oxygenase inhibitor) or BW 755C (a lipoxygenase and cyclo-oxygenase inhibitor).

The inhibiton by the steroid is prevented by actinomycin D and occurs after a 2- to 3-hour time lag which is likely required for the synthesis of regulatory proteins. Both these findings demonstrate that dextran edema is suppressed by glucocorticoids according to the suggested mode of action of steroid hormones which involves induction of the synthesis of 'regulatory' proteins.

Dextran edema is also controlled by endogenous steroids since in adrenalectomized rats low concentrations of dextran induce a much greater paw swelling (2-3 times) compared to edema formation occurring in normal animals.

Partially purified preparations of phospholipase inhibitory proteins,which greatly suppress carrageenin edema, are ineffective in dextran edema.

Therefore, dexamethasone inhibition of dextran edema depends on the induction of regulatory proteins other than the antiphospholipase ones.

PHYSIOPATHOLOGICAL RELEVANCE

In addition to their anti-inflammatory effects, glucocorticoids have many other biological actions such as promotion of cellular differentiation.

Morphological and functional differentiation of U937 cells, a human histiocytic lymphoma cell line, was observed when cells were cultured with lipomodulin[20]. Similar differentiation was promoted by dexamethasone and this differentiation was blocked by monoclonal anti-lipomodulin antibody.

Glucocorticoid treatment of rat T lymphocytes results in the formation of IgE-suppressive factors which inhibit IgE response. A glycosylation-inhibiting factor participates in the selective formation of IgE-suppressive factors. It has been shown[21] that the glycosylation-inhibiting factor is a protein with a molecular weight of approximately 16k which specifically binds to monoclonal antibody against lipomodulin. The factor exhibits phospholipase inhibitory activity after treatment with alkaline phosphatase. Therefore the glycosylation inhibiting factor can conceivably be identified as phosphorylated macrocortin.

Glucocorticoids produce beneficial effects in experimental myocardial infarction by inhibiting the early thromboxane release due to ischaemia. Macrocortin[22] appears responsible for this effect because when given intravenously to rats before coronary occlusion it is able to protect animals against sudden death due to early post-infarction arrhythmias.

The importance of phospholipase inhibitory proteins in the pathophysiology of rheumatic diseases received strong support by the reported presence[23] of autoantibodies against lipomodulin in the sera of many patients with severe rheumatic diseases such as systemic lupus erythematosus, rheumatoid arthritis and dermatomyositis.

334

Thus, in such patients, the anti-lipomodulin antibodies may increase the formation of arachidonic acid and, subsequently,the formation of inflammatory prostaglandins and leukotrienes.

Interestingly it has been reported[24] that systemic lupus erythematosus patients present disorders of arachidonic acid metabolism in the kidney, namely an increased production of renal thromboxane and PGE_2.

CONCLUSION

Glucocorticoid-induced phospholipase inhibitory proteins (macrocortin, lipomodulin, renocortins) seem to be a family of mutually related proteins which prevent the release of arachidonic acid from membrane phospholids. These proteins act as 'second messengers' of a variety of glucocorticoid effects, e.g., control of inflammation, myocardial infarction, immune response and cell differentiation. They appear also associated with the pathophysiology of severe inflammatory diseases such as rheumatoid arthritis and systemic lupus erythematosus.

However, the anti-inflammatory effect of glucocorticoids does not entirely depend on phospholipase inhibitory proteins since other regulatory proteins seem to be involved in the steroid action. Therefore it seems conceivable that the anti-inflammatory effects of steroids and probably their diverse and widespread actions throughout the organism are mediated by a pattern of proteinaceous second messengers synthesized by the target cells which translate the general biochemical message of the steroid into specific and appropriate regulatory proteins.

REFERENCES

1. J.D. Baxter and G.M. Tomkins, Specific cytoplasmic glucocorticoid hormone receptors in hepatoma tissue culture cells, Proc. natn. Acad. Sci. USA 68: 932 (1971).

2. R.E. Buller and B.W. O'Malley, The biology and mechanism of steroid hormone receptor interaction with the eukaryotic nucleus, Biochem. Pharmac. 25: 1 (1976).

3. L. Chan and B.W. O'Malley, Mechanism of action of the sex steroid hormones, New Engl. J. Med. 294: 1372 (1976).

4. A. Danon and G. Assouline, Inhibition of prostaglandins by corticosteroids requires RNA and protein synthesis. Nature, Lond. 273: 552 (1978).

5. M. Di Rosa and P. Persico, Mechanism of inhibition of prostaglandin biosynthesis by hydrocortisone in rat leucocytes,
   Br. J. Pharmacol. 66: 161 (1979).

6. R.J. Flower and G.J. Blackwell, Anti-inflammatory steroids
   induce biosynthesis of a phospholipase A_2 inhibitor which
   prevents prostaglandin generation. Nature Lond. 275: 456
   (1979).

7. R. Carnuccio, M. Di Rosa and P. Persico, Hydrocortisone induced inhibitor of prostaglandin biosynthesis in rat leucocytes. Br. J. Pharmacol. 68: 14 (1980).

8. G.J. Blackwell, R. Carnuccio, M. Di Rosa, R.J. Flower,
   L. Parente and P. Persico, Macrocortin: a polypeptide
   causing the anti-phospholipase effect of glucocorticoids,
   Nature Lond. 287: 147 (1980).

9. F. Hirata, E. Schiffman, K. Venkatasubramanian, D. Salomon
   and J.A. Axelrod, Phospholipase A_2 inhibitory protein in
   rabbit neutrophils induced by glucocorticoids Proc. natn.
   Acad. Sci. USA 77: 2535 (1980).

10. J.F. Cloix, O. Colard, B. Rothhut and F. Russo-Marie, Characte-
    rization and partial purification of 'renocortins' two
    polypeptides formed in renal cells causing the anti-
    phospholipase-like action of glucocorticoids, Br. J.
    Pharmacol. 79: 313 (1983).

11. G.J. Blackwell, R. Carnuccio, M. Di Rosa, R.J. Flower, C.S.J.
    Langham, L. Parente, P. Persico, N.C. Russel-Smith and
    D. Stone, Glucocorticoids induce the formation and re-
    lease of anti-inflammatory and anti-phospholipase proteins
    into the peritoneal cavity of the rat, Br. J. Pharmacol.
    76: 185 (1982).

12. F. Hirata, M. Notsu, M. Iwata, L. Parente, M. Di Rosa and
    J.R. Flower, Identification of several species of phospho-
    lipase inhibitory proteins by radioimmunoassay for lipo-
    modulin, Biochem. biophys. Res. Commun. 109: 223 (1982).

13. P. Coote, M. Di Rosa, J.R. Flower, L. Parente, M. Merrett and
    J. Wood, Detection and isolation of a steroid-induced
    anti-phospholipase protein of high molecular weight, Br.
    J. Pharmacol. 80: 597 (1983).

14. B. Rothhut, F. Russo-Marie, J. Wood, M. Di Rosa and R.J.
    Flower, Further characterization of the glucocorticoid-
    induced anti-phospholipase protein 'renocortin', Biochem.
    biophys. Res. Commun. 117: 878 (1984).

15. G.J. Blackwell, Specificity and inhibition of glucocorticoid-
    induced macrocortin secretion from rat peritoneal macro-
    phage, Br. J. Pharmac., 79: 587 (1983).

16. F. Hirata, The regulation of lipomodulin a phospholipase inhibitory protein in rabbit neutrophils by phosphorylation, J. Biol. Chem., 256: 7730 (1981).

17. L. Parente, M. Di Rosa, J.R. Flower, P. Ghiara, R. Meli, P. Persico, J.A. Salmon and J.N. Wood, Relationship between the anti-phospholipase and anti-inflammatory effect of glucocorticoid-induced proteins, Eur. J. Pharmac., 99: 233 (1984).

18. A. Calignano, R. Carnuccio, M. Di Rosa, A. Ialenti and S. oncada, The anti-inflammatory effect of glucocorticoid-induced phospholipase inhibitory proteins, Agents and Actions (in press 1984).

19. M. Di Rosa and D.A. Willoughby, Screens for anti-inflammatory drugs, J. Pharm. Pharmac., 23: 297 (1971).

20. T. Hattori, T. Hoffman and F. Hirata, Differentiation of a histiocytic lymphoma cell line by lipomodulin a phospholipase inhibitory protein, Biochem. Biophys. Res.Commun., 111: 551 (1983).

21. T. Uede, F. Hirata, M. Hirashima and K. Ishizaka, Modulaton of the biological activities of IgE binding factors I. Identification of glycosilation-inhibiting factor as a fragment of lipomodulin, J. Immunol., 130: 878 (1983).

22. M. Koltai, I. Lepràn, G.Y. Nemecz and L. Szekeres, The possible mechanism of protection by dexamethasone against sudden death due to coronary ligation in conscious rats, Br. J. Pharmac., 79: 327 (1983).

23. F. Hirata, R. Del Carmine, C.A. Nelson, J. Axelrod, E. Schiffmann, A. Warabi and Others, Presence of autoantibody for phospholipase inhibitory protein lipomodulin in patients with rheumatic diseases, Proc. natn. Acad. Sci. USA, 78: 3190 (1981).

24. G. Ciabattoni, P. Patrignani, P. Filabozzi, A. Pierucci, B. Simonetti, G.A. Cinotti, E. Pinca, E. Gotti, G. Remuzzi and C. Patrono, Increased renal thromboxane (TX) production in systemic lupus erythematosus (SLE), Clin. Res., 30: 445A (1982).

FORMATION AND OXIDATIVE DEGRADATION OF LEUKOTRIENES

BY EOSINOPHILS AND NEUTROPHILS

William R. Henderson

Department of Medicine
University of Washington School of Medicine
Seattle, Washington 98195

Leukotrienes, formed by the lipoxygenation of arachidonic acid, are a potent group of chemical mediators that are important in inflammation. This paper will focus on leukotriene production by eosinophils. Eosinophilic leukocytes are prominent participants in inflammatory reactions but their function in these reactions has been previously poorly understood. Also to be discussed is how phagocytic cells can inactivate leukotrienes by oxidative mechanisms. Leukotriene inactivation by phagocyte generated peroxidase and hydroxyl radical systems may serve as a host defense mechanism to limit the great biologic activities of these mediators.

LEUKOTRIENE GENERATION BY EOSINOPHILS

Eosinophils are commonly found in increased numbers in the peripheral blood and tissues of patients with tumors, parasitic infections and bronchial asthma. Other conditions characterized by eosinophilia are various immunodeficiency, pulmonary, skin and gastrointestinal disorders (Beeson and Bass, 1977; Henderson and Chi, 1984). In patients with the hypereosinophilic syndrome who have high levels of circulating eosinophils (>1500 eosinophils/mm^3 for 6 months or greater) without discernible cause, widespread organ system dysfunction occurs including endomyocardial fibrosis (Fauci et al., 1982).

Polymorphonuclear and mononuclear leukocytes after appropriate stimulation generate various lipoxygenase products of arachidonic acid metabolism. Human neutrophils (Borgeat and Samuelsson, 1979), alveolar macrophages (Fels et al., 1982, Martin et al., 1984) and monocytes (Goldyne et al., 1984; Williams et al., 1984; Neill,

Klebanoff and Henderson, unpublished observations) produce leukotriene (LT)B_4 as the predominant lipoxygenase product. LTB_4 among
other properties has potent chemokinetic and chemotactic activities
for leukocytes (Ford-Hutchison et al., 1980; Goetzl and Pickett,
1981). The sulfidopeptide leukotrienes, LTC_4, LTD_4 and LTE_4 constitute the slow reacting substance (SRS) of anaphylaxis and are thought
to play a major role in the mediation of bronchial asthma through
their potent smooth muscle contracting activity and ability to increase vascular permeability (Dahlén et al., 1980, 1981; Peck et al.,
1981; Samuelsson, 1983). The sulfidopeptide leukotrienes are major
products of stimulated peritoneal macrophages (Bach et al., 1980;
Rouzer et al., 1980; Humes et al., 1982) and mast cells (Razin et
al., 1982; Peters et al., 1984). Since leukotriene production by
eosinophils might be relevant in their action in inflammatory reactions, we investigated arachidonic acid metabolism by horse and
human eosinophils (Jörg et al., 1982; Hendersen et al., 1983b, 1984).

Horse peripheral blood eosinophils were purified to greater
than 98% (less than 2% neutrophils) using polyvinylpyrrolidone sedimentation (Jörg et al., 1982). Eosinophils after incubation with
the calcium ionophore A23187 (1-10 µg/ml) generated SRS activity
as measured by the guinea pig ileal bioassay. The eosinophils produced four to five fold more SRS on a per cell basis than similarly
treated neutrophils. Ionophore-stimulated eosinophil supernatants
then underwent high performance liquid chromatography (HPLC) for
identification of lipoxygenase products. The major product formed
by horse eosinophils was LTC_4 as identified by co-elution on HPLC
with authentic LTC_4, ultraviolet spectrum, spectral shift on treatment with soybean lipoxygenase and incorporation of radiolabeled
arachidonic acid. Other leukotrienes formed by horse eosinophils
were LTB_4, 5-(S),12-(R)-6-trans-LTB_4, 5-(S),12-(S)-6-trans-LTB_4,
11-trans-LTC_4 and LTD_4. The dihydroxy acid leukotrienes were also
identified by gas chromatography-mass spectrometry. Additional
arachidonic acid metabolites including 11-trans-LTD_4 are produced
by ionophore-stimulated horse eosinophils as resolved by ion-pair
HPLC (Ziltener et al., 1983).

Previous studies had indicated that human eosinophils stimulated with the calcium ionophore formed primarily mono-hydroxy-
eicosatetraenoic acids (HETE)s such as 5-HETE and 11-HETE (Goetzl
et al., 1980) and, if stimulated in the presence of 10^{-4}M arachidonic acid, 15-HETE was the predominant arachidonate product (Turk
et al., 1982). In the studies of Turk et al. (1982), other 15-
lipoxygenase products of arachidonic acid such as 5,15-diHETEs and
8,15-diHETEs were generated by ionophore-stimulated human eosinophils. We initiated studies to determine whether SRS sulfidopeptide
leukotrienes were also released by human eosinophils and found their
production of LTC_4 and LTD_4 (Henderson et al., 1983b, 1984).

Human eosinophils from normal individuals and patients with

340

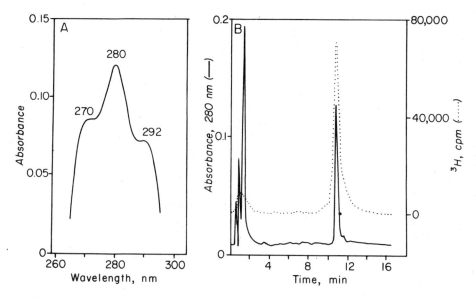

Fig. 1. Identification of LTC$_4$ production by human eosinophils. In (A) is shown the ultraviolet spectra of a compound with SRS activity obtained by reverse-phase HPLC of supernatant from 1 x 10[7] normal human eosinophils incubated with the ionophore A23187 (10 µg/ml) for 20 min at 37°C. as previously described (Henderson et al., 1984). The UV spectra of this compound dissolved in methanol/ water/acetic acid (75:25:0.01,v/v/v,pH 4.7) with a peak absorbance at 280 nm and shoulders at 270 and 292 ± 1 nm was the same as synthetic LTC$_4$. In (B), the eosinophil SRS compound (-) was identified as LTC$_4$ by its co-elution on re-chromatography with ^{3}H-LTC$_4$ (....) standard on a 3 µm Ultrasphere ODS C$_{18}$ column (4.6 x 75 mm) with the same solvent as in (A) at a flow rate of 1.6 ml/min.

the hypereosinophilic syndrome (HES) were purified to greater than 97% with less than 3% neutrophils. LTC$_4$ (Fig. 1) and LTD$_4$ were recovered from both the HES and normal eosinophils after stimulation with the calcium ionophore.

SRS sulfidopepide leukotriene formation by human eosinophils has particular relevance in the mediation of bronchial asthma in which eosinophilia is commonly noted (Beeson and Bass, 1977) and where development of clinical symptoms of wheezing and a decrease in pulmonary function has been associated with an increase in the number of eosinophils (Horn et al., 1975). LTC$_4$ and LTD$_4$ formation by eosinophils could also play a role in the host defense against tumors and parasites, conditions which are characterized by eosinophil infiltration of the inflammatory sites. Human eosinophil production of LTC$_4$ and LTD$_4$ has been subsequently reported by several groups (Weller et al., 1983; Verhagen et al., 1984; Shaw et al., 1984; Borgeat et al., 1984).

341

Normal and HES eosinophils also form LTB$_4$, the two 6-trans-isomers of LTB$_4$, 5-(S),15-(S)-di-HETE, 8-(S),15-(S)-di-HETE, 5-HETE, 12-HETE and 15-HETE after ionophore stimulation (Henderson et al., 1984). The addition of 10^{-4}M arachidonic acid prior to the addition of ionophore greatly augmented production of 15-HETE such that it became the major lipoxygenase product of both normal and HES eosinophils. These results could possibly be explained if the eosinophil 15-lipoxygenase enzyme is substrate limited in the absence of added arachidonic acid. Some of the activities of 15-HETE and its precursor 15-hydroperoxy-eicosatetraenoic acid (HPETE) include inhibition of vascular production of prostacyclin (Gryglewski et al., 1976), prevention of neutrophil formation of 5-HETE and LTB$_4$ (Vanderhoek et al., 1980) and inhibition of SRS release (Burka and Flower, 1979). The role of eosinophil generation of 15-HETE and other 15-lipoxygenase products in inflammatory reactions is unknown.

OXIDATIVE DEGRADATION OF LEUKOTRIENES

Eosinophils and neutrophils when stimulated by soluble agents (e.g. calcium ionophore A23187) or appropriately opsonized particles (e.g. zymosan) undergo a respiratory burst with an increase in oxygen consumption and formation of superoxide anion (O_2^-) (Baehner and Johnston, 1971; Babior, 1984). Two O_2^- molecules can react in a dismutation reaction in which one molecule is oxidized and the other reduced with the formation of O_2 and H_2O_2 as follows:

$$O_2^- + O_2^- + 2H^+ \rightarrow O_2 + H_2O_2$$

This reaction can be catalyzed by the enzyme superoxide dismutase or can also occur spontaneously. Hydrogen peroxide is formed both within the leukocytic phagolysosome after particle ingestion and is also released extracellularly. The toxicity of H_2O_2 is greatly augmented by interaction with peroxidase enzymes or with iron to form more reactive oxygen species such as hydroxyl radicals (OH·) and hypochlorous acid (HOCl).

Eosinophil and neutrophil activation is also characterized by the release of their cytoplasmic granule contents including peroxidase [eosinophil peroxidase (EPO); neutrophil peroxidase, myeloperoxidase (MPO)] into phagocytic vacuoles and also extracellularly (Cotran and Litt, 1969; Henderson et al., 1982). Peroxidases when combined with H_2O_2 and an oxidizable halide cofactor such as iodide, chloride or bromide form a variety of toxic molecules including HOCl. The peroxidase-H_2O_2-halide systems are toxic to bacteria (Jago and Morrison, 1962; Jong et al., 1980), tumor cells (Edelson and Cohn, 1973; Henderson et al., 1981) and helminths (Jong et al., 1981) and can induce degranulation of target cells including mast

cells (Henderson et al., 1980). The peroxidase systems can also inactivate soluble mediators including the chemotactic factors, C_{5a}
and formylmethionyl-leucyl-phenylalanine (Clark and Klebanoff, 1979),
α_1-proteinase inhibitor (α_1-antitrypsin) (Matheson et al., 1979) and
prostaglandin (PG)E_2, $PGF_{2\alpha}$ and 6-keto-$PGF_{1\alpha}$ (Paredes and Weiss,
1982). We have demonstrated that leukotrienes are rapidly and extensively degraded by the peroxidase enzyme systems and OH· generated by eosinophils and neutrophils.

Initial observations by Henderson and Kaliner (1979) showed
that mast cell granule peroxidase in the presence of H_2O_2 and chloride inactivated SRS guinea pig ileal bioactivity. Synthetic LTC_4
and LTD_4 were later found to be degraded within 1 min of incubation
with purified EPO supplemented with $10^{-4}M$ H_2O_2 and iodide or bromide
(or to a lesser degree with chloride) (Henderson et al., 1982). The
MPO-H_2O_2-chloride system also inactivated the SRS bioactivity of
these leukotrienes. The chemotactic activity of LTB_4 was similarly
decreased by the peroxidase systems although at a slower rate. Each
component of the system was required for leukotriene inactivation
and inactivation was abrogated by the addition of hemeprotein inhibitors such as azide indicating a requirement for peroxidase.
Higher concentrations of H_2O_2 ($5 \times 10^{-4} - 10^{-2}M$) alone could inactivate the sulfidopeptide leukotrienes in the absence of EPO and
halide but were without effect on LTB_4.

It was also noted that the recovery of SRS activity from A23187-
stimulated eosinophil supernatants was significantly increased by
the addition of either azide which inhibits peroxidase activity or
catalase which scavenges H_2O_2 (Henderson et al., 1982). These data
suggested that the net recovery of leukotrienes from leukocytes is
the difference between the amount formed and the amount degraded
by oxidative mechanisms. It was subsequently shown that the isolated EPO system and phorbol myristate acetate (PMA)-stimulated
eosinophils degraded exogenous LTC_4 to the 5-(S),12-(R)-6-trans-
and 5-(S),12-(S)-6-trans- isomers of LTB_4 (Goetzl, 1982). After
PMA stimulation, human neutrophils were found to transform LTC_4
into the 6-trans-LTB_4 isomers and LTC_4 sulfoxide degradation products (Lee et al., 1982); the peroxidase system and its product HOCl
were implicated in this inactivation process.

Stimulated phagocytic leukocytes also generate hydroxyl radicals (OH·). Hydroxyl radicals are formed by the iron catalyzed
interaction between O_2^- and H_2O_2 (Haber-Weiss reaction) (McCord and
Day, 1978) as follows:

$$O_2^- + Fe^{3+} \longrightarrow O_2 + Fe^{2+} \qquad (a)$$

$$Fe^{2+} + H_2O_2 \longrightarrow Fe^{3+} + OH^- + OH· \qquad (b)$$

$$\overline{O_2^- + H_2O_2 \longrightarrow O_2 + OH^- + OH·} \qquad (c)$$

When the Fe^{2+} concentration is sufficiently high, OH· are formed directly (Fenton reaction) without a requirement for O_2^- to reduce Fe^{3+}. The acetaldehyde-xanthine oxidase system which generates these same highly reactive oxygen reduction products (O_2^-, H_2O_2, OH·) has been employed in vitro as a model of the respiratory burst of phago-cytic leukocytes (Rosen and Klebanoff, 1979). Using two different iron-supplemented acetaldehyde systems we found that the SRS activity of LTC_4, LTD_4 and LTE_4 and the chemotactic activity of LTB_4 were rapidly inactivated by OH· (Henderson and Klebanoff, 1983a). At high Fe^{2+} concentration (reaction b; Fenton reaction), leukotriene inactivation was inhibited by OH· scavengers (mannitol or ethanol) as well as by catalase. When the Fe^{2+} concentration was lowered, leukotriene inactivation was also inhibited by superoxide dismutase suggesting a requirement for O_2^- in the reaction (reactions a,b,c; Haber-Weiss reaction).

In subsequent experiments, it was found that both the peroxi-dase-H_2O_2 and the Fe^{2+}-H_2O_2 systems when supplemented with iodide could iodinate arachidonic acid to form a variety of iodinated derivatives (Turk et al., 1983; Henderson et al., 1983a). Each of the double bounds of arachidonic acid was susceptible to iodination by these oxidative systems; analogous halogenation of the double bonds of leukotrienes could possibly be a mechanism for leukotriene inactivation.

The contribution of the peroxidase-H_2O_2-halide and OH· systems to leukotriene degradation by intact neutrophils was next studied (Henderson and Klebanoff, 1983b). Neutrophils were obtained from normal individuals and from patients with chronic granulomatous disease (CGD) and with MPO deficiency. CGD neutrophils fail to undergo a respiratory burst after stimulation and thus do not form H_2O_2, O_2^- or OH· (Babior et al., 1973). Patients with CGD suffer from recurrent staphlococcal and other bacterial infections of the lungs, lymph nodes, skin, gastrointestinal tract and other organs because of their failure to generate oxygen radicals during phago-cytosis (Gallin et al., 1983). MPO-deficient neutrophils which lack MPO in their cytoplasmic granules have an augmented respira-tory burst and generate OH· by the Haber-Weiss reaction (Rosen and Klebanoff, 1976). Although fungal infections such as candidiasis have been associated with MPO-deficiency (Lehrer and Clin, 1969), in general these individuals are healthy.

A23187-stimulated CGD neutrophils were found to form LTC_4, LTB_4, and the two 6-trans-isomers of LTB_4 indicating that the re-spiratory burst is not required for leukotriene formation (Henderson and Klebanoff, 1983). Since oxidative inactivation of leukotrienes is not possible by CGD neutrophils, it was anticipated that more leukotrienes would be recovered from the supernatants of A23187-stimulated CGD neutrophils compared to from supernatants of simi-larly treated normal or MPO-deficient cells that are capable of generating oxygen radicals. Consistent with this hypothesis were the findings that significantly more LTB_4 and LTC_4 were recovered from the CGD cells than from the normal or MPO-deficient neutrophils.

To further investigate the mechanism of oxidative degradation of LTC_4 by the MPO-deficient and normal cells, neutrophils from normal individuals and from MPO-deficient and CGD patients were incubated with [^{3}H]-labeled LTC_4 in the absence or presence of the calcium ionophore A23187. In the absence of ionophore, only a small conversion (<20%) of the added LTC_4 to LTD_4 and LTE_4 was noted in each of the 3 groups of neutrophils (Henderson and Klebanoff, 1983) which presumably occurs by the action of γ-glutamyl transpeptidase and aminopeptidase enzymes present in the neutrophils (Samuelsson, 1983). A23187-stimulated CGD neutrophils failed to further metabolize the added LTC_4. In contrast, complete degradation of the exogenous LTC_4 occurred when either the normal or MPO-deficient neutrophils were incubated with A23187. LTC_4 degradation by normal cells was inhibited by catalase and azide. This suggests that the peroxidase system is the predominant system for LTC_4 degradation by normal neutrophils. Degradation of LTC_4 by MPO-deficient cells was inhibited by superoxide dismutase, catalase and the OH· scavengers, mannitol or ethanol. Thus, when MPO is absent, OH· formed by the Haber-Weiss reaction can degrade LTC_4. Major degration products of LTC_4 formed by both the A23187-stimulated normal and MPO-deficient cells as well as by the isolated $MPO-H_2O_2$-chloride system and the acetaldehyde-xanthine oxidase system (which generates OH·) were the 5-(S),12-(R)-6-trans- and 5-(S),12-(S)-6-trans- isomers of LTB_4 (Henderson and Klebanoff, 1983).

These results indicate that phagocyte generation of potent oxidants may play an important modulating role in inflammatory reactions by inactivation of the biologically potent leukotrienes.

ACKNOWLEDGMENTS

The studies described here were supported in part by USPHS Grants AI17758 and AI07763. WRH is the recipient of USPHS Allergic Diseases Academic Award AI00487 from the National Institute of Allergy and Infectious Diseases. The secretarial assistance of Caroline Wilson is gratefully acknowledged.

REFERENCES

Babior, B.M., 1984, The respiratory burst of phagocytes, J. Clin. Invest., 73:599.

Babior, B.M., Kipnis, R.S., and Curnette, J.T., 1973, Biological defense mechanisms. The production by leukocytes of super-oxide: a potential bactericidal agent, J. Clin. Invest., 52:741.

Bach, M.K., Brashler, J.R., Hammarström, S., and Samuelsson, B., 1980, Identification of leukotriene C as a major component of slow reacting substance from rat mononuclear cells, J. Immunol., 125:115.

Baehner, R.L., and Johnston, R.B., Jr., 1971, Metabolic and bactericidal activities of human eosinophils, Br. J. Haematol., 20:277.

Beeson, P., and Bass, D.A., 1977, "The Eosinophil. Major Problems in Internal Medicine Series," W.B. Saunders Co., Philadelphia, 14:167.

Borgeat, P., and Samuelsson, B., 1979, Transformation of arachidonic acid by rabbit polymorphonuclear leukocytes. Formation of a novel dihydroxy-eicosatetraenoic acid , J. Biol. Chem. 254:2643.

Borgeat, P., Fruteau de Laclos, B., Rabinovitch, H., Picard, S., Braquet, P., Hébert, J., and Laviolette, M., 1984, Eosinophil-rich human polymorphonuclear leukocyte preparations characteristically release leukotriene C_4 on ionophore A23187 challenge, J. Allergy Clin. Immunol., 74(Suppl.): 310.

Burka, J.F., and Flower, R.J., 1979, Effect of modulators of arachidonic acid metabolism on the synthesis and release of slow-reacting substance of anaphylaxis, Br. J. Pharmacol., 65: 35.

Clark, R.A., 1983, Extracellular effects of the myeloperoxidase-hydrogen peroxide-halide system, in: "Advances in Inflammation Research," Vol. 5., G. Weissmann, ed., Raven Press, New York, 107.

Clark, R.A., and Klebanoff, S.J., 1979, Chemotactic factor inactivation by the myeloperoxidase-hydrogen peroxide-halide system. An inflammatory control mechanism, J. Clin. Invest., 64: 913.

Cotran, R.S., and Litt, M., 1969, The entry of granule-associated peroxidase into the phagocytic vacuole of eosinophils, J. Exp. Med., 129:1291.

Dahlén, S-E., Hedqvist, P., Hammarström, S., and Samuelsson, B., 1980, Leukotrienes are potent constrictors of human bronchi. Nature, 288:484.

Dahlén, S-E., Björk, P., Hedqvist, P., Arfors, K-E., Hammarström, S., Lindgren, J-A., and Samuelsson, B., 1981, Leukotrienes promote plasma leakage and leukocyte adhesion in post capillary venules: in vivo effects with relevance to the acute inflammatory response. Proc. Natl. Acad. Sci. USA, 78: 3887.

Edelson, P.J., and Cohn, Z.A., 1973, Peroxidase-mediated mammalian cell cytotoxicity. J. Exp. Med., 138:318.

Fauci, A.S., Harley, J.B., Roberts, W.C., Ferrans, V.J., Gralnick, H.R., and Bjornson, B.H., 1982, The idopathic hypereosinophilic syndrome: clinical, pathophysiologic and therapeutic considerations. Ann. Int. Med. 97:78.

Fels, A.O., Pawlowski, N.A., Cramer, E.B., King, T.K.C., Cohn, Z.A., and Scott, W.A., 1982, Human alveolar macrophages produce leukotriene B_4, Proc. Natl. Acad. Sci. USA, 79:7866.

Ford-Hutchinson, A.W., Bray, M.A., Doig, M.V., Shipley, M.E., and Smith, M.J.H., 1980, Leukotriene B, a potent chemokinetic and aggregating substance released from polymorphonuclear leukocytes, Nature (Lond.), 286:264.

Goetzl, E.J., 1982, The conversion of leukotriene C_4 to isomers of leukotriene B_4 by human eosinophil peroxidase, Biochem. Biophys. Res. Commun., 106:270.

Goetzl, E.J., and Pickett, W.C., 1981, Novel structural determinants of the human neutrophil chemotactic activity of leukotriene B, J. Exp. Med., 153:482.

Goetzl, E.J., Weller, P.F., and Sun, F.F., 1980, The regulation of human eosinophil function by endogenous mono-hydroxyeicosatetraenoic acids (HETE)s, J. Immunol., 124:926.

Goldyne, M.E., Burrish, G.F., Poubelle, P., and Borgeat, P., 1984, Arachidonic acid metabolism among human mononuclear leukocytes. Lipoxygenase-related pathways, J. Biol. Chem. 259: 8815.

Gryglewski, R.J., Bunting, S., Moncada, S., Flower, R.J., and Vane, J.R., 1976, Arterial walls are protected against deposition of platelet thrombi by a substance (prostaglandin X) which they make from prostaglandin endoperoxides, Prostaglandins, 12:685.

Henderson, W.R., and Chi, E.Y., 1984, In Press, Eosinophilic granuloma, in: "Progressive Stages of Neoplastic Growth," H.E. Kaiser, ed., Pergamon Press, Oxford, England.

Henderson, W.R., and Kaliner, M., 1979, Mast cell granule peroxidase: location, secretion and SRS-A inactivation, J. Immunol., 122:1322.

Henderson, W.R., and Klebanoff, S.J., 1983a, Leukotriene B_4, C_4, D_4 and E_4 inactivation by hydroxyl radicals, Biochem. Biophys. Res. Commun., 110:266.

Henderson, W.R., and Klebanoff, S.J., 1983b, Leukotriene production and inactivation by normal, chronic granulomatous disease and myeloperoxidase-deficient neutrophils, J. Biol. Chem., 258:13522.

Henderson, W.R., Chi, E.Y., and Klebanoff, S.J., 1980, Eosinophil peroxidase-induced mast cell secretion, J. Exp. Med., 152:265.

Henderson, W.R., Harley, J.B., and Fauci, A.S., 1984, Arachidonic acid metabolism in normal and hypereosinophilic syndrome human eosinophils: generation of leukotrienes B_4, C_4, D_4 and 15-lipoxygenase products. Immunology, 51:679.

Henderson, W.R., Hubbard, W.C., and Klebanoff, S.J., 1983a, Iodination of arachidonic acid by the iron-H_2O_2-iodide system, Lipids, 18:390.

Henderson, W.R., Jörg, A., and Klebanoff, S.J., 1982, Eosinophil peroxidase-mediated inactivation of leukotriene B_4, C_4 and D_4. J. Immunol., 128:2609.

Henderson, W.R., Harley, J.B., Fauci, A.S., and Klebanoff, S.J., 1983b, Leukotriene B_4, C_4, D_4 generation by human eosinophils, J. Allergy Clin. Immunol., 71:138.

Henderson, W.R., Chi, E.Y., Jong, E.C., and Klebanoff, S.J., 1981, Mast cell-mediated tumor-cell cytotoxicity. Role of the peroxidase system, J. Exp. Med., 153:520.

Horn, B.R., Robin, E.D., Theodore, J., and Van Kessel, A., 1975, Total eosinophil counts in the management of bronchial asthma, N. Engl. J. Med., 292:1152.

Humes, J.L., Sadowski, S., Galavage, M., Goldenberg, M., Subers, E., Bonney, R.J., and Kuehl, F.A., Jr., 1982, Evidence for two sources of arachidonic acid for oxidative metabolism by mouse peritoneal macrophages, J. Biol. Chem., 257:1591.

Jörg, A., Henderson, W.R., Murphy, R.C., and Klebanoff, S.J., 1982, Leukotriene generation by eosinophils, J. Exp. Med., 155: 390.

Lee, C.W., Lewis, R.A., Corey, E.J., Barton, A., Oh, H., Tauber, A.I., and Austen, K.F., 1982, Oxidative inactivation of leukotriene C_4 by stimulated human polymorphonuclear leukocytes, Proc. Natl. Acad. Sci. USA, 79:4166.

Lehrer, R.I., and Cline, M.J., 1969, Leukocyte myeloperoxidase deficiency and disseminated candidiasis: the role of myeloperoxidase in resistance to Candida infection, J. Clin. Invest., 48:1478.

Martin, T.R., Altman, L.C., Albert, R.K., and Henderson, W.R., 1984, Leukotriene B_4 production by the human alveolar macrophage: a potential mechanism for lung amplification, Am. Rev. Resp. Dis., 129:106.

Matheson, N.R., Wong, P.S., and Travis, J., 1979, Enzymatic inactivation of human alpha-1-proteinase inhibitor by neutrophil myeloperoxidase, Biochem. Biophys. Res. Commun., 88:402.

McCord, J.M., and Day, E.D., Jr., 1978, Superoxide-dependent production of hydroxyl radical catalyzed by iron-EDTA complex. FEBS Lett., 86:139.

Paredes, J-M., and Weiss, S.J., 1982, Human neutrophils transform prostaglandins by a myeloperoxidase-dependent mechanism, J. Biol. Chem., 257:2738.

Peck, M.J., Piper, P.J., and William, T.J., 1981, The effect of leukotrienes C_4 and D_4 on the microvasculature of guinea pig skin, Prostaglandins, 21:315.

Peters, S.P., MacGlashan, D.W., Jr., Schulman, E.S., Schleimer, R. P., Hayes, E.C., Rokach, J., Adkinson, N.F., Jr., and Lichtenstein, L.M., 1984, Arachidonic acid metabolism in purified human lung mast cells, J. Immunol., 132:1972.

Rosen, H., and Klebanoff, S.J., 1976, Chemiluminescence and superoxide production by myeloperoxidase-deficient leukocytes, J. Clin. Invest., 58:50.

Rosen, H., and Klebanoff, S.J., 1979, Bactericidal activity of a superoxide-generating system. A model for the polymorphonuclear leukocyte, J. Exp. Med., 149:27.

Rouzer, C.A., Scott, W.A., Cohn, Z.A., Blackburn, P., and Manning, J.M., 1980, Mouse peritoneal macrophages release leukotriene C in response to a phagocytic stimulus, Proc. Natl. Acad. Sci. USA, 77:4928.

Shaw, R.J., Cromwell, O., and Kay, A.B., 1984, Preferential generation of LTC_4/D_4 by human eosinophils and LTB_4 by neutrophils: evaluation by specific radioimmunoassay, J. Allergy Clin. Immunol., 73:192.

Turk, J., Henderson, W.R., Klebanoff, S.J., and Hubbard, W.C., 1983, Iodination of arachidonic acid mediated by eosinophil peroxidase, myeloperoxidase and lactoperoxidase: identification and comparison of products, Biochim. Biophys. Acta, 751: 189.

Turk, J., Maas, R.L., Brash, A.R., Roberts, L.J. II, and Oates, J.A., 1982, Arachidonic acid 15-lipoxygenase products from human eosinophils

Vanderhoek, J.Y., Bryant, R.W., and Bailey, J.M., 1980, Inhibition of leukotriene biosynthesis by the leukocyte product, 15-hydroxy-5,8,11,13-eicosatetraenoic acid, J. Biol. Chem., 255:10064.

Verhagen, J., Bruynzcel, P.L.B., Koedam, J.A., Wassink, G.A., de Boer, M., Terpstra, G.K., Kreukniet, J., Veldink, G.A., and Vliegenthart, J.F.G., 1984, Specific leukotriene formation by purified human eosinophils and neutrophils, FEBS Lett., 168:23.

Weller, P.F., Lee, C.W., Foster, D.W., Corey, E.J., Austen, K.F., and Lewis, R.A., 1983, Generation and metabolism of 5-lipoxygenase pathway leukotrienes by human eosinophils: predominant production of leukotriene C_4, Proc. Natl. Acad. Sci. USA, 80:7626.

Williams, J.D., Czop, J.K., and Austen, K.F., 1984, Release of leukotrienes by human monocytes on stimulation of their phagocytic receptor for particulate activators, J. Immunol., 132:3034.

Ziltener, H.J., Chavaillaz, P-A., and Jörg, A., 1983, Leukotriene formation by eosinophil leukocytes. Analysis with ion-pair high pressure liquid chromatography and effect of the respiratory burst. Hoppe-Seyler's Z. Physiol. Chem. 364: 1029.

EICOSANOIDS AND CANCER

Alan Bennett

Department of Surgery, King's College School of Medicine
and Dentistry, The Rayne Institute, 123 Coldharbour Lane
London SE5 9NU, London, England

There are many interesting and potentially important
relationships between prostaglandins and various aspects of cancer.
Associations have been found regarding cancer development, spread,
host defense mechanisms and survival, etc. These factors are
obviously relevant to the understanding of the initiation and
progress of the disease. In addition, they are of more immediate
relevance regarding the effects on cancer of common drugs such as
aspirin and corticosteroids that alter prostaglandin metabolism or
release. However, since there are so many processes involved, so
many different types of cancer, and numerous prostaglandins, it is to
be expected that the relationships are complex and often disputed.

Since the subject is vast, and the various aspects have been
discussed fairly compehensively in several recent reviews (1-6), only
a brief overview of scientific and clinical aspects is appropriate
here. Apart from the numerous experiments with prostaglandins, the
newer developments that are beginning to appear include studies on
the lipoxygenase products formed from prostaglandin precursors.
Those interested in more details than are provided here are
recommended to read the reviews listed above, together with the two
recent proceedings of meetings which contain a wealth of information
(7,8). These works (1-8) provide lists of publications for
unreferenced statements made in the text below, which focusses
briefly on many, but by no means all, scientific and clinical aspects
of eicosanoids and cancer. Because the subject is so complex, and
the interpretation of results difficult and often unclear, some
cautionary comments are included.

Eicosanoid production by tumours

The term eicosanoid includes prostaglandins, thromboxanes and leukotrienes etc. One of the factors implicating eicosanoids in cancer is the striking correlation between fat consumption and cancer incidence in man (9). Almost all tumours yield more prostaglandins than do the normal tissues in which they arise. However, the interpretation of this finding is fraught with difficulties. Are these prostaglandins the cause, the result, both or neither of cancer development and spread? To what extent are the prostaglandins produced by the malignant or the host cells? Have the substances been accurately identified: many forms of "identification" are inadequate? To what extent is the prostaglandin production by the isolated tumours equivalent to that in vivo, or is it stimulated abnormally by the tissue preparation prior to extraction, etc? Of course, the same problems apply to other substances in this and other diseases, but it is important to emphasise the difficulties of interpretation so that the evidence is put into perspective. Fortunately, some of the other aspects discussed later, such as the effects of drugs on host survival, are clearer at least in their relevance if not in their mechanism.

Release of prostaglandins into the blood

There are reports that elevated blood levels of the PGI_2 degradation product 6-keto-PGF_1alpha often occur in patients with various cancers, but there is substantial controversy about the validity of such measurements. It is now clear that normal circulating levels of this degradation product are low, but critics claim that rigorous analytical methods have not been applied to blood levels in cancer patients. It therefore remains to be verified that increased amounts of 6-keto-PGF_1alpha are present. Evidence that elevated prostaglandin formation can occur in cancer is that the urine of patients with bone metastases often contains more PGE_2 metabolite, and that blood draining breast tumours often contains more prostaglandin-like biological activity than can be extracted from the patient's peripheral blood plasma. What is the source of any prostanoids that may be released? Do they come from the malignant cells, from the endothelium of newly forming and/or established tumour blood vessels, or from other sources? Again to show the difficulties of interpretation, we should consider the possibility that blood cells of cancer patients merely release more prostanoids during blood sampling and processing.

Prostaglandin effects on blood cells

If sufficiently high concentrations of prostaglandins are released into the blood stream or come into contact with blood within

the tumour, the blood cells could obviously be affected.   The
platelets may play an important role in metastasis by protecting
malignant cells in the blood stream.   This conclusion is supported by
studies in mice with platelet anti-aggregating substances such as
aspirin, thromboxane synthesis inhibitors, PGI_2 and anticoagulants.
Many experimental tumours are immunogenic, and depressed immune
responses often accompany malignancy in patients, but the relevance
of this aspect to the growth and spread of cancer in man is not
clear.   Prostanoids can affect the leucocytes which may play
important roles in the host defense against experimental cancers,
and possibly those in man (3).   Again, controversies and opposite
findings exist, but several studies show that PGE compounds can
inhibit the activities of natural killer cells, and of T and B
lymphocytes.

Cancer promotion

Different stages have been classified in experimental
carcinogenesis.   Initiation of a cancer in mouse skin results from
the single, nontumourigenic, application of a carcinogen.   A
malignant tumour can then be produced by the repeated application of
a promoter whose action may involve prostaglandins.   The production
of free radicals formed in the generation of eicosanoids may play a
major role in the mechanism.   Free radicals contribute to many
aspects of cell damage and, for example, they are important in the
chromosomal damage by x-rays and by the tumour promoter tetradecanoyl
phorbol acetate.

Tumour cells in culture

PGA and PGE compounds can increase cell differentiation, and in
many cases various prostaglandins inhibit the proliferation of cells
in culture.   Recent work shows that this inhibition occurs with PGD
and PGJ, as well as with PGA compounds.   It may seem that these
anticancer activities contradict the anticancer effects of
prostaglandin synthesis inhibitors discussed later.   However, again
there are disagreements about the results, with some prostaglandins
such as PGF_2alpha stimulating cell proliferation and, even more
importantly, that different concentrations of PGE_2 can respectively
stimulate or inhibit cell proliferation.   We still need to know many
things such as how different cell types respond, how the results are
influenced by the experimental conditions, and what are the effects
of the numerous arachidonate and other fatty acid derivatives not yet
studied.   What responses occur when eicosanoids are combined with
each other or with different substances, and what interactions occur
when mixtures of cell types are present?

Tumour growth and metastasis in laboratory animals

Most of the prostaglandin-related work in this area has been done with nonsteroidal anti-inflammatory drugs that inhibit prostaglandin synthesis. The drug treatment usually results both in smaller tumours and in longer survival of the experimental animals. These beneficial effects seem to contradict the previously mentioned findings of a prostaglandin-induced increase in cell differentiation and a decrease in the proliferation of cells in culture. On one hand, it remains to be seen to what extent these cellular events occur in vivo. On the other hand, might the anticancer effects of anti-inflammatory drugs in vivo involve effects on nonmalignant cells; for example, the drugs might remove a prostaglandin-induced inhibition of the host immune system, reduce platelet aggregation, or interfer with tumour vascularisation. Evidence favouring a prostaglandin involvement is that PGE compounds can overcome the effects of indomethacin on mouse cancer.

Tumour size is of limited value in determining anticancer effects, and it does not take into account actions that may be unrelated to an effect on the malignant cells such as a reduction of a local inflammatory response. Although it is possible that prostaglandin synthesis inhibitors reduce the size of some tumours in this way, there is nevertheless evidence for a genuine anticancer effect in other cases. This is particularly clear in experiments which have shown complete tumour regression when the mice were treated with indomethacin.

Again it is to be expected in this complex area that not all findings agree, and some studies report no beneficial effect of prostaglandin synthesis inhibitors. However, there is little or no evidence that they have a deleterious effect. This is fortunate when considering the use of nonsteroidal anti-inflammatory drugs in man.

Some experiments show that prostaglandin synthesis inhibitors improve the response of tumour-bearing mice to chemotherapy with methotrexate and melphalan. The mechanism(s) are not clear, but in addition to the effects mentioned earlier, there might be altered penetration, binding or excretion of the cytotoxic drugs. This might be specific for methotrexate and/or melphalan since a beneficial interaction does not seem to occur with all cytotoxic drugs.

As with prostaglandin synthesis inhibitors, and seemingly in contradiction, administration of some prostaglandins can reduce tumour size. Furthermore, recent experiments in mice with cancer have shown increased survival when PGA, PGD or PGJ compounds were administered (10). The extent of any contradiction is difficult to assess. There are so many factors that may be involved, such as differences between tumour types, the ability of prostaglandins to exert a mixture of good and bad effects, the possibility that administered prostaglandins may alter the metabolism of endogenously released eicosanoids, diversion by nonsteroidal drugs of arachidonate

354

metabolism into lipoxygenase products, and actions of these anti-inflammatory drugs by nonprostaglandin mechanisms.

Human cancer

The human malignancy that has been studied most extensively with regard to prostaglandins is breast cancer. Much of this research has concerned the measurement of prostaglandin-like material (the latter term is preferable when, as in most studies, the prostaglandins have not been rigorously identified) extracted from primary tumours removed at operation, or the ability of tumour fragments to metabolise added arachidonic acid. In our own work, one of the earliest interesting findings was the higher yield of prostaglandin-like material from primary tumours of patients whose bone isotope scans indicated the presence of skeletal metastases. We thought that this might relate to the potent ability of some prostaglandins to resorb bone. However, when there were enough patients for a comprehensive analysis, it emerged that our hypothesis was wrong. The lower median value in the bone-scan-negative group was because tumours forming small amounts of prostaglandins showed no evidence of spread to bone, whereas no patient with a positive scan had a tumour producing low amounts of prostaglandin-like material. Over the rest of the range, the tumour prostaglandin values in the two groups overlapped. Other work has now been produced which indicates that bone metastasis in breast cancer does not predominantly involve prostaglandins: later skeletal recurrence in previously bone-scan-negative patients is not necessarily associated with primary tumours that produced high amounts of prostaglandins, and prostaglandin synthesis inhibitors seem mainly ineffective in treating hypercalcaemia of breast cancer.

Of more interest and potentially of greater importance are the findings that a high prostaglandin production by the primary tumour correlates inversely with recurrence (at any site) up to 18 months postoperatively, and with patient survival up to 3 years postoperatively. Despite this, however, the survival curves of patients whose primary tumours produced high or low amounts of prostaglandin-like material are similar, so that prostaglandin production on its own is not a prognostic factor. Perhaps high prostaglandin production by the tumours is associated with early death from the disease only when it occurs in conjunction with one or more other variables.

Our group has also performed similar studies with other human cancers including those of the lung, gut, and head and neck. The lung studies are even more difficult to analyse than the breast results because there are several different types of common tumour, the disease is usually very advanced at the time of surgery, and the patients are a selected group because only about 20 percent of cases are operable. In contrast to the breast studies, the measurements of lung tumour prostaglandin-like material show, if anything, an overall direct correlation with survival.

The use of anti-inflammatory drugs in human cancer

Since the possible relationships of eicosanoids to cancer are complex and unclear, what should the clinician decide about giving anti-inflammatory/analgesic inhibitors of prostaglandin synthesis to patients with cancer? Although indomethacin may be of value in head and neck cancer, there is no good general case for using prostaglandin synthesis inhibitors as therapeutic adjuvants. However, nonsteroidal analgesics effectively relieve the pain of bone metastases, and aspirin can reduce the side effects of radiotherapy. It is relevant that prednisolone is used in many regimens of cytotoxic chemotherapy. Anti-inflammatory steroids inhibit the release of prostaglandin precursors, and so reduce the formation of of prostaglandins and other lipoxygenase products such as leukotrienes. Do cancer patients need advice about whether they should take aspirin for a headache? Such medication is probably safe, since there is little or no evidence that anti-inflammatory drugs are harmful in cancer, but at the present state of knowledge we should keep an open mind. Double-blind trials of flurbiprofen in head and neck cancer and in breast carcinoma now in progress will provide further information on the utility of prostaglandin synthesis inhibitors. Hopefully other studies will examine drugs that act selectively on part of the arachidonate metabolic pathway and, in contrast, will investigate further the value of prostaglandins in cancer therapy. Perhaps the results will depend on the type of cancer and its stage of development.

References

1. Bennett A. Prostaglandins and cancer. In: Practical Applications of Prostaglandins and their Synthesis Inhibitors. Ed. SMM Karim, Lancaster, MTP Press 1979;149-88.

2. Karmali RA. Review: prostaglandins and cancer. Prostaglandins and Medicine 1980; 5: 11-28.

3. Honn KV, Bockmans RS, Marnett LJ. Prostaglandins and cancer: a review of tumor metastasis. Prostaglandins 1981; 21: 833-864.

4. Levine L. Arachidonic acid transformation and tumor production. Adv. Cancer Res. 1981; 35: 49-79.

5. Bennett A. Prostaglandins and inhibitors of their synthesis in cancer growth and spread. In : Endocrinology of Cancer, Vol. 3, Ed. DP Rose, Florida, CRC Press 1982: 113-27.

6. Bennett A. Prostaglandins and cancer. In : Handbook of the Eicosanoids. Ed. AL Willis, B Vickery, C Pace-Asciak. Florida, CRC Press, in press.

7. Prostaglandins and Cancer: First International Conference. Ed. TJ Powles, RS Bockman, KV Honn et al, New York, Alan R. Liss, 1982.

8. Icosanoids and Cancer. Ed. H Thaler-Dao, A Crastes de Paulet, R Paoletti, New York, Raven Press, 1984.

9. Carroll KK, Hopkins GJ, Kennedy TG et al. Essential fatty acids in relation to mammary carcinogenesis. Progr. Lipid Res. 1982; 20, 685-90.

STIMULATED HUMAN COLONIC SYNTHESIS OF ARACHIDONATE LIPOXYGENASE AND

CYCLO-OXYGENASE PRODUCTS BY LAXATIVES

F. Capasso*, I.A. Tavares and A. Bennett

Department of Surgery, King's College School of Medicine
and Dentistry, London SE5 8RX, England
*Department of Experimental Pharmacology, School of
Pharmacy, University of Naples, Italy

INTRODUCTION

We have recently demonstrated that rat colon can convert ^{14}C-arachidonic acid into both lipoxygenase and cyclo-oxygenase products, and that this metabolism is stimulated by the laxative phenolphthalein (Capasso et al 1984). These products can affect intestinal function. Prostaglandins (Bennett and Sanger 1982) and lipoxygenase products (Musch et al 1982) can increase intestinal motility and the secretion of water and electrolytes. Human colon forms similar products (Bennett et al 1981; Boughton-Smith et al 1983), and we have now investigated the effect of laxatives on arachidonic acid metabolism by human isolated colonic mucosa and muscle.

METHODS

The tissues were obtained from operation specimens, cut finely, and homogenised in Krebs solution to give 20 mg/ml. 5 ml aliquots were pre-incubated (20 min, 37°C) without (controls) or with the test drugs (phenolphthalein 100 µg/ml, ricinoleic acid 100 µg/ml, sodium picosulphate 125 µg/ml, sodium sulfosuccinate 200 µg/ml, or mannitol 500 µg/ml) and then futher incubated for 1 hr with [1-^{14}C]-arachidonic acid (0.1 µCi, 34 nM). The products were extracted, and chromatographed on silica gel thin layer plates together with authentic standards (hexane: diethyl ether: acetic acid, 40:60:3, 90 min) (Borgeat and Samuelsson, 1979). In 2 cases autoradiographs were prepared (Cottee et al, 1977). Comparison with the standards indicated that the products formed were PGs, 5-hydroxy-eicosatetraenoate and leukotriene B_4.

In preliminary experiments indomethacin 3 µM or the cyclooxygenase/lipoxygenase inhibitor BW755C 20 µM were incubated with the tissue for 20 min at $37^{\circ}C$ before addition of the labelled arachidonic acid.

RESULTS AND DISCUSSION

Control homogenates of human colonic muscle converted $4.0\pm0.7\%$ (mean$\pm$SE, n=8) of the added ^{14}C arachidonic acid to radioactive products (Table 1). Metabolism by the mucosa was less active, the conversion being $2.2\pm0.4\%$ (Table 2). The predominant products formed, as indicated by their chromatographic mobility, were PGs > LTB_4 > 5-HETE.

TABLE 1. EFFECT OF LAXATIVES ON ^{14}C-ARACHIDONIC ACID METABOLISM BY HUMAN COLONIC MUSCLE IN VITRO

DRUG (n)	PGs	LTB_4	5-HETE
Control (8)	0.89(.19)	0.25(.03)	0.19(.02)
Mannitol (8) 500 µg/ml	0.97(.18)	0.26(.03)	0.19(.02)
Sulfosuccinate 200 µg/ml (8)	1.24(.40)	0.22(.05)	0.25(.06)
Picosulphate 125 µg/ml (6)	1.49(.35)[a]	0.41(.12)[a]	0.27(.07)
Phenolphthalein 100 µg/ml (8)	2.10(.55)[a]	0.41(.09)[c]	0.29(.06)
Ricinoleic acid 100 µg/ml (8)	3.24(.85)[c]	0.74(.25)[b]	0.44(.10)[b]

Values are means (sem) % conversion into PGs, LTB_4 and 5-HETE. a, P<0.1; b, P<0.05; c, P<0.02.

TABLE 2. EFFECT OF LAXATIVES ON ^{14}C-ARACHIDONIC ACID
METABOLISM BY HUMAN COLONIC MUCOSA IN VITRO

DRUG	(n)	PGs	LTB$_4$	5-HETE
Control	(8)	0.38(.10)	0.13(.0003)	0.14(.02)
Mannitol 500 µg/ml	(8)	0.33(.07)	0.14(.01)	0.16(.04)
Sulfosuccinate 200 µg/ml (8)		0.63(.28)	0.15(.02)	0.22(.08)
Picosulphate 125 µg/ml (6)		0.37(.08)	0.15(.03)	0.24(.08)
Phenolphthalein 100 µg/ml (8)		0.48(.12)	0.16(.02)	0.26(.06)[b]
Ricinoleic acid 100 µg/ml (8)		0.70(.12)[d]	0.18(.01)[b]	0.27(.07)[b]

Values are means(sem) % conversion into PGs, LTB$_4$ and 5-HETE.
b, P<0.05; d, P<0.01.

Ricinoleic acid was the most potent stimulant of metabolism in both the mucosa and the muscle. Phenolphthalein and sodium picosulphate were also active while the effect of sodium sulfosuccinate was at most weak, and mannitol had no effect. Indomethacin 3 µM or BW755C 20 µM inhibited the increase in cyclo-oxygenase products, and BW775C also reduced the formation of lipoxygenase products, both in control tissues and those treated with ricinoleic acid or phenolphthalein (data not shown).

Laxatives increase the amount of PGs present in the colonic lumen of rats (Beubler and Juan 1979; Cohen 1982; Capasso et al 1983; Autore et al 1984) and increase the net secretion of water and electrolytes into the small intestine (Beubler and Juan 1979). In addition, phenolphthalein increases the formation of histamine and 5-hydroxytryptamine by the intestine (Autore et al 1984), so that these autacoids might also contribute to the cathartic effect of laxatives. The present results suggest that arachidonate lipoxygenase products may also play a part in the laxative effects, and that actions on both the mucosa and the muscle may be involved. Furthermore, 5-hydroxy- and 5-hydroperoxy acids have a strong secretory effect in the gut (Musch et al 1982) and contract isolated gastrointestinal muscle (Holme et al 1980; Goldenberg and Subers 1982).

REFERENCES

Autore G, Capasso F, Mascolo N (1984). Phenolphthalein stimulates the formation of histamine, 5-hydroxytryptamine and prostaglandin-like material by rat ileum, jejunum and colon. Br J Pharmacol 81: 347

Bennett A, Hensby CN, Sanger GJ, Stamford IF (1981). Metabolites of arachidonic acid formed by human gastrointestinal tissues and their actions on the muscle layers. Br J Pharmac 74: 435

Bennett A, Sanger GJ (1982). Acidic Lipids; Prostaglandins, in: Handbook of Exp Pharmacol 59/II, Ed G Bertaccini, Springer-Verlag, Berlin, p219

Beubler E, Juan H (1979). Effect of ricinoleic acid and other laxatives on net water flux and prostaglandin E release by the rat colon. J Pharm Pharmac 31: 681

Borgeat P, Samuelsson B (1979) Arachidonic acid metabolism in polymorphonuclear luekocytes: unstable intermediate in formation of dihydroxy acids, Proc. Natl Acad Sci USA 76: 3213

Boughton-Smith NK, Hawkey CJ, Whittle BJR (1983). Biosynthesis of lipoxygenase and cyclo-oxygenase products from [^{14}C]-arachidonic acid by human colonic mucosa. Gut 24: 1176

Capasso F, Mascolo N, Autore G, Duraccio MR (1983). Effect of indomethacin on aloin and 1,8-dioxyanthraquinone-induced production of prostaglandins in rat isolated colon. Prostaglandins 26: 547

Capasso F, Tavares IA, Bennett A (1984). The production of arachidonic lipoxygenase products by rat intestine is increased by phenolphthalein. Eur J Pharmacol, in press

Cohen HH (1982). The effect of cathartics on prostaglandin synthesis by rat gastrointestinal tract. PGs, Leukotrienes and Medicine 8: 389

Cottee F, Flower RJ, Moncada S, Salmon JA, Vane JR (1977). Synthesis of 6-keto-PGF$_1$alpha by ram seminal vesicle microsomes. Prostaglandins 14: 413

Goldenberg HM, Subers EM (1982). The reactivity of rat isolated gastrointestinal tissues to leukotrienes. Eur J Pharmacol 78: 463

Holme G, Brunet G, Hasson P Girard Y, Rokach J (1980). The activity of synthetic leukotriene C$_4$ on guinea pig trachea and ileum. Prostaglandins 20: 717

Musch MW, Miller RJ, Field H, Siegel HI (1982). Stimulation of colonic secretion by lipoxygenase metabolites of arachidonic acid. Science 217: 1253

362

CORRELATION BETWEEN K[+] FLUXES AND THE ARACHIDONIC ACID CASCADE IN

HUMAN LEUKOCYTE STIMULATED WITH A 23187 OR MELITTIN

Monique Braquet[1], Mara d'Onofrio[2], Ricardo Garay[2] and
Pierre Braquet[3]

[1]C.R.S.S.A., Division de Radiobiochimie, 1bis rue Raoul
Batany, F-92141 Clamart (France)
[2]INSERM U7, Hopital Necker, 171 rue de Sèvres, F-75015
Paris (France)
[3]I.H.B. Research Laboratories, 17 avenue Descates
F-92350 Le Plessis (France)

INTRODUCTION (*)

It is well known that leukocytes play key roles in mechanisms
of body defense against both endotoxins and exotoxins. The factors
involved in triggering such defense mechanisms involve an activation of cellular membrane processes, among which is the release
(from phospholipids) of AA and its subsequent metabolism into
various icosanoids. The liberation of such icosanoids (e.g. LTs,
PGs, HPETEs), in addition to the formation of superoxide and other
oxygen free radicals and the liberation of histamine and certain
degradative enzymes (e.g., elastase, collagenase), play key roles
not only in the destruction of suitable ingestible particles but
also in the recruitment (chemotaxic effect) of other cells for this
process. All of these events depend upon the generation and trans-
mission of a membrane signal which involves mainly membrane
metabolism and ion transport[1].

Recent studies have also revealed that K[+] might play a role
in modulating the AA cascade. In this regard, Oelz et al.[2] have
shown that certain monovalent cationophores (monensin A and

(*) Symbol: AA: Arachidonic acid; $[Ca^{2+}]$: internal calcium; $[Ca^{2+}]_i$
-dep.P_k: Calcium-dependent potassium permeability; CO: Cyclooxygenase,
HPETE: Hydroperoxyciosatetraenoic acid; HETE: Hydroxyeicosatetraenoic
acid; $[K^+]$.: external potassium; LO: lipoxygenase, pH_o: External pH;
PMNL; Polymorphonuclear leukocyte.

nigericin) stimulated prostaglandin (PG) production in rat renal medulla <u>in vitro</u>, and Dusing et al.[3] have shown that perfusion or rat aortic rings with a solution containing low $|K^+|_o$ led to an increased release of 6-keto $PGF_{1\alpha}$. A similar release of PGs has been observed in humans suffering from Bartter's syndrome, which is characterized by hypokalemia[4]. Also, in man the ratio of Na^+/K^+ intake might influence significantly the release of PGs[5]. Such effects on PG synthesis and release appear to be mediated by K^+-efflux from the cells in response to either low $|K^+|_o$ or the presence of a K^+-ionophore.

It is well known that Ca^{2+} plays a fundamental role in triggering the AA cascade[2]. Therefore, $|Ca^{2+}|_i$-dep. P_K (see fig. 1), could serve as the mechanism which links $|Ca^{2+}|_i$, K^+-efflux and AA metabolism. This phenomenon was first suspected by Wilbrandt[6] and later extensively characterized by Gardos[7] who used human erythrocytes and observed that an increase in $|Ca^{2+}|_i$ induced a loss of K^+ from the erythrocytes, and the associated increase in P_K could reach 1000 times normal with a high selectivity for K^+ over Na^+[8,9]. Since the study of Gardos[7], this phenomenon has been observed repeatedly in other systems[8,10-14].

Ca^{2+}-activated K^+ channels are considered to play a crucial role in the regulation of membrane potential (for review see[15]) and of endocrine (pancreatic β-cells)[16-18] or exocrine (parotid acini of the mouse [19], rat[19] or pig) secretions (see fig. 2.)

We have recently demonstrated that $|Ca^{2+}|_i$-dep. P_K participates in the membrane signal of the A 23187- or Melittin- stimulated rabbit platelet[21].

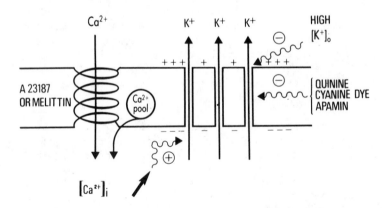

Figure 1.   A Model for Calcium-dependent Potassium Permeability

Thus we decided to investigate possible correlations between K^+ fluxes, pH and AA cascade in A 23187- and melittin-stimulated human PMNL.

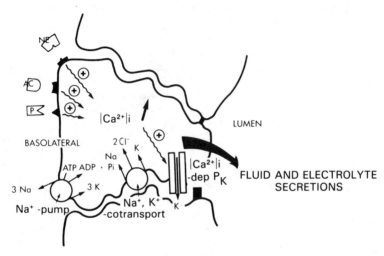

Fig. 2. A model for calcium-dependent potassium permeability in the secretory process of epithelia (this figure partially reproduces the model published in ref. 15).

MATERIAL AND METHODS

Preparation of Human PMNL

Blood samples (400 ml) were obtained from normal volunteers, 20-30 years of age. Blood was collected in the presence of CPD (citrate 0.11 M; phosphate, 16 mM; dextrose, 0.13 M), and was centrifuged at 1000 g for 25 min. The platelet-rich plasma was discarded, and the PMNL fraction was obtained following 6% dextran-500 sedimentation, centrifugation over Ficoll Paque (Pharmacia) and ammonium chloride (160 mM) + Tris (170 mM) treatment. Then, the cells were suspended in the various incubation media (see below).

Potassium Fluxes
        Measurement of K^+ fluxes. K^+ efflux was measured in PMNL

according to the following method: a suspension of 10 millions of
PMNL in 2 ml of PBS medium was centrifuged for 3 minutes at 3000 rpm
(4° C). The supernatant was removed and the cells were washed once
with ice-cold efflux medium. The composition of the efflux medium
was (mM): 140, NaCl; 10, CsCl; 1, $CaCl_2$; 1, $MgCl_2$; 10, MOPS-Tris;
0.1, ouabain; 0.02, bumetanide and 10, glucose. After washing, the
cells were resuspended with 1.2 ml of efflux medium; 0.2 ml of the
suspension were added to two tubes containing 1 ml of Acationox
0.02% for determination of cell K^+ content. The tubes were frozen
and thawed three times and K^+ content was measured by flame photo-
metry; 0.2 ml of the PMNL suspension were added to four tubes
containing 1 ml of efflux medium. All the procedure was carried
out at 4° C. Two tubes were vortexed and immediately centrifuged.
The remaining tubes were vortexed and incubated at 37°C for 10 min.
(in control experiments we observed that external K^+ increased
linearly in time over such period). After the incubation the tubes
were transferred to 4°C for 1 min and then centrifuged.

The supernatant was carefully removed from all tubes and K^+
was determined on an Eppendorf flame photometer. Rate constant of
K^+ efflux (k_K) was calculated using the equation:

$$k_K = \frac{\Delta K}{t \, (K_C)}$$

were ΔK is the difference in K^+ contents between 10 min and 0
time incubation, t is the incubation time and K_C is the reading
of cell K. In some of the experiments only ΔK is indicated.

The effects of drugs on K^+ efflux. The above procedure was
used for investigating the effect of A 23187, melittin (Sigma
Chem. C°., St Louis, Mo USA) and of some agents which inhibit
$|Ca^{2+}|_i$-dep. P_K: di-S-C$_3$(5), a cyanine dye (Molecular Probes, Junction
City, Ohio, USA), quinine and apamin (Sigma). These drugs were
added directly to the efflux medium at different concentrations.

AA Metabolism

Incubation Media. Two different buffers were used to prepare
the incubation media. The standard phosphate-buffered medium
contained (in mM): Na^+, 146; K^+, 4; Mg^{2+}, 1; Cl^-, 142; HPO_4^{2-}, 2.5;
$H_2PO_4^-$, 0.5; glucose, 10 (pH $\approx$ 7.4; determined osmolarity $\approx$ 284 mosM)
To change the Na^+/K^+ ratio, the concentrations of Na^+ and K^+ varied
inversely over the range 0 - 150 mM.

Incubation of PMNL. $CaCl_2$ and $MgCl_2$ were added to the PMNL
suspension to obtain 2 mM and 0.5 mM final concentrations,
respectively, and the suspensions were pre-incubated for 5 min. at
37°C in polypropylene tubes. The cells were then stimulated with
the Ca^{2+}-ionophore A 23187 (1.5 µM) or melittin (0.1/0.5 µM) and

incubated for a further 5 min period. In the time-course study of
the action of ionophore A 23187, incubation periods were varied
from 15 sec to 15 min. Incubations were stopped by addition of one
volume of a mixture of methanol/acetonitrile (1/1 , v/v) containing
200 ng of PGB_2 (internal standard). Ca^{2+}-ionophore was used in
ethanolic solution (0.5% maximal final concentration). In some cases,
valininomycin was used to replace A 23187 or was added together
with A 23187, either simultaneously or 5 min before the ionophore.
The possible effects on icosanoid release of the following drugs
which affect K^+ movements were determined: di-S-C_3(5), tetraethylammonium (TEA), apamin, quinine (Sigma) and 4-aminopyridine (Dept.
of organic chem., IHB Research Labs, Paris, France). Several agents
that alter pH_i were also tested: 4, 4'-diisothiocyano-2,2'-disulfonic
acid Stilbene (DIDS)(Sigma Chem.) and amiloride (a generous gift of
Merck, Sharp & Dohme, France). In general, drugs were added to the
medium 10 min. before addition of A 23187 or melittin.

Reversed-Phase High Performance Liquid Chromatography (RP-
HPLC) of AA metabolites[22]. Denatured PMNL suspensions were centrifuged at 3000 g for 15 min to remove the precipitated material.
Supernatants (2 ml) were acidified to pH 3.0 with H_3PO_4 and 2-ml
portions were then injected on a HIBAR RP 18 cartridge (125 x 8 mm,
5 μm particles, Merck) previously equilibrated with solvent A (see
below).

Table 1. Gradient Used for RP-HPLC of AA Metabolites

Time (min)	Solvent A	Solvent B	Solvent C
Initial	100	0	0
5	70	30	0
15	40	60	0
25	0	100	0
35	0	100	0
37	0	0	100
55	0	0	100

Solvent A: methanol-acetonitrile-water, 25/25/50, v/v/v, containing
0.02% H_3PO_4 and 0.0025% dimethylsulfoxide; adjusted to pH 3.1
(apparent pH) with NH_4OH
Solvent B: methanol-acetonitrile-water, 30/60/10, v/v/v, containing
0.02% of H_3PO_4
Solvent C: methanol-acetonitrile-water, 30/50/20, v/v/v, containing
0.02% of H_3PO_4, adjusted to pH 5.5 (apparent pH) with NH_4OH

The various LO products were eluted at a flow rate of 1 ml/min using the three-solvent mixture (A, B, C) shown in Table 1. All solvents were of HPLC grade. Elution of the various compounds was monitored using fixed wavelength ultraviolet photometers at 229 and 280 mm (Waters Scientific Model 441 with extended wavelength module). The pumps (Waters, model 6000 A) were controlled by a microprocessor (Waters, model 720).

Radioimmunoassay of TXB$_2$ and PGE$_2$. CO products thromboxane (TXA$_2$) and prostaglandin E$_2$ (PGE$_2$) that were released from PMNL were determined by radioimmunoassay of the stable hydrolytic metabolite TXB$_2$ and of PGE$_2$ itself.

RESULTS

Potassium Fluxes

The effect of A 23187 and melittin on K$^+$ efflux from PMNL. Figure 3 represents, in dose-response curve, the stimulation of K$^+$ efflux in human PMNL by A 23187. At 1 μM, the K$^+$ efflux was stimulated by ∿ 31% in comparison with the basal value. The maximal stimulation was observed for 50 μM (+ 200%). Half of the maximal K$^+$ efflux was observed for a concentration of ionophore equal to 8.7 μM.

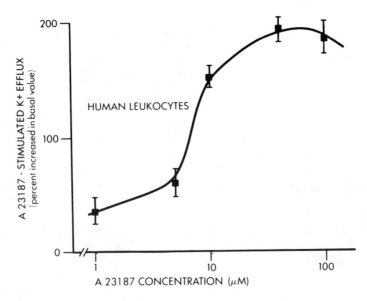

Fig. 3. Stimulation of transmembrane K$^+$ permeability by the Ca^{2+} ionophore A 23187.

Figure 4 represents in dose-response curve the stimulation of K^+ fluxes by melittin. Very low doses of this drug are able to strongly stimulate K^+ fluxes: at 0.7 µM, the K^+ efflux is 4 times the basal value and at 1.4 µM, the basal efflux is stimulated by more than 20 times. Therefore melittin is a more powerful activator of K^+ fluxes than the calcium ionophore A 23187.

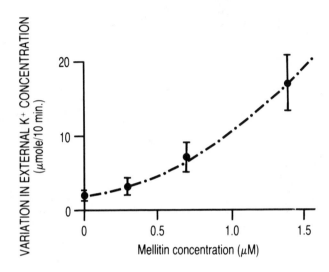

Figure 4.   Stimulation of K^+ Efflux from Human Leukocytes by melittin (mean ± SD - 5 experiments)

Effects of Drugs which alter K^+ fluxes. The highest doses of quinine (10^{-3} M, data not shown) and of di-S-C$_3$(5)(4.10^{-5} M) (Fig. 5) completely block the A 23187-stimulated K^+ efflux. Conversely apamin (10^{-8} - 10^{-5} M) failed to inhibit the A 23187-stimulated K^+ efflux (data not shown).

Table II.   Partial Inhibition by Quinine of the melittin-stimulated K^+ efflux from human leukocytes (K^+ efflux as ΔK)

Condition	Melittin Concentration (µM)		
	0	0.7	1.4
Control	2.3 ± 0.5	5.5 ± 1.5	17.5 ± 2.0
Quinine (0.25 mM)	-	3.8 ± 1.3	14.4 ± 1.4
Quinine (0.50 mM)	-	2.0 ± 1.0	10.0 ± 1.0
Quinine (1 mM)	-	1.6 ± 0.8	7.2 ± 0.7

Quinine only inhibits half of the melitin-sti,ulated K+ efflux
(Table 2).

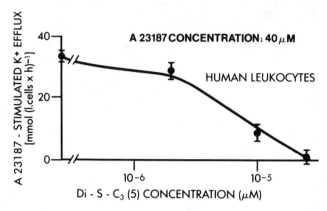

Fig. 5.   Inhibition of Calcium-dependent K+ permeability by the
Cyanine Dye di-S-C$_3$ (5)

AA Metabolism

The major metabolites that were released in the PMNL preparation
(at pH 7.4 in standard medium) stimulated with the Ca^{2+}-ionophore
A 23187 or melittin were 5 HETE (284 $\pm$ 37 ng/10^7 cells) LTB$_4$
(307 $\pm$ 32 ng/10^7 cells). 5(S) 12(S) di-HETE and the isomers of
LTB$_4$ (i.e., 20-OH LTB$_4$: 132 $\pm$ 24 ng/10^7 cells or 20-COOH-LTB$_4$) as
well as PGE$_2$, TXB$_2$ (4.3 $\pm$ 0.7 ng/10^7 cells) and LTC$_4$ (74 $\pm$ 12 ng/10^7
cells).

A time-course study (in physiological medium) of the action
of A 23187 revealed that it did not induce any significant release
of icosanoids during the first 20-30 sec after its addition to the
medium. However, icosanoid release began 30-45 sec after addition
of A 23187 and maximum stimulated release occurred generally at
3-5 min. After 5 min , the concentration of 20-OH LTB$_4$ and
20-COOH LTB$_4$ continued to increase at the expense of LTB$_4$, the
level of which decreased slowly (about half of the maximum concentration remaining after 10 min).

Effects of Modifying the External Monovalent Cation Ratio on A 23187-stimulated Icosanoid Release from Human Leukocytes:

As $|K^+|_o$ was increased from 5 to 150 mM, at the expense of $|Na^+|_o$, there occurred a progressive decrease in the release of all icosanoids that were monitored, the release being nearly abolished at 150 mM $|K^+|_o$. This effect of increasing $|K^+|_o$ was evident for both CO products and LO products. Between 5 and 20 mM $|K^+|_o$ the decrease in icosanoid release was pronounced (TXB_2: 4.3 ng/10^7 cells at 5 mM $|K^+|_o$ to 3.1 ng/10^7 cells at 20 mM $|K^+|_o$; 5-HETE: 284 ± 37 ng/10^7 cells to 184 ± 28 ng/10^7 cells; LTB_4: 307 ± 32 ng/10^7 cells to 204 ± 28 ng/10^7 cells) whereas between 20 mM and 150 mM $|K^+|_o$ the effect on release was reduced. At $|K^+|_o$ = 0 mM, the release of all icosanoids monitored was markedly reduced (TXB_2: 2.9 ng/ml; 5-HETE: 84 ng/ml; LTB_4: 102 ng/10^{-7} cells). Maximal release in phosphate buffer was obtained at about the physiological concentration of $|K^+|_o$ (4 - 5 mM). When Tris-buffered medium was used maximal icosanoid release occurred over a wide range of $|K^+|_o$ (5 - 50 mM). Rb^+ Or Cs^+, used in place of $|K^+|_o$, had essentially the same effect.

Effects of $|Ca^{2+}|_i$-dep. p_K Inhibitors on Icosanoid Release from A 23187-Stimulated Human Leukocytes:

Three inhibitors of $|Ca^{2+}|_i$-dep. P_K were used: apamin, quinine and the cyanine dye di-S-$C_3(5)$ The one considered to be the most selective is apamin even though it does not inhibit all $|Ca^{2+}|_i$-dep. P_K channels[23].

Effect of Apamin. In the standard medium, apamin produced a slight inhibition of the CO pathway, the maximal effect usually being observed at 10^{-6} M or 10^{-7} M . Thus, TXB_2 release was inhibited by 25% at 10^{-6} M and by 30% at 10^{-7} M, but the inhibition was not very evident at lower or higher concentrations. Similar effects were observed concerning PGE_2 release. A kinetic study of the release of LTB_4 (+ isomers) and 5-HETE showed that the 5-LO pathway is also slightly inhibited (- 15%) by those concentrations of apamin that inhibited the CO pathway.

Effect of Quinine. In the standard medium, quinine induced a strong inhibition of both CO and LO pathways but only at the highest concentration used (10^{-3} M). Thus, TXB_2 was inhibited by 91%, PGE_2 by 88% and LTB_4 and other LO products were not detectable on the HPLC profile. However, this effect was not evident at lower concentrations of quinine (Table 3).

Effect of Di-S-$C_3(5)$. In the standard medium, di-S-$C_3(5)$ markedly inhibited both CO and LO pathways. This effect was most evident at the highest concentrations used (10^{-4}, 10^{-3} M) in which case the release of icosanoids was only about 10% of control release (Table 4) This effect was also observed with 10^{-5} M of di-S-$C_3(5)$ where release was inhibited by about 50%. This agent did not inhibit CO activity in a microsomal preparation of ram seminal vesicle, thus supporting the view that its effect in leukocytes was indirect.

Table 3. Effect of Quinine on Icosanoid Release in Human Leukocytes

QUININE (M) (***)	RELEASE (percent of control)						
	TxB$_2$ (*)	PGE$_2$ (*)	5-HETE (**)	LTB$_4$ (**)	20-OH LTB$_4$ (**)	$\Delta^{6\text{-}t}$ LTB$_4$ (**)	12 epi-LTB$_4$ (**)
10^{-3}	9.3	12.4	≠0	≠0	≠0	≠0	≠0
10^{-4}	81.5	87.2	76.0	66.0	57.0	61.0	76.7
10^{-5}	99.3	102.1	91.4	88.7	67.4	73.8	89.4
10^{-6}	98.9	103.2	107.1	107.2	104.1	74.7	101.1

(*)   RIA determination
(**) HPLC determination
(***) mean of 5 samples

Table 4. Effect of Cyanine Dye |Di-S-C$_3$(5)| on icosanoid release in Human Leukocytes

CONCENTRATION (μM)	ICOSANOID RELEASE (percent of control)(*)		
	TxB$_2$	PGE$_2$	LTB$_4$ (**)
1	93.6	102.0	106.4
10	40.0	57.1	37.1
100	14.7	18.4	12.1
1000	16.1	25.2	17.4

(*) mean of 3 samples
(**) RIA determination

Effects of Inhibitors of Putative Voltage-Dependent K$^+$ Channels:
Two inhibitors of putative voltage-dependent K$^+$ channels were used:
4-aminopyridine and tetraethylammonium (TEA), the latter of which
has also been studied in relation to |Ca^{2+}|$_i$-dep. P$_K$ in certain
other models.

   Effect of 4-aminopyridine. In the standard medium, the lowest
concentration of 4-aminopyridine used (10^{-4} M) did not influence
LO or CO pathways (data not shown). On the other hand, 4-aminopyri-
dine (at 10^{-3} M) significantly inhibited the release of TXB$_2$ (46%
decrease) and LTB$_4$ (30% decrease).

Effect of TEA. TEA, even at the highest concentration used
(25 mM), did not influence LO or CO pathways in the standard medium.

Effect of Valinomycin on Icosanoid Release from Human Leukocytes.
The K^+ ionophore valinomycin is not able to trigger the AA cascade
in human leukocytes.

Effect of Valinomycin + A 23187 on Icosanoid Release from Human
Leukocytes: Two experiments were performed using standard medium:
(i) determination of the effect of the mixture valinomycin +
A 23187 added simultaneously; (ii) determination of the effect of
A 23187 added 10 min after valinomycin.

When valinomycin + A 23187 were added to the human leukocyte
preparation at the same time, a significant synergistic effect
appeared after 5 min of incubation for the lowest concentrations
of Ca^{2+}-ionophore used ($< 10^{-6}$ M). This effect seemed to be maximal
when the concentration of A 23187 was about $5\ 10^{-7}$ M and when the
concentration of valinomycin was 10^{-5} M. When lower concentrations
of valinomycin (10^{-7} M, 10^{-6} M) were used, the synergistic effect
was not so pronounced and a slight antagonistic effect even
appeared at the highest concentrations (10^{-4} M, 10^{-3} M). A time-
course study (0 to 180 sec) revealed that valinomycin significantly
enhanced the initial rate of AA metabolite release (Fig. 6).

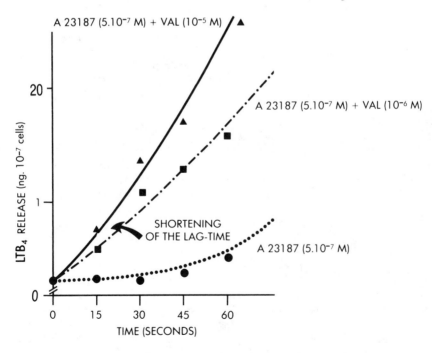

Figure 6.   Kinetic of the Release of LTB_4 rom A 23187 + Valinomycin-
VS A 23187 alone-stimulated Human Leukocytes

Conversely, when valinomycin was added <u>10 min before A 23187</u>, inhibitory effects were usually observed for all concentrations of K⁺ ionophore that were used (Table 5).

Table 5. Importance of the Time of Addition of Valinomycin to the medium

CONDITION	AA METABOLITES (percent of control) (*)				
	PGE_2	TxB_2	20 - OH LTB_4	LTB_4	5 - HETE
Valinomycin (10^{-6} M, 10 min.) then A 28187 (7.5 10^{-7} M)	47	41	27	43	74
Valinomycin (10^{-6} M) + A 23 187 (7.5 10^{-7} M)	128	154	125	134	132

(*) control : A 23187 alone (7.5 10^{-7} M), mean of 3 determinations

<u>Effects of Modifying External pH on A 23187 - Stimulated Icosanoid Release in Human Leukocytes</u>: Variations of pH_o in the MOPS-Tris-buffered medium produced profound modification in the release of both CO and LO metabolites. Thus, at all values of pH_o < 6.0 icosanoid release was abolished (Fig. 7). This effect was particu-larly evident for LTB_4: at pH_o = 6.5, LTB_4 release was about 50% of control whereas at physiological pH_o (i.e. 7.4) release was maximal. At alkaline pH_o (e.g., 8.0), LTB_4 release was slightly decreased (∿10%)(Fig. 7). In addition, alkaline conditions appeared to modify the profile of metabolites released in favor of non-enzymatic derivatives of LTA_4 (Δ6-trans-LTB_4, 12-epi LTB_4).

<u>Effect of an Anion Channel Blocker (DIDS) on A 23187-Stimulated Icosanoid Release in Human Leukocytes</u>: DIDS (10^{-5} M), in MOPS-Tris-buffered medium, profoundly inhibited icosanoid release over the whole range of pH_o studied (i.e., 6.0 - 8.0). For example regarding LTB_4, its maximal release (about 37% of control release) occurred at pH 7.5; i.e., was slightly displaced toward alkaline pH. Also, at pH_o = 8.0, LTB_4 release was markedly decreased (13% of control), which indicated a pronounced effect of DIDS under alkaline condi-tions (see Fig. 7).

<u>Effect of Inhibiting Na⁺/H⁺ Exchange with Amiloride on A 23187-Stimulated Icosanoid Release</u>: Amiloride (10^{-4} M) in MOPS-Tris-buffered medium, like DIDS, inhibited the release of all icosanoids that were monitored. Thus, inhibition was nearly complete at all pH_o values < 7.0. Here again, maximal release (40% of control) was displaced slightly toward alkaline pH . At pH_o 8.0 the inhibitory effect of amiloride on LTB_4 release was less pronounced (31% of control) than that of DIDS (see Fig. 7).

<u>Effect od DIDS + Amiloride on A 23187-Stimulated Icosanoid Release</u>:
DIDS (10^{-5} M) when used together with amiloride (10^{-4} M) pratically
abolished all icosanoid release (see Fig. 7).

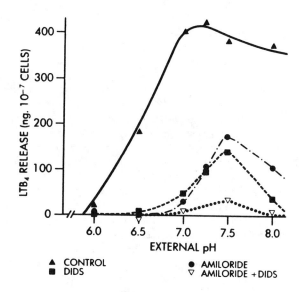

Figure 7.   Effect of DIDS, of Amiloride and of Amiloride + DIDS on
            LTB$_4$ release in Human Leukocytes at Different External
            pH Values

DISCUSSION

     The results presented herin have confirmed and extended those
of previous reports[1],[24] concerning the characterization of early
events involved in secretory phenomena associated with leukocyte
activation. We have observed here that A 23187 or melittin initiate
icosanoid release 20-30 sec after its addition to the incubation
medium. It is noteworthy that the generation of superoxide ($O_2^{\cdot-}$)
by immune complex or by concanavalin-A also had a lag period of
30-42 sec[24]. These findings thus indicate that icosanoids and $O_2^{\cdot-}$
are simultaneously released after membrane stimulation (leukocyte
activation) by agents eliciting Ca^{2+} mobilization.

     It has been previously reported that modification of $|K^+|_o$ led
to changes in icosanoid release <u>in vitro</u>[2],[3] and <u>in vivo</u> [4],[5]. This
was confirmed and extended here. Indeed, we observed that the
increase in $|K^+|_o$ results in a biphasic activation and inhibition
of icosanoid release in PMNL stimulated with A 23187. This effect

375

depends upon the buffer used in the medium, and was not always evident with MOPS-Tris. The decreased icosanoid release at $[K^+]_o = 0$ is likely due to a slight membrane depolarization that may follows the inhibition of the electrogenic Na^+ pump. The decreased icosanoid release by high $[K^+]_o$, on the other hand, was probably due to an inhibition of net K^+ efflux. This is associated with A 23187 action, as we observed here confirming previous results in erythrocytes[25] and in leukocytes[26]. This K^+ efflux could produce a transient hyperpolarization, as has been shown in macrophages[27]. In line with a mechanism by which stimulation of K^+ efflux could be due to an increased $[Ca^{2+}]_i$ which would favor opening of the K^+ channels ($[Ca^{2+}]_i$ dep P_K), Gallin et al. (26) have shown that $|Ca^{2+}|_i$ dep. P_K is involved in macrophage activation (see also OLiveira Castro and Dos Reis, Ref. 28) and it is shown herein that the inhibitors of $[Ca^{2+}]_i$ dep. P_K, quinine and di-S-C_3(5), markedly inhibited icosanoid release (both CO and LO metabolites). With further regard to the possible role of K^+ fluxes on icosanoid release, it is shown herein that K^+ ionophore (valinomycin) does not trigger the AA cascade in leukocytes, but that addition of valinomycin simultaneously with A 23187 had a synergistic effect on icosanoid reelase. This may explain a previous observation showing that valinomycin failed to induce degranulation in leukocytes. Thus, although K^+ efflux per se does not trigger the AA cascade, K^+ efflux coupled with Ca^{2+} mobilization appears to be important for this process. With regard to the mechanism involved, a kinetic study showed that valinomycin, when added together with A 23187, decreased or abolished the lag time for the stimulatory action of A 23187 on icosanoid release although maximal icosanoid release remained unaltered (Fig. 6). Evidence which indicates that the times of addition of valinomycin is important derives from our findings that an inhibition of icosanoid release occurred when valinomycin was added 10 min before A 23187 (Table 5). Thus, the hyperpolarization that is linked to K^+ efflux must occur after, rather before, Ca^{2+} mobilization. Putative voltage-dependent K^+ channels either do not exist in the leukocyte membrane or do not influence icosanoid release. The presence of external Na^+ appears to be required for leukocyte activation under several experimental conditions: Ca^{2+}-dependent, FLMP induced-enzyme release[29], $O_2 \cdot^-$ generation[30] and icosanoid release[31]. This suggests that, besides activation of K^+ efflux, the entry of Ca^{2+} into the cell interior may led to an stimulation of Na^+ influx.

The results discussed above, together with those obtained by previous workers on changes in membrane potential and Ca^{2+} efflux

that occur during leukocyte activation can be used to formulate the
following sequence of events involved in leukocyte activation (see
Fig. 8): Ca^{2+} mobilization and/or Ca^{2+} and Na^+ influxes $\longrightarrow$
increased $|Ca^{2+}|_i$ $\longrightarrow$ transient hyperpolarization via K^+ efflux

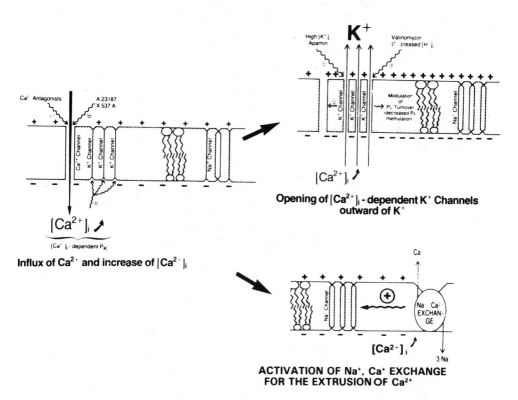

Figure 8.   A model for the initial ionic events involved in the
stimulation of leukocyte

$(|Ca^{2+}|_i$ dep. $P_K)$ and simultaneous commencement of Ca^{2+} extrusion
or sequestering mechanism $\longrightarrow$ changes in Na^+ channels $\longrightarrow$
Na^+ influx $\longrightarrow$ membrane depolarization.

REFERENCES

1. J.E.Smolen, H.M. Korchak and G. Weissmann in:Cell Biology of the Secretory Process (M.Cantin, ed), Karger, Basel, pp 517-545 (1984)·

2. O. Oelz, H.R. Knapp, H.R. Roberts, L.J.Oelz, B.J.Sweetman, J.A.Oates and P.W. Reed. Calcium dependent stimulation of thromboxane and prostaglandin biosynthesis by ionophores. In: Advances in Prostaglandin and Thrombanxe Research, Vol.3 (C.Galli, ed.) Raven Press, New York, pp. 148-158 (1978).

3. R. Dusing, R. Scherhag, R. Tippelman, U. Udde, K. Glanzer and H.J. Kramer. Arachidonic acid metabolism in isolated rat aorta. Dependence of prostacyclin biosynthesis on extracellular potassium concentration. J. Biol. Chem. 257: 1993-1996 (1982).

4. J.R. Gill, Bartter's syndrome. Annu. Rev. Med. 31: 405-419 (1980).

5. F. Skrabal, J. Aubock and H. Hortnagl, Low Sodium/High potassium diet for prevention of hypertension : probable mechansims of action. Lancet, 2 (8252): 895-900 (1981).

6. W. Willbrandt. A relation between the permeability of the red cell membrane and its metabolism. Trans. Faraday Soc.33:956-959 (1937).

7. G. Gardos. Biochem. Biophys. Acta, 30, 653-654 (1958).

8. F.M.Kregenow and J.F.Hoffman, Some Kinetic and metabolic characteristics of calcium-induced potassium transport in human red cells, J. Gen. Physiol. 60: 406-429 (1972).

9. V.L. Lew and H.G.Ferreira in : Membrane Transport in Red Cells (J.C. Ellory and V.L. Lew, eds), Academic Press, New York, pp 93-100 (1977).

10. V.L. Lew and H.G. Ferreira: Curr. Top. Membr.Transp. 20:217-277 (1978).

11. J.F. Hoffman, D.R. Yingst, J.M. Goldinger, R.M. Blum and P.A.Knauf in: Membrane Transport in Erythrocytes (U.V. Lassen, H.H. Ussing and J.O. Wieth, eds.) Munksgaard, Copenhagen, pp. 178-192 (1980).

12. W. Schwartz and H. Passow, Ca^{2+}-activated K^+ channels in erythrocytes and excitable cells. Ann. Rev. Physiol. 45:359-374 (1983).

13. G. Gardos, The role of Ca in the potassium permeability of human erythrocytes. Acta Physiol Acad.Sci.Hung. 15:121-125. (1959).

14. G. Gardos, Effect of ethylenediaminetetraacetate on the permeability of human erythrocytes. Bioch. Biophys. Acta Physiol. Acad. Sci Hung. 14:1-5 (1958).

15. O.H. Petersen and Y. Maruyama, Calcium-activated potassium channels and their role in secretion. Nature (London) 307 : 693-6 (1984) .

16. I. Atwater, C.M. Dawson, B.Ribalet and E.Rojas, Potassium permeability activated by intracellular calcium ion concentration in the pancreatic B - cell. J. Physiol. 288 :575-88 (1979).

17. W.J. Malaisse and A. Herchuelz, Nutritional regulation of K^+ conductance : an unsettled aspect of pancreatic B cell physiology . In : Biochemical actions of hormones Vol IX G.Academic Press Inc. N.Y. pub., pp. 69-92 (1982).

18. J.C. Henquin, Opposite effects of intracellular Ca^{2+} and glucose on K^+ permeability of pancreatic islet cells. Nature (London) 280 : 66-68 (1979).

19. J.A. Young, in : Membrane transport in biology Vol. IV G.Giebisch ed., Springer (Berlin) pub.,pp. 563-692 (1979).

20. W.W. Douglas and A.M. Poisner, The influence of calcium on the secretory response of the submaxillary gland to acethlcholine or to nordrenaline. J. Physiol. (London) 165 : 528-541 (1963).

21. P. Braquet, B.Spinnewyn, B.Lehuu, M.Braquet,E. Chabrier, F. Dray and F.V. DeFeudis, Prost.Leukotri.Med., in press.

22. P. Borgeat, B. Fruteau de Laclos, S. Rabinovitch, S. Picard, P. Braquet, J. Hebert and J. Laviolette, J. Allergy Immunol., in press.

23. G.M. Burgess, M. Claret, D.H. Jenkinson, Effects of quinine and apamin on the calcium-dependent potassium permeability of mammalian hepatocytes and red cells. J. Physiol.(London) 317: 67-90 (1981) .

24. H.M.Karchak and G. Weissmann, Changes in membrance potential of human granulocytes antecede the metabolic responses to surface stimulation. Proc.Natl. Acad.Sci. USA 75 : (8). 3818-22 (1978).

25. E. Edmonson and Ting-Kai Li, Effects of the ionophore A23187 on erythrocytes: relationship of ATP.2-3 diphosphoglycerate to calcium binding capacity. Biochem. Biophys.Acta.443:106-113 (1976).

26. E.K. Gallin, M.L.Wiederhold, P.E. Lipsky and A.S.Rosenthal Spontaneous and induced membrane hyperpolarizations in macrophages. J. Cell Physiol.86:653-661 (1975).

27. E.K. Callin and J.I. Gallin. Interaction of chemotactic factors with human macrophages. J. Cell Biology, 75 : 277-89 (1977).

28. G.M. Oliveira-Castro and G.A. Dos Reis. Electrophysiology of phagocytic membranes. III. Evidence for a calcium-dependent potassium permeability change during slow hyperpolarizations of activated macrophages. Biochem.Biophys.Acta,640:500-511,(1981).

29. H.J. Showel, P.H. Naccache, R.I. Sha'afi and E.L. Becker. The effects of extra-cellular K^+, Na^+, and Ca^{++} on lysosomal enzyme secretion from polymorphonuclear leukocytes. J.Immun.119: 804-811 (1977).

30. H.M. Korchak and G. Weissman. Stimulus-response coupling in the human neutrophil. Membrane potential changes and the role of extra-cellular Na^+. Biochem.Biophys.Acta, 601: 180-194 (1980).

31. M. Braquet, A. Chereau, E. Chabrier and P. Braquet. The membrane signal in human leukocyte: Evidence for a calcium-dependent potassium permeability in A23187-induced triggering of arachidonate cascade. Biomed.Biophys.Acta (in press).